Stress and Coping in Nursing

ROY BAILEY and MARGARET CLARKE

London
CHAPMAN AND HALL

First published in 1989 by
Chapman and Hall Ltd
11 New Fetter Lane, London EC4P 4EE

© 1989 Roy Bailey and Margaret Clarke

Typeset in 10/12pt Cheltenham Book by
Colset Private Limited, Singapore
Printed in Great Britain by
St. Edmundsbury Press, Bury St. Edmunds, Suffolk

ISBN 0 412 33830 0

British Library Cataloguing in Publication Data

Bailey, Roy D.
  Stress and coping in nursing.
  1. Nurses. Stress 2. Hospitals.
  Patients. Stress
  I. Title
  610.73′01′9

  ISBN 0-412-33830-0

To that professional band of carers
we know as nurses

Contents

Contents

Preface

Increasingly, stress as a concept is being used as an explanation of a wide variety of negative phenomena which are experienced by all people, but which include nurses in particular and their patients. Nursing has been identified as a 'high stress' profession and one can hardly pick up a nursing journal, or even read a newspaper article about nursing, without finding the word stress used liberally. Examples of its use are found in relation to sickness/absence rates, high level of nursing staff turnover, discontent in nursing, the effects of unemployment, the effects of overwork, having too much responsibility, having too little responsibility or control, the effects of constantly giving emotionally to others, the causes of illness, the effects of going into hospital, delayed healing, anxiety, depression and alcoholism.

Given the heterogeneous nature of these phenomena, some of which are the diametric opposite of others and that they are clearly being attributed to the one concept, stress, then that concept must necessarily be of importance within people's lives. Or is it perhaps just a fashionable, global, but ultimately empty explanation?

Roy Bailey and I believe that stress is an extremely important concept. Indeed, we would argue that it is a meta-concept rather than a concept, which does indeed serve to explain many disparate phenomena. It has also, however, become a word which is used thoughtlessly wherever negative situations arise and is in such frequent use that there is great danger that it will become meaningless. It is therefore all the more important that we are clear about definitions and meanings when we are studying stress and coping in nursing.

A major problem with the word stress and the concept underlying it is that it can take on many different meanings, even within the same conversation or written article. Lack of clarity in use may mean that two people talking together can assume they understand one another because both use the word stress. In reality they may each be meaning something very different by it and from each other, a situation ultimately leading to confusion.

The first chapter in this book focuses upon a clarification of the way the concept stress may be used, both in everyday life and scientifically. In it we also establish unequivocally, what we understand by the term and how it will be used throughout the rest of the book.

Coping is another term which is used in everyday life but has not yet acquired the same popularity as an explanation, as has the word stress. However, we believe that coping is inextricably linked with stress and is every bit as important as an explanatory concept. Since, in contrast to the way in which some people conceptualize stress, as something that happens to a passive sufferer, we take the view that stress provokes coping and is the outcome of inadequate coping, hence the title of the book. The second chapter is devoted to a consideration of the ways in which the concept 'coping' may be defined and understood. Again we state our own understanding of the term for use in the remainder of the book which is concerned with the part stress and coping play in the lives of nurses, patients and their relatives and friends.

Incidentally the popular view of stress is as a negative experience, but we also aim to show that it is also a positive experience and promotes satisfaction as well as dissatisfaction.

The book is somewhat unusual since we have chosen to discuss stress and coping in relation to nurses themselves and their patients within the same book. This is not only because stress and coping applies to all human beings and thus to patients and nurses, but because patients and their carers form a system in interaction. Stress and coping affecting one part of an interactional system will affect all other parts as well. Therefore the stress and coping of nurses will affect their patients and vice versa.

As John Donne said so long ago:

No man is an iland, intire of itselfe; everyman is a peece of the continent, as part of the maine; if a clod bee washed away by the Sea, Europe is the lesse, as well as if a Promentorie were, as well as if a mannor of thy friends or of thine owne were; any man's death diminishes me, because I am involved in Mankinde; And therefore never send to know for whom the bell tolls; It tolls for thee. (1624)

Acknowledgements

In spite of the frustrations of events which intervened and prevented work upon this book, it was a great comfort and support to work in partnership with Roy Bailey. We would both like to thank the editorial staff at Chapman and Hall for their patience with us and their encouragement.

Eileen Lee did a great deal of the typing of draft chapters and diagrams and we owe her a great deal for her speed and accuracy.

We would like to thank both W.B. Saunders Company and the nursing journal R.N. for permission to reproduce *Guidelines for the development of sensory messages*, included in the chapter on Hospital Admission: Coping and Recovery. We would also like to thank the following people for their advice and support; Hans Selye, Richard Lazarus, Hazel Allen, David Chiriboga, Pat Shipley, June Bailey and Anne Baldwin.

M. Clarke
University of Hull

PART ONE

UNDERSTANDING THE APPROACH

CHAPTER ONE

Meanings and models of stress and coping

'Then you must say what you mean', the March
Hare went on. 'I do' Alice hastily replied; 'at least – I
mean what I say – that's the same thing you know'.

Lewis Carroll (1832–1898)
Alice's Adventures in Wonderland

There are two ways in which a knowledge of stress and coping can help a
nurse in her day-to-day work. First it can help directly in patient care.
Research has suggested that stress adversely affects healing and recovery
rates (Boore, 1978). A nurse who knows the circumstances under which stress
is likely to occur can help to prevent dysfunctional stress. One who can recognize signs of stress can help by teaching the patients to cope. For those
patients who have developed their own coping strategies, a knowledgeable
nurse can give reinforcement and support. Secondly, nurses themselves are
by no means immune to stress. Learning to cope not only gives them control
over their own lives and well-being but leaves them free to concentrate on
helping patients.

In this book we hope to provide the answers to some of the questions nurses
might ask about stress. What is stress? What sorts of stress directly associated
with being or working in hospital may be experienced by patients and nurses?
Do nurses cope adequately with discomforting and disabling levels of stress,
associated with emotions such as anger, anxiety and depression? How may
stress relate to somatic complaints? Under what circumstances and in which
situations does stress occur? What coping behaviour may nurses adopt in a
working context? How effective is nurse coping? How do patients who are
suffering from physical illness cope? Can we appreciate the complex nature of
stress and coping and the role it plays in maintaining human health? Is stress
always a bad thing?

A thorough understanding of the concepts of stress and coping is necessary
as a basis for the answers to such questions (McGrath, 1970). So first we must
examine the main models of stress used by social scientists to promote clarity
in the use of the term. An understanding of these models gives a firm basis on
which to build when looking at research on stress and coping in hospital

patients and helps in understanding how people use the term 'stress' in everyday life.

1.1 CLASSIFICATION OF MODELS OF STRESS

There are three broad approaches to defining stress.

1. Stress may be defined as something outside an individual in the environment, which impinges on him. A clear example is that of an extreme environmental temperature. Another example might be the threat of being made homeless. It is the stimulus to which the individual responds which is considered to be the stress and this approach is called a **stimulus-based model**.

2. In everyday language, however, we often talk about the person as being stressed. When the term is being used in this way it is the individual's physiological response to an extreme environmental temperature or his psychological response to threat which comprises the stress. Using the term 'stress' in this way is the basis of the **response-based models**.

3. The third way of looking at stress is that it is the result of an interaction between the environment and the person who perceives or appraises the situation. This is the **transactional model of stress**. To give an example of what this means in practice we can again think of extreme environmental temperature or the threat of being made homeless. Using a transactional model of stress either example becomes stressful through the individual's interpretation of the situation as threatening and one in which his own efforts will make little or no impact on the outcome.

The majority of writers on stress today subscribe to the transactional model. Nonetheless it is helpful to consider both the stimulus and the response models of stress, as much of the research into stress was based on one or other of these theoretical positions. Data obtained from these studies provide the basis of our present knowledge, but some of the data proved incompatible with theory and thus provided a stimulus for modification of the theory. Through this continuing process the transactional models were formulated.

Brief explanations of the stimulus and response models of stress will be presented here, together with a critique of each model before the authors outline their own preferred model, a transactional one. Examination of the earlier theories and the reasons why they were modified help our understanding of the concept 'stress'. A thorough knowledge of the different ways of looking at stress also helps in reading research reports in which the theoretical position of the researcher has not been made explicit. Finally, it provides a framework for understanding how people may use the word 'stress' in everyday life.

Stimulus models of stress

When writers imply that stress is something applied to an individual, then they are using a stimulus model of stress. An explicit example of such use can be quoted from the first paragraph of a study by MacPherson (1974): 'Stress is best considered to be an attribute of the environment and strain an attribute of the individual – the change – physiological or otherwise induced in the individual by exposure to the environment.' Holmes and Rahe (1967) were said by Pilowsky (1974) to 'consider the term stress as consisting simply of a stimulus which requires the organism to change'. A stress–strain model is illustrated in Fig. 1.1

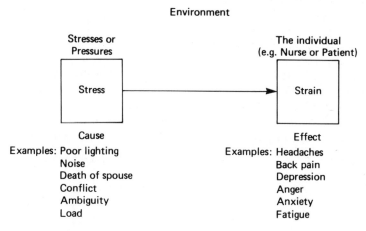

Figure 1.1   The stimulus-based model of stress.

Cox (1978) in discussing stimulus models of stress states: 'Such an approach usually treats stress as an independent variable for study and demands consideration of what stimuli are diagnostic of stress.' Problems with the stimulus model of stress arise at the very point where one starts to consider the stimuli which comprise stress.

The stimulus model of stress arose from a misunderstanding of Hooke's Law of Elasticity (*International Dictionary of Physics*, 1961). MacPherson (1974) stated 'The analogy with Hooke's Law . . . is at once apparent'. This law describes how loads produce deformation in metals. Commonly, those who use this analogy declare that stress is the load which when placed on the metal produces deformation in the material. However, a true reading of Hooke's Law shows that there is no claim that the load is the stress, but that stress exists within a body (the metal). Strain results when forces from outside exert such pressure that resistance breaks down along the lines of stress. (It is worth noting that a good analogy in nursing is the pressure sore which develops due to shearing force. This originates in the tissue layer which is the most vulnerable to tearing).

In any case, to compare a behaving, intelligent human being with an inert piece of metal does not seem to be a particularly fruitful line of enquiry.

Research using the stimulus model of stress has shown that typical strains produced are anxiety, depression, headache, diarrhoea and fatigue. Identification of the stimuli which reliably produce these effects has proved more difficult. Such stimuli as extreme heat, extreme cold, extreme noise and extreme hunger are perhaps the best examples. Even with such stimuli there are problems, however. MacPherson (1974) was reviewing the literature on thermal discomfort as a function of environmental temperature (stress) using a stimulus model. One of the properties of a stimulus model should be the ability to relate the degree of stress with the degree of strain and to relate the two mathematically. On attempting to do this MacPherson found that

> no measure of heat stress can be expected to provide, except in the most general terms, a measure of the physiological strain produced in any particular individual. . . . Intolerable conditions for some may mean only serious discomforts for others. Even the same individual may vary from time to time in his reaction to a standard heat stress.

The Hooke's Law analogy broke down even further, as MacPherson went on,

> There is for each person, however, a third level – the affective – at which he becomes aware of discomfort and resents his environment. This level like all responses to heat stress, differs from person to person and for the same person from time to time depending upon a host of physical and psychological factors such as health and degree of motivation.

Here then, a writer who adheres to the stimulus view of stress finds that even for a physical stimulus such as heat, a simple model of stress–strain is inadequate, and account must be taken of psychological factors. This is even more the case with psychological stimuli. Another worker, Ferguson (1974), who investigated the high sickness absence rates (i.e. strain) amongst telegraphists in Sydney concluded

> Any adverse influence of the physical work environment appeared to have come less from physiological load than from its contribution to general dissatisfication. The physical environment was similar in three geographically separated offices, yet attitudes to it varied greatly.

Ferguson, who started his study with an explicitly stated stimulus model of stress, appears to find the model so inadequate at one point in his report that he refers to stress as an intra-psychic phenomenon – a position similar to that of the transactional model.

Nowadays it is impossible to ignore psychological stimuli as factors causing strain, yet they are so subject to individual variation that it is impossible to provide a list of such stimuli that cause strain in all individuals.

Implicit in the stress–strain model is the expectation that strain increases in proportion to the strength of stimulus. In metal, the greater the load, the greater the strain, and the lighter the load the less likely is resistance to break down, causing strain. Here, the analogy with human strain is poor. One of the most disagreeable situations known to man is the complete absence of stimuli. Even monotonous stimulation is unpleasant. Welford (1974) has found that for maximum efficiency, man requires a moderate stimulation level and that either insufficient or excessive stimuli can be considered as stress.

In discussing human stress and strain, whilst we can identify the effects that occur we cannot relate cause and effect with any great reliability. For example, we can identify a raised temperature as a response to an adverse stimulus but that adverse stimulus might have been an infection, an excessive environmental temperature, or a deep-vein thrombosis. On the other hand, we have already noted that an identical stimulus may have widely divergent effects on two different individuals or even on the same individual on two different occasions. A further example of the latter is the effect on respiration of being at a high altitude. After acclimatization the high altitude ceases to increase the respiratory rate to anything near the initial level. What does this tell us about human beings? It shows that in humans the response to stress is to some extent adaptable, malleable and plastic and there is a degree of tolerance or even acclimatization. This degree of tolerance may be high in some people and low in others. Variation in levels of tolerance to stress occurs within the same individual from occasion to occasion and may be affected by learning and motivation. From this we may conclude that in relation to humans, stress cannot be explained in terms of simple ideas of cause and effect. An example illustrates the complexity. Bereavement may be followed by illness in one individual whilst another picks up his life again and copes, hardly showing grief to the casual onlooker. The major problem with the stress–strain model is the underlying assumption that all effects have the same cause and conversely that all causes are specific and have the same effects on different individuals.

A final criticism of the stress–strain approach to stress is the omission of any reference to the coping ability of human beings. The concept of resistance of the material to stress is used in mechanical engineering. However the concept of resistance in humans does not equate in any way to coping. Resistance is a rather passive term whilst coping implies active dynamic behaviour (Lazarus, 1981). Examples of coping include the actions engaged in by nurse or patient to avoid or reduce anticipated stressful situations. When a theatre nurse takes time to visit a patient before his operation, or a ward nurse stays with a patient who is having an operation until he is completely unconscious, these actions are helping to reduce the degree of strain for the patient of going to the operating theatre.

A nurse in training who is frequently changing wards may develop a strategy for learning the names of permanent ward staff quickly; their likes and dislikes; and the ward routine. In this way she is reducing the potential stressfulness of the new ward environment and actively coping.

A patient going to the operating theatre for operation may practise active relaxation techniques to prevent anxiety. This also is a way of coping. Such methods cannot be explained within a model of stress which implies a simple causal relationship between stressful stimuli and the individual's response.

To sum up this brief account and critique of the stimulus model of stress: Any reference to stress being a property of environmental stimuli which impinge on humans implies that the speaker or writer subscribes to a stimulus model of stress. Such models characterize the stimulus as the independent variable to which the individual responds with strain. The model is a simple cause and effect one.

Problems with the model are:

(a) It is impossible to identify stimuli which cause strain in all individuals or even in the same individual on all occasions.
(b) The model does not account for research findings which show that both very excessive and very low levels of stimuli cause strain.
(c) Human ability to cope is not allowed for in this model.

Response models of stress

Whilst the search for stimuli which have a simple causal relationship with strain has proved illusory, it has been possible to identify the response of the individual who is suffering strain and to argue from that that the circumstances which caused the strain must have been stressful. However, the individuals who use this line of reasoning call the person's response 'stress' and that which caused the response a 'stressor'. It is important to be clear about this as the word 'stress' means something very different in the stimulus as opposed to the response models. We now adopt the definitions appropriate to the response model in the discussion which follows.

Hans Selye and the general adaptation syndrome

Rather than discuss response models in general we focus upon the work of Hans Selye who developed the most influential model of stress as a response phenomenon. Selye, an endocrinologist, is acknowledged as 'the father of the stress syndrome'. As an endocrinologist he studied the physiological components of stress which he suggested form a syndrome of highly stereotyped sequences of physiological response. The syndrome is non-specific, however, in the sense that it is evoked by many different demands made on the body, ranging from acutely physiological, such as haemorrhage, to purely psychological, such as bereavement. Selye called this non-specific stereotyped response of the body **The General Adaptation Syndrome (GAS)**. The General Adaptation Syndrome comprises three stages: (a) the alarm reaction; (b) the stage of resistance; (c) exhaustion. The GAS can be triggered by any demand from the environment and Selye coined the term 'stressor' for such demands.

Before describing the physiology of stress it will be useful to give a historical account of how Selye formulated his concepts of stress. This should help to dispel any incredulity felt by the reader, since Selye (1980) confided after more than fifty years of work on the GAS that:

> I have found it hard to convince people that the body can respond in the same manner to things as different as a painful burn and the news that you have won the jackpot of a lottery. All of the influences and changes individuals encounter present them with the same problem, namely adaptation in the interests of continued well-being.

What led this eminent endocrinologist to concern himself with stress when we would assume his work would centre on the endocrine system? A brief history shows how Selye's scientific training in observation and asking questions led him to spend his life's work on studying stress.

EARLY OBSERVATIONS AND FIRST QUESTIONS

It was soon after his graduation from the University of Prague that Selye had a hint of his future discovery. He described observations of human patients made under the direction of his professor (Selye, 1956, p. 15):

> As each patient was brought into the lecture room, the professor questioned and examined him. It turned out that each of these patients felt and looked ill, had a coated tongue, complained of more or less diffuse aches and pains in the joints, and of intestinal disturbances with loss of appetite. Most of them also had fever (sometimes with mental confusion), and enlarged spleen or liver, inflamed tonsils, a skin rash, and so forth.

Even at this early point Selye began to question the clinical significance of the *common* features displayed by patients with different diagnoses alongside their avowed individual medical conditions. However, there was no experimental evidence to suggest a common syndrome at that time. Moreover, Selye's contemporaries were inclined to encourage him to pursue his search for a new sex hormone – perhaps politely 'guiding him' out of his absurdity into productive and scientifically respectable research. Selye did apparently surrender his ruminations about a common stress response and embarked on a series of experiments with rats. The search for a new hormone had begun. Paradoxically, it was these early experiments in the 1930s which led to Selye's discovery of the stress syndrome – the basis for the later development of the General Adaptation Syndrome. The first findings were submitted in a letter to *Nature* in 1936 entitled 'A syndrome produced by diverse noxious agents'. Later he found that a whole variety of substances injected into rats could produce the GAS. To begin with, he injected ovarian and placental extracts, and observed the series of changes in the organism of alarm, resistance and exhaustion which characterize the GAS.

What typical effects did this have on the organism? Selye noted four main results.

1. Adrenal enlargement and discolouration (he inferred this was due to congestion, fatty secretion, and build up of granules).
2. Shrinking of the thymus.
3. Shrinking of the lymph nodes.
4. Numbers of blood-coloured ulcers located in the stomach.

These experiments provided the foundation for Selye's future views on stress which remain much the same today, with some important modifications to include psychological influences on the GAS (Selye, 1980).

SELYE'S THEORY OF STRESS

Selye's very early observation of the non-specificity of the physiological response (GAS) has remained the cornerstone of his work. He has defined the stress syndrome in the following terms:

> Stress is the state manifested by a specific syndrome which consists of all the non-specifically induced changes within a biological system. (Selye, 1956, p. 54)

> The non-specific response of the body to any demand made upon it. (Selye, 1975, p. 14)

> For scientific purposes, stress is defined as a state which manifests itself by the GAS. (Selye, 1956, p. 47)

This view suggests that many causes (or stressors) can have the same physiological effects (stress). Studies both of patients and people in general tend to support this view.

It is obviously appropriate now to describe in detail the physiological mechanisms said by Selye to be triggered by stressors. As he was an endocrinologist it is perhaps not too surprising to learn that his experiments have led him to the view that the GAS is mediated by the hypothalamus, pituitary

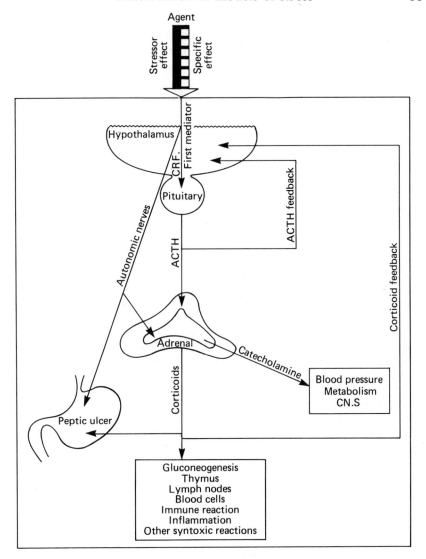

Figure 1.2 The hypothalamic–pituitary–adrenal cortex axis (HPACA) (modified slightly from H. Selye (1976) *Stress in Health and Disease*, Butterworth).

and adrenal glands. These work together as a control system which Selye termed the hypothalamic–pituitary–adrenal cortex axis (HPACA for short). Figure 1.2 shows this system and how Selye claims it operates in the presence of 'stressors'.

The HPACA as a physiological system functions in a way which enables the individual to survive by contributing to the maintenance of a stable internal environment. The important function of maintaining a stable internal environment was described by Walter Cannon (1932) as 'homeostasis'. Homeostasis is an extremely important physiological concept. Other endocrine glands, the central nervous system and the autonomic nervous system also have a major role in the maintenance of homeostasis.

Selye described how a stressor triggers a response. A stressor can be a physical agent (e.g. heat, cold, trauma) or the individual's interpretation of experience (e.g. a nurse's view of a ward sister as extremely threatening). The response to the stressor is said to be transmitted to the hypothalamus via the first mediator. This first mediator stimulates the hypothalamus to secrete corticotrophin-releasing factor (CRF). On reaching the anterior pituitary gland, CRF in its turn stimulates a discharge of the adrenocorticotrophic hormone (ACTH) into the bloodstream. ACTH stimulates the cortex of the adrenal gland to secrete hormones which Selye collectively termed corticoids. These:

> ... elicit shrinkage of the thymus simultaneously with many other changes, such as atrophy of the lymph nodes, inhibition of inflammatory reactions, and production of sugar (a readily available source of energy). Another typical feature of the stress reaction is the development of peptic ulcers in the stomach and duodenum, a process facilitated through the increased levels of corticoids in the blood and mediated in part by the autonomic system. (Selye, 1980, p. 127)

This process is clearly associated with some of the physical changes Selye noted following the injection of noxious substances into rats.

The quotation from Selye's work given above shows how it is possible to describe the events which have occurred in a single moment of time. However, the GAS is not a static phenomenon but a dynamic process occurring over time as it serves different survival functions. Selye himself drew attention to the concept of the GAS as a process.

> Now we shall have to bring the important element of *time* into our considerations of non-specific responses. While stress is reflected by the sum of the non-specific changes which occur in the body at any one time, the general adaptation syndrome (or GAS) encompasses all non-specific changes as they develop throughout time during continued exposure to a stressor. One is a snapshot, the other a motion picture of stress. (Selye, 1956, p. 64)

The inferred phases of the GAS were (a) alarm reaction, (b) stage of resistance and (c) exhaustion (Figs 1.3 and 1.4). The non-specificity of GAS according to Selye is shown in Fig. 1.5.

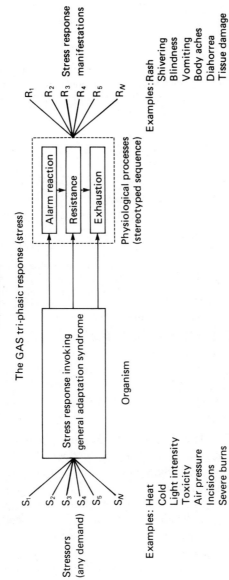

Figure 1.3 The General Adaptation Syndrome (GAS) response-based model of stress.

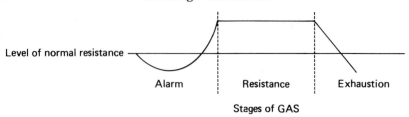

Stages of GAS

Figure 1.4 Sequence of GAS showing alarm reaction, stage of resistance and exhaustion. (From Hans Selye, 1975 *Stress without Distress*. Cygnet Books, New York.)

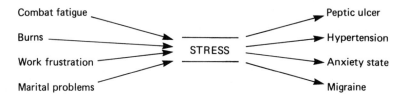

Figure 1.5 Selye's view of non-specificity. Each result (notice this on the left and not the right as in most conventional representations of causality) is a specific manifestation and each causative agent (on the right) is also specific. Yet they are all simultaneously non-specific. The reason for this is that they must all travel through a common pathway (the GAS). No direct connection between cause and effect is possible. This phenomenon is illustrated in the diagram.

Alarm reaction
This reaction appears on sudden exposure to noxious stimuli or any demand to which the organism is not properly adapted. It consists of two phases:

(a) The Shock Phase: This is an initial and rapid reaction to the stressor. A variety of responses may be observed such as tachycardia, reduction of muscle tone, depressed blood pressure and body temperature; all typical signs of the alarm reaction.

(b) The Countershock Phase: This consists of a counter-action phase, characterized by the mobilization of the body's biological mechanisms to combat the stress response induced by the stressor. It is this pháse which overlaps into the resistance phase of the GAS, resulting in adrenal cortex enlargement and increased adrenocorticotrophic hormone secretion.

Resistance
The continued presence of a stressor stimulates the resistance phase of the GAS. This phase is evidenced by a full adaptation to the stressor. When this

occurs the symptoms of the alarm reaction either improve or disappear. Simultaneously however, there is a marked decrease in the capacity of the organism to deal with other demands. This means that the vulnerability of the organism to other stressors is increased.

Exhaustion

Prolonged exposure to stressors puts unrelenting demands on the organism's capacity for adaptation. Since the energy and adaptation of the organism is finite, exhaustion usually follows under these conditions. Where the stressor is continuous and severe enough to induce these stress responses in the GAS, symptoms *reappear* followed by the death of the organism. Hans Selye has illustrated how the GAS might be understood (Fig. 1.4). It will be noted that Selye implicates both the sympathetic nervous system and corticoids in the stress reaction.

Action of the sympathetic nervous system brings about the release of the hormones adrenaline and noradrenaline (catecholamines). Although Selye mentioned the role of adrenaline when discussing the GAS (Selye, 1956), his writings are concerned to a far greater extent with the role of the corticoids. Nonetheless the role of the sympathetic nervous system is known to be important in the response to a stressor, particularly as part of the alarm reaction, since it is the sympathetic division of the autonomic nervous system which initiates the physiological adjustments underlying the behavioural response of 'flight or fight'. The actions of corticoids and catecholamines are summarized in Tables 1.1 and 1.2, respectively. However in real life the

Table 1.1   Physiological and pharmacological actions of glucocorticoids

---

Physiological
  Stimulates the breakdown of protein molecules
  Stimulates the uptake of amino acids by the liver and their conversion to glucose (gluconeogenesis)
  Assists the stimulation of gluconeogenesis by other hormones (e.g. glucagon, growth hormone)
  Inhibits glucose take up and oxidation by many cells (brain cells are an exception)
  It is essential for the cardiovascular response to stress mediated by the sympathetic nervous system
  It may enhance learning
  An anti-inflammatory effect

Pharmacological (when administered in large doses)
  Profoundly reduces the inflammatory response to injury or infection
  Can accelerate the development of hypertension, atherosclerosis and peptic ulcers
  Can interfere with the menstrual cycle
  Can cause bone dissolution

Based on Ganong (1975) and Vandor et al. (1975).

Table 1.2   Actions of adrenaline and noradrenaline (catecholamines)

1. Increases the hepatic and muscle breakdown of glycogen to form glucose
2. Increases the breakdown of triglycerides from adipose tissue providing a supply of glycerol for conversion to glucose and fatty acids for use in metabolism
3. Increases skeletal muscle contractility and decreases muscle fatiguability
4. Increases cardiac contractility and increases the heart rate, which combined with increased venous return leads to an increased cardiac output
5. Constricts arterioles in the skin and visceral organs, together with arteriolar dilatation in skeletal muscle
6. Increases respiratory ventilation
7. Increases the coagulability of blood
8. Increases central nervous system arousal
9. Dilates the pupils

Based on Ganong (1975) and Vandor et al. (1975).

Table 1.3   Joint action of catecholamines and glucocorticoids

1. Mobilize nutrients to increase the blood sugar
2. Increase respiration
3. Re-distributes blood away from skin and visceral organs to the heart, muscle and brain
4. Increases blood coagulability
5. May increase the extracellular fluid volume
6. Central nervous system is aroused with possibly increased learning

Based on Ganong (1975) and Vandor et al. (1975).

hormones may be released together and their actions reinforce one another (Table 1.3).

LOCAL ADAPTATION SYNDROME (LAS)

Selye also described a **Local Adaptation Syndrome (LAS)** which occurs in a specific part or tissue of the body and is determined by the nature or site of the stressor. The LAS is also a process in time characterized by three stages. These are (a) inflammation, (b) degeneration, and (c) death of cells. A good example of a local adaptation syndrome is the progress of a boil or abscess. The inflammatory process may effectively seal the affected part from the rest of the body and then the GAS arises only in an attenuated form. The LAS may proceed through all stages to exhaustion or death of cells. Selye illustrated this by reference to exhaustion of eye muscles after prolonged reading in poor light, but another example would be someone who has 'lost his voice' following excessive speaking or singing. A number of LASs may occur together, as anyone who has had multiple boils can witness, or a cold at the same time as an injured hand. Selye stated,

Several of these may go on simultaneously in various parts of the body, and in proportion to their intensity and extent, they can activate the GAS mechanism. (Selye, 1956, p. 65)

The GAS and LAS mutually influence each other, in that local injury activates not only the local, but also the systemic non-specific defense mechanisms while the resulting GAS can, in turn, regulate the course of topical reactions to stress. (Selye, 1979, p. 19)

It may be worth noting here that differential signs and symptoms of disease reflect the LAS whilst the signs and symptoms which diverse diseases have in common reflect the GAS.

The relationship between LAS and GAS is a complex and intricate one. Selye claimed that they both use up adaptive energy. He postulated that each person has a finite amount of adaptive energy and when it is depleted death ensues. Selye also suggested that the process of ageing may be seen as prolonged GAS. However, the nature of adaptation energy has never been established. Obviously, then, it cannot be measured and used to help promote patient recovery.

STRESS AND DISEASE

Selye supported a view taken by other writers that the stress response participates in the pathology of every disease. On the other hand, he also stated that no disease is ever due to the general stress response alone.

Thus we may classify diseases into two categories:

1. Those in which the signs and symptoms are due to both the effect of the disease agent (stressor) (e.g. microorganisms) and the body's adaptive coping response to that agent. The outcome may be successful coping and cure or it may be less satisfactory than that.
2. Those in which the signs and symptoms are due only tenuously to a stressor but to a large extent to a maladaptive stress response.

Perhaps a more accurate idea is to view illness on a continuum according to the role played by the stress response. At one end of the continuum would be conditions which were so severe that the stress response failed to come into operation at all in the maintenance of homeostasis, e.g. the massive, instant, physical damage caused by a fatal road traffic accident (RTA). At the other end of the continuum would be illness in which there is no physical damage from a stressor which is objectively present, but a maladaptive GAS comes into play as a result of psychological factors and assumes major importance in the pathology of the disease. Somewhere between these extremes would lie illness in which the GAS came into play in response to physical or psychological stressors and brought about a return to homeostasis and thus a satisfactory outcome.

Selye clearly implicated psychological factors in both the causation and the progress of disease.

> From the foregoing it should now be evident that psychological factors can often be the decisive influence both in the *causation of disease and in the course taken by an established disorder*. In fact, this is where the profession of nursing can make a special contribution, since its practitioners are in direct control of such variables [italics added]. (Selye, 1980, p. 130)

Thus Selye reached a position of acknowledging the importance of mind influencing the body and vice versa. Within the discipline of medicine this can be characterized as a holistic position. Within a broader framework it is a psycho-biological view of health and stress, a view to which the authors of this book subscribe. Indeed we would go further to suggest that the essential factors in stress and coping are nearly always psychological in nature.

CRITICAL ANALYSIS OF SELYE'S VIEWS OF STRESS

Within Selye's theory of stress, adaptation plays the vital role in the maintenance of a steady state within the internal environment (homeostasis). Adaptation can thus be seen as preventing excessive deviations from normal physiological parameters in response to a stressor. Walter Cannon first developed the idea of homeostasis, which is necessary for a proper understanding of GAS (*homos* = the same; *stasis* = state). Cannon's work has not received sufficient acknowledgement in Selye's work and neither has Selye paid enough attention to the role of the central nervous system (CNS) in the maintenance of homeostasis. Indeed the CNS plays a primary role in adaptation. Mason (1975) has criticized Selye for his lack of acknowledgement of Cannon's work. Yet Selye obviously placed high value on homeostasis in regard to adaptation:

> Regardless of the specific natures of the demand and response, however, the work of the body is the same; to preserve *homeostasis*, the harmonious balance of the organism, through compensatory adjustments. (Selye, 1980, p. 128).

Another area which is underplayed in Selye's work is also related to Cannon who made the exciting discovery of the fight–flight mechanism of the organism to attack or withdraw from contact with stressors. Selye has indeed implicated the autonomic nervous system in his 'alarm reaction' and this is the system which underlies the fight or flight response. The sympathetic response of the system within the GAS and in fight or flight are almost identical but Selye emphasized the adrenal cortical hormonal responses in the GAS almost to the exclusion of the adrenal medullary hormonal responses mobilized concurrently with the sympathetic nervous system in flight or fight. In experimental work it has been shown that adrenaline and noradrenaline (catecholamines) are secreted in response to environmental threat. Indeed to isolate one hormone system (HPACA) as Selye has done as underlying the GAS, has been to ignore the way in which one hormone can affect the secretion of all other hormones in the body. It has been shown since Selye's original work in 1956 (Levine *et al.*, 1978) that catecholamines, prolactin, luteinizing hormone and growth hormone, *all* appear more responsive to stressors than ACTH itself. Selye also completely ignored behavioural components of the alarm reaction which he might have described had he given greater emphasis to the role of fight or flight in adaptation. Indeed, Pavlov's orienting response to novel stimuli includes aspects of the fight-or-flight response and it might have been possible to bring together many aspects of psychology and physiology had Selye paid more attention to the role of the autonomic nervous system (ANS). However Selye's special contribution has been the elucidation of the role of the adrenal cortex in stress.

THE MYSTERY OF THE 'FIRST MEDIATOR'

One of the disappointing aspects of Selye's work is that he apparently developed his theory without linking it to discoveries being made in other fields whilst he was still building up his own work. An example of this is the idea of a 'first mediator' which links the stressor to the release of CRF by the hypothalamus. There are plenty of candidates for this role of the CNS in the light of our current knowledge which could have been incorporated into Selye's work. Mason carried out work which suggests that activation of the HPACA system is due to psychological factors labelled by the organism as unpleasant or threatening and working through the nervous connections from the cerebrum to the hypothalamus.

Further support that stress originates from perceived threat to the organism has come from Wolff's study of patients.

> Man is vulnerable because he reacts not only to the actual existence of danger, but to threats and symbols of danger experienced in his past. (Wolff and Goodall, 1968, p. 3)

and

> Sometimes threat evokes reactions of long duration and even of greater magnitude than the assault itself. The resulting protective adaptive reaction, when sustained, may be far more damaging to the individual than the effects of the noxious agent *per se*. (Wolff and Goodall, 1968)

Wolff and his co-workers also clearly appreciated that the first mediator was psychological in nature. In doing so they provided us with two important guidelines for the study of stress and by implication, coping. First, stress does not exist independently in the environment as stressors or a noxious stimulus, but 'can be defined as noxious only if they are so *perceived* by the individual implicated [italics added] (Wolff and Goodall, 1968). Second, and more importantly, an individual's stress and disease cannot be properly understood without reference to his psychology, and the meaning he gives to his experience and the actions which arise from it. The present writers would suggest the same is true for the study and understanding of coping. Thus there is a subtle integration of psychology and physiology in stress and coping. But the emphasis should be on the psychological processes which induce unbearable or discomforting levels of stress, and how individuals cope with them.

Lacey (1967) questioned the basic assumptions underlying the GAS. For instance, Lacey reported evidence which shows the tri-phasic nature of the GAS is not immutable. In certain cases a patient suffering from extreme stress (e.g. severe burns) may just pass straight into exhaustion and death. Selye has acknowledged this difficulty in his later speculations about the stress response syndrome.

One of the more attractive, but under-emphasized, aspects of Selye's views on stress is that it need not necessarily be negative or pathological for the organism. This was evident even in his early formulations about stress:

> Stress is not even necessarily bad for you; it is also the spice of life, for any emotion, any activity causes stress. But of course we must be able to take it. The same stress which makes one person sick can be an invigorating experience to another. (Selye, 1956, Preface)

Selye has recently called the more pleasant, enjoyable, ecstatic and fulfilling aspects of experience **eustress**, and the more unpleasant, damaging and pathogenic disturbances **distress**. It is interesting that Selye distinguished these different forms of stress psychologically. For there is nothing in his biological view of stress which permits the differentiation of various stress states. Once more it is implicit, if not explicit, that the understanding of stress in the GAS can be greatly enhanced by psychological explanations.

Selye's response-based model of stress has been presented here in some detail. His work is important in its own right and it is particularly relevant to nursing which is concerned with the care of ill people who display features of the stress response.

Whilst accepting that the stress process does consist of many fundamental physiological changes, the response model of stress still presents man as a passive being reacting to a hostile environment.

The cognitive–phenomenological–transactional model of stress and coping to which we turn now, largely overcomes many of the criticisms made of both the stimulus and response-based conceptualizations of stress. The model presented is a generally accepted one, but a few minor modifications have been made by the present authors. We believe that this model holds great promise for the applied study of stress and coping in nursing.

The cognitive–phenomenological–transactional (CPT) view of stress and coping

The cognitive–phenomenological–transactional (CPT) (Fig. 1.6) view of stress and coping which will be described here owes much to the thinking and experiments of the psychologist Richard Lazarus (1966). The model is **cognitive** because it contains the assumption that thinking, memory, and the meaning or significance of events to the individual experiencing them, are the central mediators and the immediate causal agents in determining stress and coping. That is, whether stress or coping occur, and in what form, depends on each individual's way of appraising his relationship to environmental events. Such appraisal is a function of past experience and memory. The approach is **phenomenological** because it is the individual's own highly individual and often idiosyncratic appraisal which is seen as the crucial factor in his response. For instance, one nurse may appraise the apparatus in an intensive care unit as 'aggravating' and 'gets on my nerves', whereas another may find it 'comforting' and 'reassuring' that efforts are being made to help patients. The phenomenological view permits an appreciation that on yet other occasions, the nurse who was aggravated may now report feeling comfort from the apparatus, whilst the once reassured nurse is now aggravated. Moreover, the phenomenological view of stress and coping makes it perfectly tenable to have both these nurses feeling the same way as each other, or different from each other, under objectively identical circumstances.

The **transactional** aspect of this model of stress and coping emphasizes the interaction between the appraisals made by the individual and the environment in which they find themselves. For a nurse or patient many of these appraisals will take place in the social environment of the hospital. Appraisal is said to lead to evaluation of the degree of threat, harm, loss or challenge perceived as actually taking place or anticipated as likely to occur. For example, a patient about to undergo surgery may appraise it as 'harmful' and this then induces anxiety. Another patient may see himself as 'fortunate to get the operation' and so be relaxed and trusting. Whether either of these responses is optimum for effective coping and patient rehabilitation is another matter.

However, the concept of coping is an essential one in relation to threat. If we could use Selye's term of stressor, it is obvious that whether a potential stressor is actually perceived as threatening or not, depends on whether the individual also appraises himself as able to cope. An example comes to mind here: a recent victim of a car bomb suffered severe injuries to both legs. However, he appraised the situation as one with which he could cope, since he was

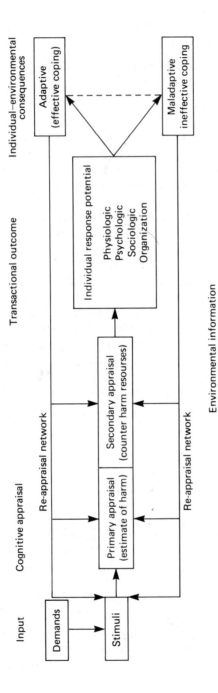

Figure 1.6 Cognitive–Phenomenological–Transactional model of stress and coping (based on Lazarus, 1966, 1976, 1979).

physically fit, highly trained and his morale was good. Later he attributed his survival to this appraisal. So in any model of stress we need to include not only the person's appraisal of the situation but also his appraisal of his ability to cope. Lazarus (1966) conceptualized three types of appraisal. **Primary appraisal**, i.e. when the individual assesses the challenge or demand made by the situation. **Secondary appraisal** is the individual's estimate of his ability to cope or his 'counter-harm' resources. **Reappraisal** entails a check on the relative effectiveness of any coping behaviour adopted by the individual to reduce or remove the source of threat. Nurses may like to note the similarity of this model with the nursing process (assessment of problems, planning to cope with problems, carrying out plan, reassessment.) When this view of stress and coping is presented, its application and elegance as a practical model for nurses to guide them in coping both with their own and patients' stress becomes evident.

Some general points will now be made about this model. Lazarus was one of the first people to draw attention to the problems associated with the definition of stress and stressors. He did this through a series of experiments in which films of gruesome accidents and initiation ceremonies were shown to subjects (Folkman *et al.*, 1979). He found that not only reported feelings but also physiological indicators of the stress response were influenced by the way in which the films were introduced to the subjects. The manner of introduction had altered their perception and led them to qualitatively different ways of appraising what they saw. These experiments were reported in a seminal book *Psychological Stress and the Coping Process*, where Lazarus has made quite clear his view on stress.

> One of the fundamental features of stress (and emotion) as a concept is that it refers to relations between an organism and the environment, rather than to either the organism or the environment alone. (Lazarus, 1971, p. 54)

Therefore in the transactional view, stress can only be defined, if at all, by the relationship between the individual and his surroundings. A point which arises from this is that the individual is not just at the mercy of stressful situations in which he finds himself as many of the studies of stress within nursing imply. Rather the individual is seen as a dynamic system attempting to control levels of threat or demand to which he or she is exposed by effective coping. This is an absolutely vital point for anyone concerned with health. As Moos points out:

> The understanding of any one person's behaviour or in an interpersonal situation solely in terms of the stimuli presented to him gives only a *partial and misleading* picture for, to a very large extent, these stimuli are created by him. They are responses to his own behaviors, events he has played a role in bringing about, rather than recurrences

independent of who he is and over which he has no control [italics
added]. (Moos, 1976, p. 127)

Lazarus suggested that stress should be considered as fitting in a broad
rubric of a collection of related problems rather than a single narrow concept.
The CPT model proposed allows the incorporation of physiological, psychological and sociological factors and so fits well with current theories of
nursing. However, physiological and sociological factors are considered to
exert their impact on the individual through individual psychological factors
which determine not only how he appraises both sociological and physiological factors in his environment, but also physiological aspects of his body,
together with his own coping strategies and resources. One of the assumptions made in the CPT model is that stress is negative or damaging to the
individual.

To speak of something as falling within the rubric of stress presumes a
damaging transaction between some specific type of organism and
some particular condition of the environment [italics added]. (Lazarus,
1971, p. 94)

Lazarus' work, with some modifications, seems to the present authors to be
far more useful as a framework for clinical nursing practice and nursing
research than the stress as stimulus or stress as response models.
Two examples show how the CPT model can be applied in nursing.

EXAMPLE NO 1

Individual in transaction:	Staff nurse
Behaviour setting:	Oncology Ward
Environmental demand:	Patient with cáncer insults nurse
Primary appraisal (threat significance):	Nurse assesses demand as patient's response to pain and his hopeless future
Secondary appraisal (coping or counter-harm resources):	Nurse overcomes initial feeling of anger and bases coping on the view that the patient requires counselling. She sits beside patient and asks if there is anything she can do which might 'help'
Reappraisal (check on efficacy of coping):	Nurse waits for patient to reply and does not interrupt patient. Patient apologizes for being 'cruel' but is not 'comfortable' and that is 'your job'. In any event 'I feel useless now'

EXAMPLE NO 2

Individual in transaction:	Adolescent male patient in traction after RTA
Behaviour setting:	RTA Ward
Environmental demand:	Nurse prepares to give patient bed-bath

Primary appraisal (threat significance):	Patient anxious at 'the thought' of having his body washed by a 'stranger'
Secondary appraisal (coping or counter-harm resources):	Closes eyes, and imagines it is his mother who is bathing him
Reappraisal (check on efficacy of coping):	Under the circumstances, patient regards this as a good way of 'getting over' his anxiety. Decides it was not as bad as he feared, and will use this coping strategy for the next bed-bath

These are only two short examples out of the many which occur daily in hospital. It is a particularly useful way of analysing episodes as it allows nurses to see the multitude of coping strategies that can be used in different situations. They can then become skilled in using them to cope with threat they see aimed at themselves on primary appraisal. More than this, it gives them a method of helping patients by suggesting coping strategies.

The attractiveness (appeal) of the CPT model of stress and coping

The main appeal of this model is the way in which it can be applied to real life. Not only that, but it provides a framework for strategies which can help individuals, especially in the face of unavoidable threat or demand. This latter property is its advantage over previous formulations of stress which leave the individual responding rather passively or even helpless in the face of threat. Using a CPT model, the perceived source of threat can be identified, and coping strategies can be planned. The relationship between threat and coping can be made explicit and the individual may be helped to gain personal control over threat or demands imposed by the physical and social environment. An individual who understands the model gains the knowledge to analyse the situations they judge threatening; to gain insight into the characteristics of threatening situations; and also to develop a range of coping strategies. Finally, it allows him continually to evaluate the efficacy of the coping strategies he uses. For a nurse who understands the model, she can use it not only to help herself to cope in the face of the environmental and social pressures inherent in the nature of the job, but by using the model, can identify situations patients find threatening, help them to cope, or better still help them to develop their own strategies for coping, and finally evaluate the outcome of the coping.

Theoretically the model can account for individual variation in stress and coping, unlike the stress as stimulus and stress as response models. Lazarus has said,

It soon becomes clear that stress cannot be defined exclusively by situations because the capacity of any situation to produce reactions also depends on the characteristics of the individual. Similarly, stress reactions in an individual do not provide adequate grounds for defining the situation associated with it as a stress, except for that individual or individuals like him. (Lazarus, 1966, p. 5)

Some recent studies of patient stress and anxiety have been based on Lazarus' work (Wilson-Barnett, 1980) but have not explored the full implications of the CPT model which has the virtue of avoiding a narrow or restricted definition of stress. The emphasis is placed on the relationship between the individual and the environment, and this is in line with current concerns in nursing. It supposes an ecological relationship between man and his environment. It is when this relationship is disturbed by the individual's appraisal of threat that stress responses may follow. However these are then proportional in severity, not necessarily to the degree of threat, but to the individual's capacity for coping.

A final point in favour of the model is that it allows intervention not only at the point of secondary appraisal, but also at the point of primary appraisal by allowing that a different interpretation of the potentially threatening event will show that it is not threatening at all. This aspect of the model is elaborated further in Chapter 2.

Internal–external events

So far we have emphasized the view that threat is focused out in the environment. The model does however allow for the individual to make primary or even secondary appraisals about potential threat from within his body. For example, a patient who experiences pain after operation will primarily appraise it differently if he knows it is normally to be expected than if it is completely unexpected. Similarly, the secondary appraisal will be different if he knows that a prescription is available to allow nurses to administer a powerful analgesic. His final reappraisal will be in terms of how well the analgesic has worked. Another example is a person who experiences ventricular extrasystoles. On primary appraisal he will not see this as threatening if he knows that they have been caused by excessive drinking of coffee. A person who is not able to interpret missed heart beats in this way may respond with anxiety which increases the heart rate and on secondary appraisal he will interpret this as even greater threat. A nurse can help the patient to cope by giving him information and by assuring him that professional help is at hand. In this way the CPT model is able to explain people's individual responses to internal events, and even such things as individual differences in seeking medical help in the face of apparently identical symptoms.

Stress in the absence of threat

In order to see how robust the CPT model is, it is worth checking whether it can account for circumstances in which an individual feels threatened although there is objectively nothing in the environment or his internal state to justify such an appraisal. Two examples will illustrate the point.

1. A nurse is allocated to a ward in charge of which is a sister who is constantly 'picking on' the nurse. The nurse feels threatened by this, not only when she is on duty but also her off-duty times are made miserable by anticipation of the next time she has to work with the sister.
2. A patient is much more anxious than his apparently minor operation would warrant. On exploring this, the nurse discovers that his anxiety is due to fear about his family business and the care of his family whilst he is in hospital.

In each case the individual was affected by threat which was not present in the immediate internal or external environment. However the CPT model states that it is the individual's cognitive appraisal (or thinking and perceiving) which determines threat for him. Therefore, appraisal of threat from remembered or anticipated events can be accommodated within this model. This is something which the stress as stimulus and stress as response models cannot account for. Use of the CPT model directs a nurse's attention to the possibility of sources of threat to the patient from the external world as well as from within the hospital environment. This allows for a broader framework in assessment.

The cognitive orientation – a model for individuals

One of the biggest advantages of the CPT model, both for theoretical and practical purposes lies in its cognitive and individual orientation. It takes account of the fact that the identical situation will be threatening to one person but not another, and that the situation may change so that a person who did not find a situation threatening on one occasion finds it extremely threatening a week later. The key to the model is that it is the individual's way of seeing the situation at that precise moment, and the coping resources he/she has available at that same moment which determine the stress experienced. Five minutes later and the person's perception, or coping resources, may have changed. It is one of nursing's tasks to ensure that this change takes place for the patient in the direction of preventing or alleviating stress.

The model also applies to nurses themselves and gives nurses a framework in which they can investigate their own appraisal of sources of threat and coping mechanisms. It gives a tool for counsellors to help nurses through the application of the model. Throughout this book the writers are as much concerned with the psycho-biological health of the nurse as with the patients whom she nurses.

'Harmless' stimuli

The CPT model also enables us to appreciate how apparently benign or 'harmless' stimuli can be appraised as significantly threatening. For example, a patient's primary appraisal of a priest visiting the hospital bedsides of many patients in his ward may be alarming, especially when the priest is approaching nearer and nearer to his bed. He may have appraised the visit as highly threatening, 'because priests always visit dying patients'. The patient's inference from this may be 'am I dying?' or more stressful still, 'I am dying!' The nurse should remember the significance of such an event for the patient, and help him to cope with it. In the case of the patient asking a question, the nurse may ask a question in return such as 'What makes you think that?' When the source of the threat has been established the nurse would be in a position to provide the patient with correct information. This should then influence both his original appraisal of the situation and how he copes with it. For example, when it became clear that the patient's discomfort was rooted in the priest 'threat', the nurse could explain that he visits to provide some companionship and conversation and that very few patients die on that particular ward. Next time the priest arrived the patient's primary appraisal would be different and coping would be unlikely to come in the form of alarmist questions. Obviously what the nurse should not do in such a situation is to prevent the patient explaining his fears by telling him 'not to worry'. This is a sign that the nurse is not listening with understanding, something which has been of considerable concern in recent research on communication between nurse and patients and carried out by Jill MacLeod-Clark (1981).

Conditioning and the CPT model

Some readers may be thinking that many of the examples we have mentioned could be explained by conditioning. The two main types of conditioning in psychology are classical conditioning (Pavlov, 1928) and operant conditioning (Skinner, 1953). Classical conditioning is the type most relevant to stress reactions. Reflexes subserved by the autonomic nervous system have been used to demonstrate classical conditioning. It will be recalled that the autonomic nervous system has an important underlying control function in the many physiological components of stress. The famous example of classical conditioning comes from Pavlov's work. He presented a neutral stimulus such as the sound of a bell at the same time as he placed dried meat powder in a dog's mouth. After several such paired presentations of stimuli the sound of the bell came to elucidate the response of salivation. These events were now called the conditioned stimulus and the conditioned response respectively. Classical conditioning has been implicated in the learning of unpleasant emotional responses, such as anxiety and fear, in the presence of neutral objects. This produces what we call phobias. Anxiety and fear are common emotional components in stress reactions (Spielberger, 1970). Is it necessary then to evoke a relatively complicated explanation such as the CPT model when conditioning might be the real process that goes on? Such a question shows a misunderstanding of the relationship between classical conditioning and the CPT model. Almost certainly some stress reactions result from classical conditioning. This does not however invalidate the approach from the point of view of the meaning of the threatening stimulus to the person, and an attempt to strengthen his coping resources in dealing with the threat.

An example illustrates the point: If a nurse suffers from haemophobia (fear of blood) it may have arisen from the fear and pain experienced during a childhood accident. Seeing blood has become conditioned to fear, nausea and physical discomfort, which she experiences whenever she sees blood. The crucial factor here is the meaning which became attached to the incident during the original conditioning and which has been strengthened since. The sight of blood has acquired great significance to the nurse and a simple stimulus response explanation is only a partial one. For humans, conditioning explanations may be a necessary but certainly not a sufficient explanation for those circumstances in which they apply. It is far more difficult to apply a conditioning explanation to a person's fear of something which they have never previously experienced whilst the CPT model can account for this.

How realistic is the CPT model?

A possible criticism of the CPT model lies in its apparently lengthy processes of primary appraisal, secondary appraisal and reappraisal. Faced with threat, have people got time for all this? Lazarus anticipated such a criticism by saying,

> As in the case of the primary process of threat appraisal, there is no implication that in secondary appraisal the individual engages in a lengthy reflection about the situation although this may indeed occur. The process is often nearly instantaneous, although it is also often a symbolic process, especially in higher mammals. Similarly, the individual need not be fully aware of the evaluation he is making of the factors that enter into them. (Lazarus, 1966, p. 161)

The nurse, patient or any other individual can engage in this process rapidly. Indeed an example shows how it is necessary to go through such a process rapidly if one is to survive. A person who is driving a car round a bend, and is suddenly confronted with a lorry on his side of the road overtaking another car goes through a process of primary appraisal ('Threat of crash and my car will come off worse than the lorry'). Secondary appraisal ('Can I drive on to the verge?') and reappraisal ('Thank God, he missed me by inches. If I hadn't driven on to the verge I would probably have been dead by now'). The reader will appreciate how rapidly and almost automatically such a process takes place.

On another occasion the process may take much longer. Even primary appraisal may take a while in particularly ambiguous circumstances. An example is the friend who uncharacteristically speaks to one in anger. Should this be interpreted as a threat against oneself, or an expression of the mood of the moment? i.e. the friend is feeling under threat for some reason. Primary appraisal may continue until further information is provided to allow the event to be evaluated in terms of the degree of threat posed.

In summary, the activities involved in cognitive appraisal occur on a continuum from fast-instantaneous to slow, deliberate assessment of events, their significance in terms of threat and the resources available for coping. A nurse should understand this since she may be called upon to assess a patient's condition instantaneously if he has ceased to breathe and to set in motion the coping mechanisms of resuscitation whilst she may take twenty-four hours to record another patient's nursing history and assessment.

The present authors find they cannot agree with one aspect of the CPT model as developed by Lazarus. That is its sole concern that stress is a negative or damaging transaction with the environment. Clearly there are many kinds of individual–environment transactions which nurses and patients carry out in their daily commerce with each other in the hospital setting. However, these are not necessarily damaging or unhealthy for patients or nurses. On the contrary, these same transactions in health care delivery are largely responsible for nurse satisfaction with their work (Bailey, 1980) and successful patient rehabilitation (Moos, 1979).

Lazarus' view of stress is that stress always impairs human functioning. Indeed the vast literature on stress in nurses, patients, and other populations, although not necessarily defining stress in the same way, present their clinical-research reports of stress as being antithetical to psycho-medical health. We are unable to support this position, for a number of reasons. In the first instance, since transactions between the individual and the environment are essentially continuous rather than discrete, it would seem that stress is more or less present all the time during the human lifespan. Wolff and Goodall in their valued book *Stress and Disease* have highlighted a similar view of stress from a biological perspective:

> Since stress is a dynamic state within an organism in response to a demand for adaptation and since life itself entails constant adaptation,

living creatures are continually in a state of more or less stress. [italics added] (Wolff and Goodall, 1968, p. 4)

The present authors would argue that a psychology of stress and coping which is linked to physiological and biological functioning must take into account the relative nature of stress, and its intrinsic necessity for the survival of the human species. In its simplest form stress entails life and its absence, death. Put into nurse and patient terms it suggests they are not either under stress or stress-free. Rather it means trying to appreciate, that in a subtler way, we function psychologically, physiologically and biologically, in states relative to the meaning different environments have for us at different times in our lives. This seems nearer to our experience of daily living as nurses, patients or whatever our personal life circumstance. However, it is a conceptualization which raises a problem for the CPT model of stress and coping. It is this. How can the nurse or patient apply the model so as to differentiate between those states which are pleasant and exhuberant and those which are regarded as unpleasant, debilitating and damaging to psycho-medical health? Selye has attempted to overcome this problem by calling the former 'eustress' and the latter states 'distress'. But we have evaluated the GAS response-based approach to stress and found it inadequate for the study of stress and coping in nursing – which we regard primarily as a psychological matter.

The remaining question might be: 'Can the CPT model of stress and coping be applied to those relative states of stress found in everyday life?' No change is required of the model in this respect. For the appraisal which nurses and patients make of the environment will still be made relative to the degree of threat, loss or challenge they perceive and the coping they assume to deal with the environment. However because a situation is appraised in this way it does not mean that a negative stress reaction should follow. For example the student may find the threat of a first medical ward exhilarating and a challenge to show the sister and her colleagues she is a 'born nurse'. Whereas threat, loss and challenge seems to be used by Lazarus to mean a damaging or negative transaction with the environment, we use it here in a more technical sense, namely that they are defined as the degree to which demands from the environment alter the psycho-biological homeostasis of the individual. The way in which the nurse copes with appraisal of threat, loss or challenge may range from obvious incompetence to complete mastery. In this way we can account for the thrill of threat, relief of loss (death of a suffering patient) and joy of challenge, in one nurse or patient, to the fear of it in others.

The CPT model, with these minor modifications, presents an attractive theoretical and practical approach to stress and coping in nursing. Although many of the studies of nursing stress and patient coping with physical illness employ the stress–strain model, nurses should find the CPT approach to stress and coping fruitful in future research. Moreover, it has substantial promise for the practical understanding and self-regulation of the nurse's own health and those in her charge, coping with physical illness.

1.2 SUMMARY

We have considered stimulus, response and transactional meanings and models of stress. The stimulus approach to stress seems an unsatisfactory model for nursing. The main reason is its simplistic view of causality. Furthermore, it gives no help in predicting which stimuli will cause stress. It does not permit us to understand the rich range of individual differences in stress and coping. The model is also limited in that it does not suggest how people cope. Finally, it can be criticized for being a passive model and not dynamic enough to account for human activity. The response-based approach to stress and coping developed by Hans Selye has been outlined and the processes of the General Adaptation Syndrome described. This model too, although helpful in general to appreciate the physiological functioning of stress reactions, is not thought to be fruitful to apply in most studies of stress and coping in nursing. Its main weakness is the limited place given to psychological factors influencing stress and coping. Although the GAS has been amended to account for these, it is firmly based in physiological assumptions about stress. A cognitive transactional model of stress and coping was then discussed. It is based on ideas formulated by the psychologist Richard Lazarus. This model is essentially psychological in nature. Apart from minor changes, it is strongly supported by the present authors as a valuable model to apply both theoretically and practically in clinical nursing.

REFERENCES

Bailey, J. T. (1980) Job stress and other stress-related problems, in *Living with Stress and Promoting Well Being* (eds K. E. Claus and J. T. Bailey), Mosby, St. Louis, MO.

Boore, J. R. P. (1978) *Prescription for Recovery*, Royal College of Nursing, London.

Cannon, W. B. (1932) *The Wisdom of the Body*, Norton, New York.

Cox, T. (1978) *Stress*, Macmillan Press Ltd, London.

Ferguson, D. (1974) A study of occupational stress and health, in *Man Under Stress* (ed. A. T. Welford), Taylor and Francis, London, pp. 83–98.

Folkman, S., Shaefer, C. and Lazarus, R. (1979) Cognitive processes as mediators of stress and coping, in *Human Stress and Cognition: an Information Processing Approach*, (eds V. Hamilton and D. M. Warburton), J. Wiley, New York.

Ganong, W. F. (1975) *Review of Medical Physiology*, 7th edn, Lange, Los Altos, CA.

Holmes, T. H. and Rahe, R. H. (1967) The social readjustment rating scale. *J. Psychosomatic Research*, **11**, 213.

International Dictionary of Physics (1961), 2nd edn, Van Nostrand, Amsterdam.

Lacey, J. I. (1967) Somatic response patterning and stress: some revisions of activation theory, in *Psychological Stress*, (eds M. H. Appley and R. Trumbull), Appleton Century Crofts, New York.

Lazarus, R. (1966) *Psychological Stress and the Coping Process*, McGraw-Hill New York.

Lazarus, R. (1971) The concept of stress and disease, *Social Stress and Disease*, **1**, 53–60.

Lazarus, R. (1976) *Patterns of Adjustment*, McGraw-Hill, New York.

Lazarus, R. (1979) Positive denial: the case for not facing reality, *Psychology Today* (November), 44–60.

Lazarus, R. (1981) The stress and coping paradigm, in *Theoretical Bases for Psychopathology*, (eds C. Elsdorfer, D. Cohen, A. Kleinman and P. Maxim), Spectrum, New York.

Levine, S., Wunberg, J. and Ursin, M. (1978) Definition of the coping process and statement of the problem, in *The Psychology of Stress: A Study of Coping Man*, (eds H. Ursin *et al.*), Academic Press, New York.

Macpherson, R. K. (1974) Thermal stress and thermal comfort, in *Man Under Stress*, (ed. A. T. Welford), Taylor and Francis, London, pp. 45–56.

Mason, J. W. (1975) A historical view of the stress field, Part 1. *J. Human Stress*, **1**, 6–12.

McGrath, J. (1970) *Social and Psychological Factors in Stress*, Holt, Rinehart and Winston, New York.

McLeod-Clark, J. (1981) Communicating with cancer patients: communication or evasion?, in *Cancer Nursing Update*, (ed. R. Tiffany), Baillière Tindall, London.

Moos, R. (1976) *The Human Context: Environmental Determinants of Behaviour*, Wiley, New York.

Moos, R. (ed.) (1979) *Coping with Physical Illness*, Plenum Press, New York.

Pavlov, I. (1928) *Conditioned Reflexes*, OUP, Oxford.

Pilowsky, I. (1974) Psychiatric aspects of stress, in *Man Under Stress*, (ed. A. T. Welford), Taylor and Francis, London, pp. 125–32.

Selye, H. (1956) *The Stress of Life*, 2nd edn, McGraw-Hill, New York.

Selye, H. (1975) *Stress without Distress*, Cygnet Books, New York.

Selye, H. (1976) *Stress in Health and Disease*, Butterworth, London.

Selye, H. (1979) The stress concept and some of its implications, in *Human Stress and Cognition: An Information Processing Approach*, (eds V. Hamilton and D. M. Warburton), J. Wiley, New York.

Selye, H. (1980) Stress and a holistic view of health for the nursing profession, in *Living with Stress and Promoting Well Being*, (eds K. E. Claus and J. T. Bailey), Mosby, St. Louis, MO.

Skinner, B. F. (1953) *Science and Human Behaviour*, Macmillan, New York.

Spielberger, C. (1970) *Anxiety and Behaviour*, Academic Press, New York.

Vandor, A. J., Sherman, J. H. and Luciano, D. S. (1975) *Human Physiology: the Mechanisms of Body Function*, 2nd edn, McGraw-Hill, New York.

Welford, A. T. (1974) Stress and performance, in *Man Under Stress*, (ed. A. T. Welford), Taylor and Francis, London, pp. 1–14.

Wilson-Barnett, J. (1980) Prevention and alleviation of stress in patients, *Nursing*, (1st series) No. 10, pp. 432–6.

Wolf, F. S. and Goodell, H. (1968) *Stress and Disease*, 2nd edn, Charles C. Thomas, Springfield, IL.

CHAPTER TWO

Coping

Coping is one component of the individual's transactions with his internal and external environment. It is the means by which he attempts to control perceived levels of demand or threat. A dictionary definition of the verb to cope is 'to contend evenly' or 'to grapple successfully'. Our definition is somewhat broader than this as it includes *all* attempts by the individual to reduce the impact of perceived threat or demand upon himself whether or not they are successful in reducing demand. We believe that for nurses an understanding of coping is crucial. One way of conceptualizing the role of the nurse is that it involves: (a) identifying, strengthening and reinforcing of coping strategies used by the patient; (b) teaching patients new coping strategies; and (c) acting for the patient who is unable to cope for himself. As many nurses work in an extremely demanding social environment it is likely also to be personally helpful in both their working and private life for them to have a thorough understanding of coping.

Four main approaches to the interpretation of coping can be identified in the literature. These may be classified and characterized as:

1. Ego-defensive coping
2. Coping as a personality trait
3. Situation grounded coping
4. Phenomenological–transactional coping.

As in the previous chapter, we think it helpful to analyse each approach critically, and by doing so, contribute to a greater understanding of the dimensions of coping. We can then bring together several approaches and use them within a discussion of the phenomenological–transactional view, which is the one we favour.

2.1 EGO-DEFENSIVE COPING

This view of coping comes mainly from the psycho-analytical school of psychology. Freud and his followers have described a number of defence mechanisms which occur unconsciously and protect the ego or rational self-image from threat (Coleman and Hammen, 1974). Ego-defence mechanisms include denial, repression, displacement, reaction formation, sublimation and

Table 2.1 Summary chart of ego-defence mechanisms

Denial of reality	Refusing to perceive or face unpleasant reality
Repression	Preventing painful or dangerous thoughts from entering consciousness
Regression	Retreating to earlier developmental level involving less mature responses and usually a lower level of aspiration
Fantasy	Gratifying frustrated desires by imaginary achievements
Rationalization	Attempting to prove that one's behaviour is rational and justifiable and thus worthy of the approval of oneself and others
Projection	Placing blame for difficulties upon others or attributing one's own unethical desires to others
Reaction formation	Preventing the expression of dangerous desires by exaggerating the opposite attitudes and types of behaviour
Identification	Increasing feelings of worth by identifying oneself with some outstanding person or institution
Introjection	Incorporating into one's own ego structure the values and standards imposed by others
Emotional insulation	Reducing ego involvement and withdrawing into passivity to protect oneself from hurt
Intellectualization	Suppressing the emotional aspect of hurtful situations or separating incompatible attitudes by logic-tight compartments
Compensation	Covering up weakness by emphasizing some desirable trait or making up for frustration in one area by over-gratification in another
Displacement	Discharging pent-up feelings, usually of hostility, on objects less dangerous than those which initially aroused the emotions
Undoing	Counteracting 'immoral' desires or acts by some form of atonement
Acting out	Reducing the anxiety aroused by forbidden desires by permitting their expression

Source: From Contemporary Psychology and Effective Behavior *by James C. Coleman and Constance L. Hammen (1974).*

identification. (For a complete list with descriptions see Table 2.1.)

An example of denial often given in the literature is that of a patient who denies he is at all anxious about his forthcoming operation. Following our earlier discussion of stress, it is interesting to note that there is an implicit assumption here that a forthcoming operation inevitably causes anxiety and that someone who claims not to feel anxious is employing a defence mechanism. Repression occurs when an individual forgets a distressing experience through an unconscious process which results in an inability to recall the experience directly. This becomes accessible, if at all, through the interpretation of dreams, hypnosis, word association or some other psycho-analytic technique. Displacement means diverting the aggression felt toward a power-ful but threatening person onto someone who is less powerful ('kicking the cat') and toward whom it is safer to show aggression. Reaction formation occurs when an individual compensates for physical or psychological inade-quacy not merely by overcoming it but by becoming more than adequate in that quality. An example would be a person who was afraid of heights but overcame this to the extent of becoming a mountaineer. Sublimation is used when an individual's desires are antisocial or otherwise unattainable. The individual compensates by using his energy in a socially acceptable substitute activity. In this case the individual's own superego (conscience) is what deter-mines whether or not an activity is acceptable. Examples which are fre-quently cited are people who have a desire to kill but instead become surgeons, using the scalpel to heal; others with strong maternal feelings may become nurses. Identification is when an individual having identified a simi-larity between himself and a person of higher status, then assumes that other qualities are also similar and acquires status himself through this perceived relationship.

Knowing that people may use one or more of these defence mechanisms as a means of coping with threat to the self-image is helpful in understanding the behaviour of some patients. On the whole, however, nurses cannot make use of such knowledge therapeutically. First, there is real difficulty in identifying the defence mechanism which is being used by a patient when staff do not know the patient well. It may be difficult to be certain whether or not a patient is using a defence mechanism at all. To go back to our first example; if a patient denies feeling anxious in the face of an impending operation is this because he genuinely does not feel anxious or is it because he consciously rather than unconsciously does not wish to confess what to him appears a weakness? If a patient appears aggressive toward a nurse, is this because the nurse has annoyed him or is it because the consultant was the source of the irritation? The difficulty is a real one (Folkman and Lazarus, 1980).

Another problem is in determining whether or not such mechanisms are helpful to the patient or not. If they were known to be helpful perhaps staff could encourage patients to use them. Unfortunately there is some evidence that whilst the use of ego-defence mechanisms might be helpful in the short term, it might pose a threat to health in the long term. Such methods fall into the category of palliative coping which will be discussed later in this chapter. Evidence that defence mechanisms are threatening to physical health comes from a study by Janis (1958). He found that patients who denied feeling anxious prior to operation showed longer recovery times than patients who said they felt moderately anxious pre-operatively. As far as a threat to mental health is concerned, evidence comes from the study of patients by Freud which led him to describe ego-defence mechanisms in the first place.

Accepting that psycho-analytical theory is valid, this brings us to another reason why a knowledge of defence mechanisms is of limited help to nurses and that is because nurses have very limited acquaintance with psycho-analytical techniques. Training in such techniques is specialized and lengthy.

Our major criticism of the ego-defensive approach to coping is that it ignores other types of coping, whilst in itself it is only a partial explanation of some types of coping.

Whilst it may be possible to identify behaviour related to the use of mental mechanisms currently, there is no way of controlling their use since essentially they are unconscious processes. We should not however ignore the temporary usefulness of ego defence (Kubler-Ross, 1973) but interpret this within a broader theoretical framework. Lazarus (1976) has described a further defence mechanism within his phenomenological–transactional view of coping. This is intellectualization which he describes as occurring among medical students, for example. Through intellectualization a person gains emotional detachment by isolating his own or a patient's problem from the full complexity of implications and treating it as a one-dimensional problem to be solved cognitively. In this way a medical student (or anyone else) protects himself from the full impact of the demand presented by the human dilemma of the person with a (medical) problem.

It is possible to characterize defence mechanisms as valuable short-term forms of coping which allow the individual to deal with what might otherwise be overwhelming levels of threat. They act as holding devices to allow time before proceeding to alternative forms of coping. It may be that it is only if such devices are maintained over a long period of time that they are associated with psycho-pathology.

Colin Murray Parkes's classical work on bereavement (1972) illustrates how in extreme loss widows may cope initially by adopting defence mechanisms. It is worth quoting him in full as his view on defence mechanism coincides with our own views on the positive role defence mechanisms may have as short-term coping devices in the face of extreme loss of control (Parkes, 1972, pp. 71–72).

> A subtle ethic has crept into much of our thinking, which seems to imply that ego defences are a 'bad thing' and that we would be much better off without them.
>
>   Studies of bereavement throw doubt on this assumption. In short, it seems to me that most of the phenomena we lump together as defences have an important function in helping to regulate the quantity of novel, unorganized, or in other respects disabling, information an individual is handling at a given time. We see this most clearly in the nursery when the young child is scanning, manipulating and exploring an environment whose complexity varies greatly. In the face of new or large or threatening stimuli he withdraws or hides, or calls upon his mother for

support; then gradually and warily, he begins to make familiar those very stimuli he at first found alarming.

In a similar way the widow, whose world has suddenly changed very radically, withdraws from a situation of overwhelming complexity and potential danger. Lacking her accustomed source of reassurance and support, she shuts herself up at home and admits only those members of her family with whom she feels most secure.

At the same time, and to an increasing extent as time passes, she begins, little by little, to examine the implications of what has happened, and in this way to make familiar and controllable the numerous areas of uncertainty that now exist in her world.

Thus we have two opposing tendencies: an inhibitory tendency, which by repression, avoidance, postponement, etc., holds back or limits the perception of disturbing stimuli. At any given time an individual may respond more to one of these tendencies than to the other, and over time he will often oscillate between them.

Viewed thus, 'defence' can be seen as part of the process of 'attacking' a problem, of coming to grips with it in a relatively safe and effective way. That it may not always enable the individual to succeed in mastering the problem, and may at times become distorted or pathological, does not detract from its biological function, which is the maintenance of appropriate distancing.

These observations may be generalized to apply to some patients in hospital. Parkes (1972) has shown how defence mechanisms may be used in the face of personal loss by amputation patients before they come to acceptance and make the transition to an altered life style. There is much support for the view that defence mechanisms are important in the process of coping after severe injury, surgery and illness, especially when there is an accompanying change of body image.

Defence mechanisms may be seen as part of the psychological armamentarium which patients use to deal with levels of demand which for the moment cannot be resolved by other forms of coping. Obviously the use of defence mechanisms is available to all human beings including nurses themselves when confronted with levels of demand which amount to threat. Leaving aside the difficulty of identifying and defining defence mechanisms, it would be useful to have further research to show what positive function defence mechanisms play in the processes of coping, and therefore in the maintenance of health. At the same time it must be recognized that defence mechanisms may be effective only in the short term and that used as a long-term strategy or inappropriately they may themselves lead to long-term health problems. In other words, unless they form only a minor part of a changing dynamic process used by an individual they may outlast their therapeutic value as a palliative form of coping.

2.2 COPING AS A FUNCTION OF PERSONALITY

Another way of viewing coping is that there is a characteristic style of coping used by any one individual and this style is determined by the individual's personality. Any given person can be placed at a point on several personality dimensions concerned with coping. Personality traits or dimensions are usually characterized by their extreme poles and theoretically each individual could be described on these personality dimensions by their position between each pair of extremes as determined by measurement. The usual method of measurement is by questionnaire.

Examples of personality dimensions relevant to coping are:

(a) self-reliant versus dependent;
(b) introversion versus extroversion (Eysenck, 1947);
(c) problem confrontation versus problem avoidance (Coelho et al. 1974);
(d) repression versus sensitization (Byrne, 1964).

Taking each of these in turn:

(a) An individual at the self-reliant pole would always seek to cope with demand personally and independently, whilst a person who was extremely dependent would always attempt to cope with demand by seeking help from others.
(b) Someone who was an extreme extrovert would find solitude and lack of stimulation much more threatening than would an extreme introvert. Their styles of coping would also differ; an extrovert coping by seeking company, whilst an introvert would cope by shunning company; an extrovert using physical practical coping methods, an introvert using intellectual, more abstract coping.
(c) A person who confronts problems actively and 'head-on' can be contrasted with the person who delays coping with problems until action is forced by events.
(d) In relation to coping, repression versus sensitization describes at one extreme the person who subconsciously represses knowledge of problems, thus appearing not to perceive them. At the opposite pole is the individual who not only perceives problems but is abnormally sensitive to them, perceiving problems which do not exist for others.

One useful aspect emerging from this school of thought is the suggestion that individuals differ both in the way they perceive threat and the way in which they cope. However, there is the less useful assumption that a person's method of coping is relatively stable and that he copes in the same way in all situations he perceives as threatening regardless of the objective characteristics of the situation. This somewhat simplistic view ignores the considerable mounting evidence of the complexity of coping (Lazarus, 1983) and that any one individual varies his coping according to the situation (Antonovsky, 1979). Personality influences upon coping are probably strongest where the situation is ambiguous. In general, personality measures are poor at predicting the coping processes used and their outcomes (Ekehammar, 1974; Blass, 1977, Magnusson and Endler, 1977). They may be occasionally useful in predicting the coping style of an individual in the light of a specific situation and at a particular time. However, this undermines the whole personality trait view of coping.

2.3 SITUATION GROUNDED COPING

In criticizing the personality trait approach to coping we mentioned coping methods arising from the characteristics of the situation to which coping is a response. This is what we mean by situation grounded coping. Using this approach coping becomes specific and appropriate to the situation and differences in coping style between individuals are played down. A good deal of human learning is devoted to the development of coping strategies appropriate to the situation. Nurse education and training equips nurses with the skills to cope with a multitude of threatening situations, each defined by its characteristics, e.g. how to recognize cardiac arrest and how to cope, how to recognize skin breakdown in a patient and how to cope with this. For further examples see Table 2.2. The nursing process is concerned with the identification of potential and actual threats (problems) to the patients and deciding on

Table 2.2   Situation-grounded coping

	Situation	*Coping*	*Result*
Patient	Wound	Sutured	Wound closed
	Operation	Asked for information about operation and how long it would take, and recovery chances	Given information session by nurse about operation
	Staff nurse off-hand	Patient spoke to her about her attitude	Staff nurse more pleasant and sociable
Nurse	Patient has cardiac arrest	Resuscitation procedure	Patient recovered usual breathing pattern
	Exam to sit	Study and plan for anticipated questions	Marks within top 5% for class

the best coping strategy. The evaluation phase of the nursing process allows examination of the efficacy of coping. What has been less evident in nurse training in the past is any emphasis on the nurse's own feelings of threat and methods of coping. Another neglected area has been the patient's experience of psychological threat, its alleviation or prevention. We hope to include a great deal about these areas of concern in this book. Research has been carried out to identify specific ways in which patients cope with a particular illness or injury, such as cancer (Mages and Mendelsohn, 1979), spinal cord injury (Bulman and Wortman, 1977) and burns (Andreasen and Norris, 1972).

Situation grounded coping is functional. Its purpose is to change the situation, reducing inherent threat and so reducing the stress which is experienced. It is worth noting in this connection that by coping successfully with life-threatening events experienced by the patient, a nurse reduces not only the patient's stress but also the stress which is inherent for herself.

However, as with the approaches discussed earlier the situation grounded approach to coping also has its limitations. The first is that this approach is at its most useful in relation to situations which are objectively extremely threatening and where the threat is of a physical nature (Visotsky *et al.* 1961; Lazarus, 1966; Cohen and Lazarus, 1979). There is little in this approach for situations of an objectively trivial or apparently harmless nature which a particular individual may find extremely threatening. It fails to take account of the individual differences in coping between people and of differences in the way the same person may cope with identical-appearing situations on two different occasions. There is an underlying assumption that a person always deals with a given situation in an identical way because the characteristics of the situation are always the same (Folkman and Lazarus, 1980), but of course the individual who is coping may have changed in the meantime, and so may perceive the situation differently, or may have decided to try a different method of coping.

The situation grounded approach contains an implication that direct coping is always appropriate, but there are many situations in which indirect coping may be the most appropriate method. Another implicit assumption is that threatening situations occur one at a time when real life may be more complex and present several threatening situations at a time.

As with other approaches to coping we have described, this approach deals well with a single aspect of coping but fails to account for the entire complexity of events and people's behaviour (Hinkle, 1974).

It is particularly important for a nurse to understand the complexity of behaviour. Otherwise he or she will assume that a patient will behave in the same way on the second occasion a threat occurs as on the first occasion this particular threat was met. The assumption that all patients behave in the same way on meeting similar threats is equally dangerous. Both assumptions lead to stereotyped care which fails to deal with patients' needs in precisely the way that task assignment has failed. Coping, like stress, is complex and involves many aspects of human functioning in relation to the physical and social environment.

Moos (1979) has pointed out in an excellent review of coping with physical illness, that a patient must deal with many sources of stress which are highly individual. Such sources are manifold. For example, pain and disability, aspects of the ward or hospital environment, relationships with members of staff, treatment procedures, home problems. To one or all of these potential sources the patient must make coping attempts, preserve his emotional balance, maintain a satisfactory self-image, and remain on good terms with staff, family and friends. These multitudinous demands require an arsenal of coping strategies of a breadth and complexity not explained by any one of the approaches we have described so far. An approach is needed which includes relevant aspects of the views discussed but which allows in addition an appreciation of the way an individual perceives threat, and copes with it as well as the way in which his perception and coping may change over time. The phenomenological–transactional approach to coping fulfils these requirements and it is to this approach that we now turn.

2.4 PHENOMENOLOGICAL–TRANSACTIONAL APPROACH TO COPING

Within the phenomenological–transactional approach coping is viewed as a transaction between the individual and his environment as he perceives it. The behaviour of the individual is variable. Sometimes he actively copes, successfully dealing with demands. At other times he decides not to act upon demands but to wait. He may cope by adjusting his perception of the demands so that he no longer experiences them as threatening. Another individual may have learned methods of psychological and/or physiological relaxation in the face of the type of demands for which active coping is unrealistic. Yet another person may use a palliative method of coping which permits a putting aside of the threat for the time being without changing the threat in any way or altering his own tolerance in the long term.

Above all, the phenomenological–transactional view of coping describes how a person may change over time in the way in which he copes. It acknowledges that some people learn apparently improved ways of coping with threat from their past efforts whilst others fail objectively to improve their coping. Some people cope in a way which is objectively sound and realistic, whilst others cope in a way which is objectively unsound and unrealistic. A person's style of coping is a function of the circumstances, his perception of the circumstances and what he brings to the situation in terms of his past history of coping and general predisposition for action (personality). This approach above all emphasizes individuality. It fits well with the way in which nurses are beginning to approach the planning of patient care.

Since this view of coping emphasizes the complexity of the process it is helpful to classify methods of coping in some way. We can classify them as:

(a)   direct coping;
(b)   indirect coping;
(c)   palliative coping.

These classes of coping are implicit within the transactional model of stress and coping which are outlined in Chapter 1. We have taken our definition of coping as a transaction between an individual and his environment from this model.

> The individual's attempts or efforts to manage, master, tolerate or alter events so that the demands on him are not so threatening. (Lazarus and Launier, 1978)

We will now discuss each type of coping in turn, using examples relevant to nursing.

Direct coping

In this form of coping the individual concerned perceives the demands of the situation in a similar way to the perception of hypothetical onlookers (reality grounded perception) and attempts to deal with the demands by direct action with the intention of changing the situation into one which is less demanding. However, even in such an apparently clear-cut situation, individuality of perception, background and predisposition play an important role as illustrated in this example.

Nurse example

> A nurse who is alone in the ward at night whilst her colleague is away having a meal, suddenly notices the empty bed belonging to a patient who had been transferred from the cardiac monitoring unit that day. The nurse deduces that he must have got up whilst she was busy giving an injection to someone else. She finds the patient sitting in the day room in a state of distress and she discovers that he was worried by the new surroundings, the lack of lights, and the fact that there was only one nurse on duty. The nurse feels his pulse which is rapid but regular and helps him back to bed. She then phones for the doctor. Whilst waiting, she sits and listens to the patient talking about his worries and then tells him that he has been transferred to this ward because he is doing so well. By the time the doctor arrives the patient is calm, his pulse has returned to the rate which was recorded at 10 p.m., and he is

ready to settle to sleep. The doctor is full of praise for the nurse and reassures her that she acted promptly and correctly. However, the nurse herself is unhappy. She feels she should have identified the possibility of the patient being upset earlier and given him the opportunity to talk about his anxieties.

This example shows direct coping in the way the nurse acted. It also shows that the coping was perceived as satisfactory by one person (the doctor), but not by the nurse herself. The example also shows that perception of demands varies according to culture and training. The situation was demanding by virtue of the fact that the main 'actor' was a nurse who had been given responsibility for other people which she had accepted. Finding someone out of bed in the night is not a threatening situation unless that person is ill and one has accepted responsibility for him. Neither is it a direct physical threat in any way. However, the demands made on that nurse not only included demands from the patients, but from the doctor, the day staff, night nursing officer, and above all, her expectations of herself, i.e. her self-image. Her expectations of self had derived partly from the theory she had learned in the school of nursing where she had been taught to identify potential patient problems and to plan the appropriate care. However, there was a discrepancy between the theoretical teaching and the facilities and opportunities to practise in the ward (e.g. insufficient staff). This is a common source of stress for student nurses.

Patient example

A patient realizes that there is the demand from his business colleagues to know if he intends to retire since he has had an acute coronary attack. The fifty-one year old stockbroker reviews his health over the past ten years, and discusses the matter with physicians and nurses. After a further period of thought and some worry he writes to all of his business associates assuring them of his intent to carry on. This letter is the first evidence of his decision. He also informs them that medical opinion supports his decision, and that increased exercize and selective diet are now part of his lifestyle. Finally, he explains this is likely, if anything, to enhance his health and alertness for business activities and life in general. A month later, his secretary confirms the confidence in his coping by showing him copies of renewed contracts and fresh business orders. The stockbroker communicates his relief and confirms his decision to commit himself to his altered lifestyle.

In this example the stockbroker mastered the situation as he saw it using many coping skills. By taking the direct action of writing to his colleagues he reduced the demands being made on him. However, he also used other people to help him to cope by asking the advice of doctors and nurses. In taking their advice he would also be attempting to prevent the threat from another coronary attack in the future.

Both these examples show the complexity of direct coping. Coping actions may change over time as the appraisal of demands changes. As an individual's actions bring about a change in the demand he is able to perceive these changes and change his actions. Successful direct coping should result eventually in diminished stress.

Indirect coping

There are many circumstances in which people may feel that they cannot or should not attempt to cope directly with demands. A quotation from Moos (1979) is apt:

> Environments congruent with certain behaviour make behaviours more likely to occur. But one of the characteristics that distinguishes man from animals is his ability to adapt to hostile environments and to change them to meet his demands. Thus, people will attempt to modify incongruent environments. *If they cannot, as is often the case* they may cope by changing their mental images of the environment, or by dropping out and selecting a more suitable setting. [emphasis added]

People are often confronted with situations which have to be endured since they cannot be altered by direct coping. An example is the death of a loved one. No amount of action will change the situation and so any coping will have to be indirect. By indirect coping is meant (a) a change in the individual's perception of the threat, or (b) the use of methods which actually change the individual's experience of the physiological or psychological components of stress through relaxation, imagery etc. An example of the first type of indirect coping follows:

> A first-year student nurse discovered that a male patient whom she liked had an inoperable brain tumour. At first she felt helpless, angry and frustrated. She felt that there was nothing she could do for the patient. During a conversation with him, he said he felt that he had lived a satisfying life and on the whole thought he had achieved as much as was possible. He had also found that he could accept the thought of his tumour. He considered himself lucky. He had lived a satisfying life, whilst so many people seemed miserable. The doctor had told him that he was unlikely to suffer pain at all.
>
> The nurse asked him how he could be so accepting. He said he lived by a philosophy which ran something like this: 'God grant me the sere-

nity to accept the things I cannot change, courage to change the things I can, and the wisdom to know the difference'.

After this conversation, the nurse's view of the patient and her own feelings of impotence changed. She felt closer to him and was able to spend time listening to him. This gave her the feeling that she was helping. She also perceived the situation afresh. As she changed her mental image of the patient so the situation became less threatening.

Similar instances can be found by contrasting nurses who feel helpless, sad and depressed when a patient dies with those who experience tranquility and relief that the patient has escaped further pain.

The example serves to illustrate that nurses' and patients' perceptions of the same events may be very different from each other. In this example it was the nurse who learned and gained a new perspective from the patient. This helped to restructure her understanding of events and her indirect coping.

The second type of indirect coping is illustrated by the following example:

> A patient was experiencing 'unbearable' pain post-operatively. He had already been given as much analgesic as the doctor would allow. He was obviously in great distress and was lying with tensed-up muscles. A nurse approached him. She had spent some time studying and practising different relaxation techniques. She suggested that the patient was increasing his own pain by being so tense. She told him that he could control his tension by imagining relaxing scenes and breathing slowly and easily. This would make his pain more tolerable. The nurse instructed him to concentrate on breathing deeply and with an even rhythm. With each inhalation he was to imagine that he gained strength to tolerate the pain and with each exhalation he was blowing the pain away. The patient did this. He relaxed, his pulse rate slowed and his pain eased. Furthermore, he used this technique the next time the pain began. In this way the normal dose of analgesic was able to control his pain.

This example shows that indirect coping can be used to alter the physiological effects (muscle tension) of demand (pain). The breathing control and imagery brought about relaxation of the tense muscles and this reduced the pain the patient experienced. In addition the technique altered his perception of the threat indirectly by helping him to feel he could help himself and thus had some control over events. Breath control and visualization (commonly called 'guided visual imagery techniques') are two ways in which pain tolerance can be increased (Bakal, 1979). The use of these, and similar techniques under the general heading of 'relaxation methods' is supported by a growing body of research evidence and will be discussed in greater detail later in this book. They act by reducing the negative psychological and physiological consequences which the individual may experience in circumstances of threat.

Palliative coping

Like indirect coping, palliative coping does not lead to mastery over the sources of threat. It is a term which covers actions which reduce temporarily the threat perceived or experienced by the individual. This temporary relief may be at the expense of greater stress at a later date. Some forms of palliative coping may lead to less efficient coping even in the short term. Several may be associated with increased risk of psychological or physical illness. Examples of palliative coping are given in Table 2.3.

The significance of delay in palliative coping

On studying Table 2.3, an important point emerges; the difference between the immediate outcome and the long-term effects of palliative coping upon mental and/or physical health. Immediate effects of palliative coping appear to be that it helps to reduce or eradicate feelings of psychological and/or physical discomfort associated with perceived threat. There is evidence of this. Lower anxiety scores may be shown on self-report measures of anxiety (Mackay, 1980). Objectively there may be signs of physical relaxation, lowered heart rate and blood pressure.

Some individuals suggest that, for them, smoking, drinking alcohol and eating snacks may each be effective under different circumstances.

Logically, how can we claim that coping behaviour which has short-term benefits in alleviating stress can have long-term ill effects, especially ill effects which themselves may cause stress? This apparent paradox can be overcome when considered within the phenomenological framework, since time is an important dimension to be considered within the total dynamic transaction between the individual and his environment. It is likely that a person may well adopt palliative coping in the full knowledge of the possible long-term outcomes. This statement finds support in the research showing that although smoking is generally on the decrease (or more precisely that fewer people are starting to smoke), there is still a high level of smoking amongst patients. Perhaps the greatest irony is the relatively high incidence of smoking amongst nurses (Spencer, 1982). Nurses above all, should be aware of the long-term consequences of smoking on health.

The phenomenological–transactional approach to coping allows for changes in outcome over time to be incorporated into the model of stress and coping. The role of time is not relevant exclusively to palliative coping, of course, but to all forms of coping. Time and its relationship to processes of coping is an area in which there is a need for further research. One of the

Table 2.3 Examples of palliative coping

Threat to individual	Palliative coping	Short-term effect	Long-term effect
Boss angry	Individual expresses his anger in turn by being angry with his children when they are noisy	Relief from frustration	Destructive relationship with his children
Doctor tells an individual there is something seriously wrong with her breast. She must see consultant	Avoids telling anyone. Fails to keep appointment with consultant	Forgets about problem	Carcinoma spreads
Individual anxious when mixing socially	Smokes in company	Gains confidence	Increased anxiety in company unless smokes. Develops cough. Bronchitis
Boredom and depression from being alone all day	Eats snacks and sweets	Less depressed Less bored	Weight gain. Unattractive. Less inclined to go out. More bored and depressed
Worried about meeting workmates socially, as they are competing for promotion	Drinks alcohol to gain confidence	Feels more confident	Feelings of remorse. Worries about slips of the tongue. Depression, lapses of memory

authors of this book has been engaged in research into stress and coping among student nurses over a period of time (Bailey, 1985).

Among the methods of coping which are classified as palliative are included the psychological defence mechanisms described earlier in this chapter. Their use is usually considered to have deleterious effects not only in the long term but also in the short term, although this is not our view. Lazarus (1979) has suggested that the use of at least one of these defence mechanisms (denial) may be essential to health for some people and in some situations. Even so, he does not suggest that it is healthy to continue to use denial to shield oneself from reality over a long period of time. Examples he gives of the usefulness of denial are mainly from the world of medicine. For that reason they are of particular interest to nurses. Researchers studying the victims of severe burns and of paralysis from polio found that initial denial of the severity of the disease was the valuable first step to coping. It 'buys time', allowing the individual to face demands at a more gradual and manageable pace. Lazarus suggests that such denial aids morale at a time when high morale is essential to the individual who must work toward his own recovery.

2.5 THE PURPOSE OF COPING AND PERSONAL CONTROL

We have argued that coping can take different forms: direct action; indirect methods; and palliation. What then are the functions or purposes of these various forms of coping? Used singly or in combination with each other they all serve the purpose of helping the individual to gain personal control over internal or external threatening events. A nursing example may be given: direct coping occurs when a nurse learns to judge accurately when to call a doctor at night to see a patient whose condition is deteriorating. In turn the doctor praises the nurse instead of being angry at being called up unnecessarily, or not being called up when he should have been. The nurse feels she has gained control over the situation. Our definition of coping can be refined, and becomes any activity by the person which changes his perceived relationship with his environment (internal or external) to the point where he no longer regards it as threatening, whilst the attainment of personal control is the outcome of successful or effective coping.

However, to reduce perceived threat the individual may use subtle combinations of direct, indirect and palliative coping and thus achieve personal control. The relationship between the use of direct coping actions and indirect strategies such as relaxation, visualization of calm scenes etc. has yet to be investigated, but an example may serve to illustrate the interaction between methods of coping in real life:

The situation arises from the promotion to nursing officer of a ward sister who is at least one year the junior of another ward sister. This will be analyzed from the point of view of the more senior ward sister who has not been promoted.

The perceived threat to our informant arises from her feeling that she has been judged less competent than her colleague. She feels she has been unfairly treated. Her self-esteem has been injured and she fears that her relationship with her own ward staff and consultants will be affected.

She uses the coping methods in Table 2.4. Although looking through Table 2.4 this example may appear complex, it is probable that it has been simplified in the analysis and the real life situation would be even more complex.

Table 2.4 Coping methods

Method	Classification of type of coping	Outcome
1 She analyzes the situation to determine how to handle similar situations in the future	Direct	Perceives she will cope better in future
2. She decides that the crucial difference between herself and her colleague is that her colleague is more 'pushy' and sucks up to people and she herself would never do that	Indirect – changes perception of situation	Restores her self-esteem by boosting her self-image in important areas of value
3. In order to sleep on the night she had heard the news she listened to calm serene music and practised relaxation	Indirect	Felt calmer but still could not sleep
4. She resorted to taking a sleeping pill	Palliative	Slept well
5. She publicly congratulated her colleague but also made it clear to everyone that she had made a conscious decision not to apply for the post of nursing officer which she could easily have got if she wanted. She herself valued the patient contact in being a ward sister	Direct	Perceived restoration of self-esteem in the eyes of valued colleagues

Overall outcome: Personal control

Personal control as a function of level or degree of threat and level or degree of coping

Whilst the style of coping may be unique to each situation a person finds himself in, there is also a relationship between the degree, level or amount of threat and the level of coping resources available to the individual at the time the threat is present. The achievement of personal control depends upon this relationship. For example, a patient who has been told he has an inoperable tumour may find this poses a threat for which he has insufficient coping resources. This results in stress which may manifest itself both physically and psychologically. He may break down and start crying whilst at intervals he asks for more information about his condition and also makes arrangements to alter his will. Physically he may become restless and sleepless and his pulse rate and respiration may rise.

The degree of stress experienced (lack of personal control) can be viewed as an outcome of the relationship between degree of threat and degree of coping available, although the relationship is not necessarily a simple one. A person's feeling of control depends on his perception of both the strength and the importance of the threat on the one hand and his perception of his coping strengths and weaknesses on the other hand. His perception of the importance of coping also influences control, although this is usually a function of the perceived importance of threat. It may also vary with the individual's self-image and value system. Logically, a number of different threat–coping relationships are predictable which affect levels of personal control. These are illustrated in Table 2.5

Table 2.5   Relationship between threat, coping and control

Perceived level of threat	Perceived level of coping	Experienced control
Low	High	High
Low	Low	Low
High	High	Low
High	Low	Low

To all intents and purposes it is often the perceived level of threat which is the crucial factor in determining the level of control which is experienced. An example might be a nurse who regarded herself as being generally able to cope with running the ward on which she was working. However, circumstances may change in spite of her high level of skill by the introduction of a high level of threat into the situation. The admission of a confused patient who shouts the whole time is such a change. Under this circumstance the nurse may experience a lack of personal control and stress. Thus even a high degree of coping skill cannot guarantee high personal control the whole time; such skill will be challenged by perceived threat from time to time. Indeed coping efforts in the face of acute perceived threat may actually *increase* stress in the attempt to gain personal control.

One of the authors has suggested that effective coping in conditions perceived as highly threatening leads to feelings of reward and increased self-esteem (Clarke, 1984). Conversely, in conditions of low demand, and especially where the situation is one which is familiar, coping becomes routine and does not contribute to reward and self-esteem although it does lead to personal control. However under conditions of high threat, routine may help to compensate to some extent for lack of personal control in other areas. To illustrate this we give an example of the wife of a patient who has just been told he has an incurable disease. This poses a major threat to them both. The wife continues to carry out her normal day-to-day housework activities and derives comfort from this as it helps her to feel more in control.

Personal Control and Psycho-biological equilibrium

Personal control as an outcome of effective coping is often experienced by the individual in terms of a return to psycho-biological equilibrium. For example, a nurse may become anxious when abused (threatened) by an angry patient. The nurse's pulse rate and respiration may rise and he or she may flush or become pale. These are early signs of Selye's (1956) alarm reaction discussed in Chapter 1. By learning to listen to angry patients and not challenging or confronting them the nurse finds that his or her own signs of distress become less noticeable. This is an indication of a maintenance of, or return to, psycho-biological equilibrium, derived from mastery of the situation. Mastery of the situation is the essence of personal control. In the example above the nurse used direct coping methods. The same effect on psycho-biological equilibrium can be derived from indirect methods of coping. For example, in the case of noisy, confused patients the nurse may be in no position to change the patient into a quiet, rational one which would be a way of direct coping. Instead he/she can learn to perceive the situation differently, as one in which the noisiness is explained by the patient's diagnosis of cerebral atrophy and is no longer seen as threatening. A return to psycho-biological equilibrium occurs.

Many of the indirect methods of coping have as their primary aim the maintenance or return to psycho-biological equilibrium, either as an adjunct to direct coping or in circumstances where direct coping is impossible or inappropriate. For example, relaxation, meditation, and autogenic therapy are specifically designed to reduce rapid heart beat and respiration, muscle tension and disturbing thoughts.

Palliative methods of coping also act upon psycho-biological equilibrium. Sleeping tablets in particular will lower anxiety and restore to normal the associated physical signs. Alcohol and smoking affect psychological equilibrium but both may actually increase the heart rate, for example, and so their effects are somewhat different.

However, in our view it would be a mistake to assume that the achievement of personal control should always be associated with the maintenance of a harmonious homeostatic state. Control does not always imply equilibrium, and equilibrium does not always imply control. For example, a nurse may expend considerable effort in coping with an extremely busy ward during a night shift. Coping is effective and personal control is maintained but psycho-biological equilibrium is lost and a sleepless day follows. The nurse then develops a cold.

In this example the cost of maintaining control has exceeded the nurse's capacity to remain in psycho-biological balance.

On the other hand, there are circumstances where psycho-biological equilibrium is maintained but not through gaining control over a major source of threat. An example is the patient who has been told he is dying but who engages in denial as a defence mechanism. To the observer his psychological equilibrium is greater than one would expect from a seriously ill patient, whilst his physiological state is no worse than expected from a knowledge of the disease process. In this case the patient has not gained control but has maintained equilibrium (at least for the time being).

So we can see through these examples that personal control and psycho-biological balance may not always correspond directly with one another, particularly in respect to time. One may follow the other rather than both occurring together. Time may be a particularly important dimension for consideration in terms of control and effective coping. Sometimes viewing the situation at one point in time it looks as if coping is unsuccessful, whilst at a later point personal control has been gained and we can declare coping as effective. For example, to go back to our instance of the nurse on night duty it is likely that at many points during the shift she would have perceived the situation as one with which she was unable to cope and therefore very stress-ful. Personal control was gained by the time the shift ended. On the other hand someone who uses a palliative method of coping may perceive that he has gained personal control only to find at a later date that the threat is as great as ever, if not worse.

Personal control and psychological coherence

Earlier it was suggested that effective coping at a high level of demand or threat was rewarding. This can also be termed psychological coherence (Antonovsky, 1979) and it develops from a consciousness of increased mastery over threat. Coherence is not merely a sense of a job well done. It goes further than this and entails a psychological shift in the individual's view of himself. In relation to a nurse it may be typified by the development of a general confidence in his/her own ability to overcome difficulties which may arise, for example, in patient care, running a ward or interpersonal relation-ships. There are three typical signs which are indicators of a high personal control over threat. These are: (a) considerable self-esteem; (b) a person's belief in their own competence (White, 1959); and (c) a sense of their own autonomy to influence events.

Personal control and health

The converse is also true: absence of control or very low levels of personal control leads to stress. Specifically, individuals who feel a sense of personal helplessness to overcome threat to their psychological or physical well-being are likely to show more stress-related problems such as anxiety, depression and somatic complaints than those individuals who believe in their own ability to influence events.

This is particularly important for patient care, especially when patients are admitted to hospital. In hospital, patients are able to exert little or no control over their environment, the structure of their day and time of treatment, for example. It could well be that such lack of control leads to a longer recovery period. Conversely, there is accumulating evidence to suggest that the enhancement of his personal control whilst a patient is in hospital is not only associated with fewer emotional problems but with a shorter recovery period (Boore, 1978). One way in which a patient could achieve greater personal control is by the staff giving greater choice in such areas as clothing, waking times and exercise times. Where choice cannot be given, detailed information may act to make events more predictable allowing a greater feeling of control. Literature under the heading of health psychology points to the relationship outlined above, but what is not yet clear is whether increased control has a direct bearing on health or whether it acts by reducing emotional problems which in turn allows the natural healing processes of the body to bring about recovery.

It does mean however that nurses should address themselves to the promotion of greater patient control over areas which have traditionally been within the control of nurses. As such, it may seem to threaten the professional role of the nurse. However, we feel that rather than bringing conflict the nurse should look at this as fulfilling a higher professional objective; that of primary responsibility to the patient and his well-being. As part of the nursing process, nurse and patient together could identify areas where they can (a) share control over discomforting events, (b) accept that some aspects should be entirely within the control of patients and (c) accept that other aspects will have to be entirely in the hands of the nurse. Rather than giving up areas of professional skill it adds a new dimension of responsibility to nursing. That is: the assessment and teaching of patients in the skills of identifying and gaining control over threatening aspects of the environment. This might not only help patients to cope with the present but also give them new coping skills for the future. Given that this is successful in helping patient recovery it will have a positive effect upon the nurse's feeling of control and self-image.

Helplessness

There is evidence to suggest that people experience a sense of helplessness (Seligman, 1975) with emotional upset where their efforts at personal control are thwarted or have no apparent effect upon outcomes. A growing literature on occupational stress endorses this view for a large number of occupations including business executives (Cooper and Marshall, 1978; Cooper and Payne, 1978).

The concept of helplessness has received attention in both animal and human studies, confirming that depression and anxiety frequently occur when subjects are unable to influence important outcomes in their environment. Full-blown helplessness is manifested by the individual having bouts of sadness or longer uninterrupted periods of depression. His mood is 'flat' and motivation extremely low. Early indicators of loss of personal control include frustration, anger and general irritability.

Sometimes, to combat severe loss of personal control and chronic helplessness the individual becomes sick as the only coping alternative available. This may be relevant to nurses, and if so, then more research is needed to compare those nurses who cope and maintain sufficient personal control under threat with those who do not but become sick. By becoming sick they leave the stressful situation in order to recover. Seen in this light, going off sick for short periods may be a reasonable alternative to leaving the job or even the profession and/or becoming severely depressed. It allows a period during which personal control could be recovered, mood lightened, and interest gained with renewed commitment to nursing.

We may note that becoming sick as a strategy when faced with low personal control is a palliative method of coping. Perhaps we should also point out that there is no implication that this is a deliberately thought out strategy. The individual may be only too unaware of the problem. As with other palliative coping methods the individual gains time. It may be that in the rapidly-changing ward environment some of the threatening aspects have changed for the better whilst the nurse is recovering.

As we have already discussed, similar problems occur for patients. They too may become depressed, lackadaisical and withdrawn. There is substantial evidence from studies of both adult and child patients that this is indeed the case. Unfortunately they may be seen as 'good patients' when in fact they are showing the symptoms of reduced personal control and helplessness. The most striking evidence for this view may be observed in patients who apparently give up further attempts at living (Seligman, 1975). The belief that helplessness leads to death through the inability to affect outcomes through one's own efforts is a far from novel idea. It has been reported in anthropological studies under such headings as 'voodoo death'.

2.6 THREAT, COPING AND LEARNING

Consideration of time as a dimension in coping leads us to examine concepts of habituation and learning in relation to threat. From animal and human studies we know that with repeated exposure to threatening stimuli the response becomes less and less marked, provided that physical or psychological harm has not arisen from exposure to the threat. This attenuation of response is known as habituation and it acts to reduce the impact of environmental events which are no longer novel. Another result of repeated exposure to a threatening event may be the learning of the skills of direct coping, specific to that event, these becoming more effective on each occasion the threat occurs. In human beings, each presentation of a threat stimulus which leads to habituation or skill learning will also lead to changed perception of the stimulus. The individual will perceive the stimulus as less threatening. That is there is a cognitive change. Meichenbaum (1979) has shown how altered levels of experienced stress can result from changing the meaning of events for individuals so that they perceive the events as less threatening. This is a cognitive approach to coping.

There may be circumstances in which the stimulus retains its potency as a threat but the individual learns to relax in its presence. We have already classified this as a form of indirect coping and it may be a useful method when a threatening event cannot be avoided, e.g. a forthcoming operation for a patient or an examination for a nurse.

Taking the example of a nurse sitting an examination, a relaxation technique may restore calm (psycho-biological equilibrium) to a point where direct coping can come into play. Further research is needed into the relationship between indirect coping methods and examination performance. Charlesworth et al. (1981) show that relaxation may improve examination performance. However, this may not be the case in all individuals. On theoretical and empirical grounds, some people perform better given a certain amount of anxiety and stress. In the study referred to above, some nurses in the central group gained better grades than those in the experimental group, suggesting that for them, some anxiety was beneficial. Sarason (1977) has presented evidence that for different individuals there is a different optimum level of anxiety to produce the best examination performance. It follows that for some people, stress-control techniques might render them too relaxed for optimum performance in examinations. This reinforces Selye's (1956) position that extremely low levels of stress are not desirable since they may be associated with low levels of performance.

To return to a consideration of a change in one's perception of threat as a method of indirect coping, this can be contrasted with direct coping which means perceiving and responding actively to threat and mastering it. There is evidence that a certain degree of stimulation or demand from the environment is necessary for optimum performance. Perhaps for some individuals in some situations, indirect methods of coping reduce environmental demand below the optimum level and so the balance between direct and indirect methods of coping may be crucial.

As far as nursing is concerned it appears that direct coping methods are favoured in the training programme and that nurses in general tend to gain greater relief from anxiety by direct physical actions. Unfortunately as we have said before, it is not always possible to deal directly with threat and indirect methods of coping certainly have a place in helping nurses to deal with the demands placed upon them. Nurses also need to know about indirect methods to be capable of teaching them to patients who have fewer opportunities to use direct coping to gain personal control.

Problem-focused coping versus emotion-focused coping

Much of our discussion has related to direct and indirect methods of coping and psycho-physiological equilibrium. A different way of conceptualizing these has been proposed by Lazarus (Lazarus and Launier, 1978) based on research. Two fundamental dimensions of coping are proposed, problem-focused coping and emotion-focused coping.

Problem-focused coping refers to the individual's attempts to overcome anticipated or experienced threat by thinking, planning and putting their coping plan into action. The efficacy of this coping strategy can then be reappraised for its influence upon the individual. The nursing process is analogously a typical example of the problem-focused approach to nursing. Some examples of the problem-focused dimension of coping applicable to nurses and patients are shown in Table 2.6. Notice the similarity to aspects of the nursing process involving identification, assessment, direct action and evaluation. These examples show problem-based methods of dealing with sources of threat. Coping is providing action answers to problems, and the nurse or patient engages in the processes of primary and secondary appraisal and reappraisal. But there may be occasions when direct coping is not available to the nurse or patient. At other times direct problem-focused coping may not be appropriate, even though it is readily available or within the competence of the individual nurse or patient. In such instances, emotion-focused coping may be the dimension on which nurses and patients base their efforts at personal control and psycho-biological equilibrium. Some examples illustrating the content of emotion-focused coping are shown in Table 2.7.

Clinical aspects of problem-focused coping and emotion-focused coping

Further research is needed to consider more closely the relationship between problem- and emotion-focused coping (see e.g. Lazarus et al., 1980). However, we wish to draw attention to the clinical aspects of these dimensions of coping. Conceptually; problem- and emotion-focused coping are two separate dimensions. The problem-focused coping examples show how much of this dimension is closely associated with direct coping, and the processes of primary and secondary appraisal and reappraisal. Similarly, emotion-focused coping seems linked with indirect coping and the various stages of appraisal and reappraisal for each individual. In other words, problem-focused coping and emotion-focused coping fit nicely into the transactional model of stress and coping developed by Lazarus (1966, 1976, 1978, 1980; Lazarus et al.,

Table 2.6 Examples of problem-focused coping

| Source of threat | Primary (appraisal/assessment identification) | Problem-focused coping | | Reappraisal (evaluation/review) |
		Secondary appraisal		
Patient: John *Condition*: Spinal injury	1. Lonely. Decides relatives are not visiting him often enough	1. Telephones 2. Writes to them to see him on Wednesdays and Saturdays for next 2 months 3. Confirms this is OK with Sister		1. Visits made as requested 2. Sister well informed 3. John satisfied with new visiting arrangements
Patient: Liz *Condition*: Lump in breast	1. Feels panicky and anxious at thought of losing breast	1. Asks for information about her diagnosis/prognosis 2. Wants the facts in layman's terms; not jargon, so she understands		1. Information given – exploratory operation 2. May not be malignant, so she might not lose breast, or only part of it 3. Liz still has some concern but less, and no panic
Nurse: Erica, Student Nurse	1. Worried because she has missed two lectures and practical demonstrations on coronary care	1. Asks 'best' note-taking colleague for summaries of lectures 2. Seeks advice from tutor on areas to study 3. Visits library and follows up coronary care references 4. Attends coronary care ward in off-duty time and observes coronary care procedure in practice		1. Obtains all notes on subject 2. Tutor advises refs and CC ward visit 3. Librarian has key references made available 4. Sister glad Erica is taking such interest and makes special effort to demonstrate CC procedures

Table 2.6 *continued*

Source of threat	Primary (appraisal/assessment identification)	Problem-focused coping	
		Secondary appraisal	Reappraisal (evaluation/review)
Nurses: Paul and David, Charge Nurses	1. Anger at conflicting ward management practice resulting in confusion for patients	1. Set time aside to view different approaches to managing ward 2. Specifically consider areas of agreement/ disagreement 3. Canvas opinions of trained staff and patients 4. Outline hospital policy on ward management – if there is one	1. Series of three meetings arranged between two charge nurses 2. Clarified and itemized areas of agreement/ disagreement in principle and practice 3. Shared positions on staff and patient opinions of management 4. Discovered no explicit hospital policy on ward management 5. Practice combination of best new ward management policy and practices from each charge nurse taking into consideration other's opinions 6. Conflict reduced between charge nurses 7. Confusion largely overcome 8. But new ward management policy to be monitored and evaluated now for its suitability

Table 2.7 Examples of emotion-focused coping

Source of threat	Emotion-focused coping	
Patient: Sylvia Pre-operation anxiety	1. Practice relaxation exercises in muscle groups around legs, arms, shoulders, neck, face and spine 2. Employ restful, peaceful images 3. The thought 'calm' with each exhalation and 'ready' with each inhalation 4. Adopts emotion-focused coping prior to experienced discomfort, or when pain occurs	1. Muscle tension in affected groups decreased 2. Tranquil images replaced fear-impression of surgery 3. Feels calm but 'ready' for operation 4. Can produce effective emotion-focused coping leading up to operation, and to deal with unpredictable episodes of reported spinal pain.
Patient: Mike, RTA Amputated right leg above knee. Emotionally flat Denying and refusing to accept loss of leg	1. Gradual course of autogenic relaxation training 2. Symbolic introduction of 'letting go' in relaxation sessions. 3. Sessions practised with guidance of competent therapist	1. Autogenic relaxation given over 8-week period 2. 'Letting-go' established, and crying episodes appear. Beginning of mourning for lost leg 3. Sessions covered by therapist intensively for 8 weeks – involving Sister and Staff Nurses
Nurse: Margaret Feels nauseous and anxious at thought of nursing dying children (is sick on ward on first day)	1. Enrols in cognitive desensitization programme run by clinical psychologist and nurse counselling service	1. Reports no further vomiting episodes – respiration lower, less sweating

Table 2.7 *continued*

Source of threat	Emotion-focused coping	
		2. Nausea manageable, even in presence of unexpected contact with a dying child
		3. Some anxiety remaining but does not interfere with nursing proficiency
Nurse: Paul Depressed. Considers patient's poor response to treatment is due to his professional incompetence. Has recently taken this view of patient care in general	1. Confided his problem to close colleague	1. Cried and felt relief at sharing the burden of patient care and responsibility for their health – recovery
	2. The colleague invited him to attend clinical psychologist's well-nurse clinic	2. Kept clinic appointments for 4 weeks. Then dropped in for coffee and informal discussions occasionally
	3. Attended clinic	3. Reported a more informed and realistic picture of patient response to illness and nursing care
	4. First shown facts that not all patients make same or rapid recovery from illness	
	5. Second, reviewed first two years of training. Agreed that his overall performance in class, tutorial and ward reports above average	4. Has confirmed his professional competence as judged by his tutors and senior nurses
	6. Third, reduced the high expectations he was putting on himself as the 'healing nurse'	5. Has altered expectations of himself. But still sometimes tends to blame himself for patient's poor response to treatment. No longer depressed

2. Learns to label dying as 'nature taking its course'

3. Practises stress-relief programme in counselling service and on own two sessions prior to work

1981). How does it help us in understanding nurse or patient stress and coping? Clinically it is important for a number of reasons.

In clinical practice, as most nurses would be quick to point out, combinations of problem- and emotion-focused coping are engaged in by nurses and patients. Being aware of this should help patients and nurses to analyze their coping strategies for dealing with threat and experienced threat. Additionally, it appears to us at least, to be a helpful way of conceptualizing the transaction between threat and how people cope. For instance, at least five possible combinations are feasible between problem-focused coping and emotion-focused coping. These can best be illustrated by a simple coping dimension window. (Fig. 2.1)

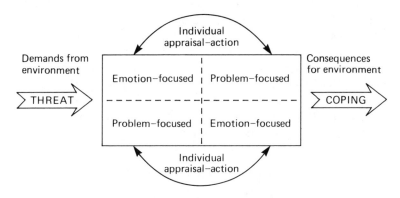

Figure 2.1 Coping combinations dimension window.

First, coping is engaged to deal with the primary appraisal of threat. If the threat is emotion-based, then emotion-focused coping seems an appropriate form of coping. Similarly, a problem-based threat may usefully be overcome by problem-focused coping, resulting in mastery over threat. These seem to be the most elementary associations between threat and problem-focused or emotion-focused coping. But notice the way coping exchanges may take place in the coping dimension window. Other combinations are possible, and indeed, we would argue, reflect what takes place in human transactions in nursing. For instance, emotion-based threat may be overcome by adopting problem-focused coping and direct action. The nurse who is anxious over carrying out a new procedure may find her anxiety becoming progressively lower as she successfully carries out each step. Thus, problem-focused coping by direct actions may serve to compete with anxiety and bring about lower levels of experienced stress. Donald Meichenbaum's (1979) work on cognitive behaviour modification in coping with stress supports this view of coping.

Both Meichenbaum (1979) and Zastrow (1979) have shown how talking one-self through stressful episodes leads to effective coping. Other coping permu-tations are made possible too. Emotion-focused coping may be enlisted to deal with problem-based threats. The nurse who cannot solve every patient's problems with nursing procedures may resort to coping with this difficulty by relaxation training or relabelling those patients who can be helped and those who cannot. A further observation of the dimensions in the coping window shows how it is perfectly feasible for a nurse or patient to switch from one coping dimension to another, or to combine both in different sequences in an attempt to cope with stress. This is indeed what happens in practice for many people. When one mode of coping does not work, they adopt another, or combine different dimensions of coping to overcome threat.

Another attractive aspect of the coping dimensions window is it can also account for maladaptive coping in, and over, time – for the same and diffe-rent situations. For example, because a nurse or patient adopts emotion-focused coping to deal with a problem-based threat, it is unlikely to lead to satisfactory coping outcomes. The same point holds for all coping dimensions and the possible combinations in theory and practice. The implications of problem-focused and emotion-focused coping dimensions identified in Lazarus et al.'s. (1980) research are consistent with, and can be interpreted within, the CPT model of stress and coping.

The complexity of coping

From our consideration of coping we have endorsed the three main types of coping propounded by Lazarus and Launier (1978), i.e. direct, indirect and palliative. It is an over-simplification, however, to claim that that is all that coping amounts to. Coping is a response but also a product of the actions of an individual in attempting to maintain personal control and psycho-equilibrium within the duration of a lifespan. Forms of coping may change and improve over time as a result of earlier coping efforts. Coping may also stay fixed in form although we would suggest that this is pathological and likely to cause psychological or physical ill health. Thus we would emphasize again the importance of time as a dimension. Our view of the efficacy of coping may depend upon our time scale. From this perspective, coping can be appre-ciated as a dynamic process rather than a fixed-state entity. This has an important bearing upon nursing practice. For by seeing that coping may change with situation and time it raises the hope that control and equilibrium will return for patients (and for nurses themselves). An understanding of coping and personal control can help nurses to intervene to give greater control to patients. In turn, the patients will become less irritable, anxious or depressed, complain less of physical ailments and make a more rapid recovery, or achieve a higher level of rehabilitation. As nurses become more competent in direct nursing actions, in listening to and communicating with patients, their efforts become rewarded and their feeling of professional competence and individual self-esteem is enhanced. Conceptually it is of limited value to define rigidly the cause–effect relationships in such a dynamic view of coping. Just as the static view of stress was shown to be misleading in our previous chapter, so we believe the static view of coping is also misleading. Coping is not necessarily a synonym for satisfactory achievement. We have defined coping as the individual's attempts to reach goals of personal control.

When this has been achieved it may last only for a moment in time or much longer. In nursing, coping takes the form of attempts to reach the goals of recovery, rehabilitation, and comfort for the patient. These goals may not be achieved but in attempting to reach them some personal control and psychobiological equilibrium will be achieved both for the patient and for the nurse.

The transactional model of stress and coping allows for an individual to follow explicitly and consciously, or automatically, a general procedure of appraisal to identify sources of threat and to assess the efficacy of their coping. Whilst a nurse will do this in personal terms for herself, as a result of her nursing experience she will also develop a knowledge of sources of threat for patients and methods of helping patients to build their own coping strategies. This will include the assessment of levels of threat and levels of coping which should always be seen in relation to one another. If coping is inadequate to deal with threat this leads to failure in personal control. If the level of coping is too great for the level of threat, it means wasted effort. It is important to remember that the optimum condition for patient recovery is not the absence of demand, but a level of demand which is manageable. The object of care is to provide for patients to gain or maintain personal control. Where a patient is dying, personal control over the way in which the remaining time is used must be considered. This means telling the patient he is dying when he indicates a desire to know. By providing this information openly the patient is in a position to exercise control and choice over aspects of his life in the time remaining. He can put his affairs in order, plan for the future of his dependants and so on. This gives him personal control in a very real way.

Threat or demand is far from a negative concept under all circumstances. It can play a catalytic role in the recovery of patients by bringing about coping and control. Threat is negative or destructive only when psychological or physical resources are insufficient to maintain or gain control and stress is experienced. This experience may in turn bring about greater and more effective coping. A transactional approach to stress and coping does not assume a one-way relationship between cause and effect. Rather it suggests that threat can influence coping and coping can influence threat. It is then a short step to the suggestion of psychosomatic interaction. At times perception of bodily dysfunction influences psychological levels of threat and coping whilst at other times or the same time, psychological experiences influence the duration and direction of physical health and illness.

Given an insight into stress and coping, nurses can begin to help patients who have had limitations placed upon their personal control by the very nature of their condition. For example, they can encourage spinal injury, amputation and stroke patients to relinquish unrealistic hopes of pre-injury levels of functioning. Instead new areas of personal control can be gained to facilitate effective coping.

Evaluation of the transactional model of coping

Like other formulations of coping, the transactional model does have a number of limitations. First, it is a very general approach to the way people cope and as such is better for analysis than prediction. However, it has the great advantage of flexibility over other models of coping. It can be employed to understand what disturbs patients and nurses and how well they cope in any one or more given situations at any one time and over time. A second criticism, however, is that the approach does not allow prediction of indivi-dual behaviour. That is, who will cope in what way and to what effect. This is a criticism in no way unique to the transactional–phenomenological view of coping and it could be said of many other areas of psychological, nursing and medical knowledge. Thirdly, little work has been carried out to investigate which forms of coping best serve to give psychological equilibrium in nursing and in the best interests of their patients. Similarly, more clinical and field-based research is urgently required into the relationship between patient coping and physical recovery or rehabilitation. The transactional frame-work would seem to be a useful theoretical base for studies of this kind, since it does suggest the kind of psychological process of appraisal and the behavioural actions likely to be involved in coping with hospitalization and illness.

Although this framework is concerned with the individual patient or nurse, through its emphasis on individual appraisal and perception it can be adapted to an application to groups since an individual's appraisal and perception may be influenced very strongly by both present group membership and past groups (culture). The transactional framework also makes possible the investigation of a rich variety of coping rather than the narrow range implied in other approaches.

2.7 SUMMARY

We have considered four fundamental approaches to the study of coping. These are ego-defensive coping, coping as a personality trait, situation grounded coping and the transactional–phenomenological view of coping. Each approach has been discussed and evaluated. The case for preferring the transactional–phenomenological view has been argued. This is based on both the conceptual and practical implications (its usefulness) of the transactional view when applied to the study of stress and coping in nursing.

REFERENCES

Andreasen, N. J. C. and Norris, A. S. (1972) Long-term adjustment and adaptation mechanisms in severely burned adults. *J. Nervous and Mental Disease*, **154**, 352–62.

Antonovsky, A. (1979) *Health, Stress and Coping*, Jossey-Bass, San Francisco, Washington, London.

Bailey, R. (1985) *Autogenic regulation training. Sickness absence, personal problems, time, and the emotional-physical stress of student nurses in general training*. Thesis submitted for degree of PhD, University of Hull.

Bakal, D. (1979) Pain and pain patients, in *Psychology and Medicine: Psycho-biological dimensions of Health and Sickness*, Ch. 5, Tavistock Publications, London, pp. 139–71.

Blass, T. (ed.) (1977) *Personality Variables in Social Behaviour*, Lawrence Elbaum Assoc., John Wiley, Chichester.

Boore, J. (1978) *Prescription for Recovery*, RCN, London.

Bulman, R. J. and Wortman, C. B. (1977) Attributions of blame and coping in the 'real world': severe accident victims react to their lot. *J. Personality Soc. Psych.*, **35**, 351–63.

Byrne, D. (1964) Repression–sensitization as a dimension of personality, in *Progress in Experimental Personality Research* (ed. Brendam A. Maher), Vol. 1, Academic Press, New York, pp. 170–220.

Charlesworth, E. A., Murphy, S. and Beutler, L. E. (1981) Stress management skill for nursing students, *J. Clinical Psychology*, **37** (2), 284–90.

Clarke, M. (1984) 'Stress' and 'coping': constructs for nursing. *J. Adv. Nursing*, **9**, 3–13.

Coelho, G., V., Hamburg, D. A. and Adams, J. E. (eds) (1974) *Coping and Adaptation*, Basic Books, New York.

Cohen, F. and Lazarus, R. (1979) Coping with the stresses of illness, in *Health Psychology: A Handbook*, (eds George C. Stone, Frances Cohen and Nancy E. Adler), Jossey-Bass, San Francisco, Washington, London, pp. 217–54.

Coleman, C. and Hammen, C. L. (1974) *Contemporary Psychology and Effective Behaviour*, Scott Foresman.

Cooper, C. and Marshall, J. (1978) *Understanding Executive Stress*, Macmillan, London.

Cooper, C. and Payne, P. (1978) *Stress at Work*, John Wiley, Chichester.

Ekehammar, B. (1974) Interactionism in personality from a historical perspective. *Psychological Bulletin*, **81**, 1–26.

Eysenck, H. J. (1947) *Dimensions of Personality*, Kegan Paul, London.

Folkman, S. and Lazarus, R. (1980) An analysis of coping in a middle-aged community sample. *J. Health and Social Behaviour*, **21**, 219–39.

Hinkle, L. E. (1974) The effect of exposure to culture change, social change and changes in interpersonal relationships on health, in *Stressful Life Events: Their Nature and Effects* (eds B. S. Dohrenwend and B. P. Dohrenwend) John Wiley, Chichester.

Janis, I. L. (1958) *Psychological Stress*, Academic Press, New York.

Kubler Ross, E. (1973) *Death and Dying*, Social Science Paperback edn, Penguin, Harmondsworth.

Lazarus, R. S. (1966) *Psychological Stress and the Coping Process*, McGraw-Hill, New York.

Lazarus, R. S. (1976) *Patterns of Adjustment*, McGraw-Hill, New York.

Lazarus, R. S. and Launier, R. (1978) Stress related transactions between person and environment, in *Perspectives in Interactional Psychology* (eds M. Pervin, and M. Lewis), Plenum Press, New York.

Lazarus, R. S. (1979) Positive denial: the case for not facing reality, *Psychology Today* (November) 44–60.

Lazarus, R. (1981) The stress and coping paradigm, In *Theoretical Bases for Psychopathology* (eds C. Eisdorfer, D. Cohen, A. Kleinman and P. Maxim), Spectrum Publications, New York.

Lazarus, R. (1983) The cost and benefit of denial, in *The Denial of Stress* (ed Reznitz) International University Press, New York.

Lazarus, R. Kanner, A. and Folkman, S. (1980). Emotions: A Cognitive–Phenomenological Analysis in *Theories of Emotion*. (eds R. Plutchik and H. Resuormann), Academic Press, New York, pp. 189–217.

Mackay, C. (1980) The measurement of mood and psychophysiological activity self-report measures, in *Techniques in Psychophysiology* (eds I. Martin and P. H. Venables), Ch. 9, pp. 501–62, John Wiley, Chichester.

Mages, N. L. and Mendelsohn, G. A. (1979) Effects of cancer on patients' lives: a personalogical approach, in *Health Psychology: A Handbook* (eds G. C. Stone, F. Cohen and N. E. Adler), Jossey-Bass, London.

Magnusson, D. and Endler, N. S. (1977) *Personality at the Crossroads. Current Issues in International Psychology*, John Wiley, New York, London.

Meichenbaum, D. (1979) (1st edn. 1977), *Cognitive-Behaviour Modification*, 2nd edn, Plenum Press, New York.

Moos, R. (1979) *Coping with Physical Illness*, 2nd edn, Plenum Press, New York.

Parkes, C. M. (1972) *Bereavement: Studies of Grief in Adult Life*, Tavistock, London.

Sarason, S. (1977) *Work, Aging and Social Change*, Free Press, New York.

Seligman, M. E. P. (1975) *Helplessness: On Depression, Development and Death*, W. H. Freeman, San Francisco, CA.

Selye, H. (1956) *The Stress of Life*, McGraw-Hill, New York.

Spencer, J. (1982) *The Postal Survey of Nurses' Smoking Behaviour*, Nurses' Smoking Behaviour Research Report No. 1, Institute of Nursing Studies, University of Hull.

Visotsky, H. M., Hamburg, D. A., Goss, M. E. and Lebovitz, B. A. (1961) Coping behaviour under extreme stress, *Archives General Psychiatry*, **5**, 423–48.

White, R. W. (1959) Motivation reconsidered: the concept of competence. *Psychological Review*, **66**(5), 297–333.

Zastron, C. C. (1979) Talk to Yourself: Using the Power of Self Talk, Spectrum Books, New York.

PART TWO

NURSES – STRESS AND COPING

The responsibility of caring for and interacting with people who are ill or infirm can be emotionally demanding, subjecting the health professional to considerable stress.

Colligan, Smith and Horrel, 1977

CHAPTER THREE

Pupil and student nurse stress

3.1 INTRODUCTION: NURSING – A STRESSFUL PROFESSION

Stress has become a watchword for nurses. Even the more carefully researched studies seem to confirm the view that nurses can expect to experience stress at one time or another during their career. As Marshall (1980) has noted, the studies of stress and nurses suggest that nurses may be particularly prone to stress. The studies assume that stress is a bad thing, and that stress is intrinsic to nursing. Marshall observed:

> the job pressures identified in the literature tempt me to conclude that the job of nurse incorporates several distinctive features which set it apart as a special case in the stress literature. It appears to take to extremes certain aspects of experiencing stress which usually operate more moderately and are thus more subject to variability from individual and environmental differences. (Marshall, 1980, p. 20)

Clearly nursing makes demands on nurses that are not applicable to the population at large (Bailey, 1986). What are these job demands? Are there distinctive features of the nurse's job which inevitably lead to stress? Are there extremes of stress and variability related to different aspects and types of nursing and the demands made on nurses? How do these relate to the experience of nurses in different work settings and the roles they occupy? Even more questionable is the apparent assumption in some studies of stress and nurses that there is none or little satisfaction to be derived from nursing. Is this so? These and other questions concerned with stress and nurses have been investigated in the literature on the subject. Studies of stress and nurses range from the anecdotal and descriptive, to empirically-based research. These studies have attempted to discover if stress is an inevitable consequence of:

(a) becoming a nurse;
(b) practising nursing; and
(c) exposure to unusual occupational demands.

These general points are all important for us to understand if we are to get a better understanding of stress amongst nurses. However, as we shall see the problem of stress and nurses is sometimes a highly specific and often complex phenomenon. We would also like to show that some of the evidence on stress amongst nurses is questionable, subject to alternative interpretations, and amenable to more plausible accounts of the data such as the application of a cognitive–phenomenological–transactional (CPT) approach to stress and coping (Lazarus 1966, 1976; Lazarus and Launier, 1978; Folkman and Lazarus, 1980), which we outlined in Chapter 1. This will become more apparent as we progress through the consideration of nurse studies. We begin with some anecdotal and individual reports of stress, and then continue to an evaluation of work relating to groups of nurses.

3.2 POPULAR ANECDOTAL AND DESCRIPTIVE ACCOUNTS OF STRESS

Nurses in Britain have become more outspoken in presenting their opinions on 'the problem of stress' (Haynes, 1978). The respected nursing press and popular magazines alike have all carried articles which suggest nurses are ill-prepared to deal with the demands of nursing – particularly the highly dependent patient, (Dosett, 1978, Bailey, 1983) and the demands made on nurses in accident and emergency services (Thomson, 1983). For instance Dosett claimed that 'One cause of stress in a conscientious nurse is insufficient knowledge to deal with the situation' (Dosett, 1978, p. 88). Yet it is not clear what knowledge this should be or if indeed knowledge would be enough to alleviate stress related to the demands of nursing. More recent research by Sellek (1982) investigating anxiety and satisfying incidents for nurses, shows that insufficient knowledge of nursing procedures is not a source of anxiety for student nurses. We would also add that a knowledge of nursing practice need not necessarily result in the nurse practising what is regarded as the appropriate nursing procedure in any particular case. Finally, knowing what patient procedures to adopt and carrying them out may not lead to a reduction of experienced stress for nurses. Hay and Oken (1972) make this point vividly clear in their poignant descriptive account of nurses employed on the intensive care unit.

Individual reports

The publication of highly personalized views of stress has helped to draw attention to the diverse range of demands, stress and difficulties of coping experienced by nurses (Hawkins, 1979; Bailey, 1983; Thomson, 1983). We would suggest that the most obvious way to find out if nurses experience stress and what it is like for them, is to ask them. One of the present authors showed how valuable this can be, by collating a number of revealing cameos from nurses (Clarke and Montague, 1980). Three of them are presented here in detail, and illustrate the relevance of interpreting them within a cognitive–transactional model of stress and coping for individual nurses.

Cameo 1

Bob, a State Registered Nurse (SRN) observed:

> When my brother was 20 he developed a bad attack of renal colic. Apparently he had a congenital defect of his left ureter. When they operated, they found that the kidney was so badly diseased that it had to be removed. When he regained consciousness he was told he had lost his kidney. I went to see him 24 hours later. He looked dreadful. It upset me, even though I am a nurse. His breathing was so fast, and he looked semi-conscious. He wouldn't speak to me. Luckily, the next time I went to see him a nurse had explained you can live a perfectly normal life with only one kidney. He was looking so much better you wouldn't have known it was the same person. It really brought home to me the importance of giving patients information.

Christine, another SRN, shows how sources of stress-inducing threat need not only be generated from the care of patients but also by other colleagues in her own profession.

Cameo 2

Christine, SRN, related:

> In my old hospital I had been taught that dying patients need to talk to a sympathetic nurse. Shortly after I came to my present hospital, I was on a general surgical ward and there was a dying patient in a cubicle. She must have felt I was sympathetic because she kept pleading with me with her eyes for me to stay with her. I couldn't just leave her so I used to sit and listen. It caused so much trouble with the rest of the staff though, that I got quite desperately depressed. They said I was lazy, and too involved emotionally with my patient. One nurse even accused me of being a 'ghoul'. I think I would have given up nursing if I hadn't been moved from that ward.

Another typical source of threat is examinations (Mechanic, 1962; Sarason, 1972, 1980; Birch 1978, 1979; Lazarus and Launier, 1978). Many nurses will be able to recall their experience of anxiety or panic during, or preparing for, State examinations, Jenny, a student nurse summarizes neatly her own appraisal of an examination paper, the influence of the threat on her and what happened as a consequence.

Cameo 3

Jenny , Student Nurse, noted:

> My mind just went completely blank when I saw the examination paper.
> I must have panicked because the next thing I knew I was bolting
> straight out of the hall.

These three cameos are interesting in their own right for a number of very
important reasons. First, three different sources of threat have been identified
by three different nurses. Second, three different outcomes are associated
with the three sources of threat. Third, even this small sample of simple
individual cameos illustrates nicely the potential unsuitability of adopting
simplistic cause–effect models in our efforts to understand stress. The application of the CPT model of stress and coping here is clinically more helpful,
practical and revealing. Analysing stress in terms of threat appraisal and the
transactional outcome for the nurse also permits us to view the relationship
between threat, stress and coping as a *dynamic* rather than a *static* phenomenon. We claim the value of the CPT model is further emphasized when we
consider that in nursing, the nurse may experience a *continuous* stream of
satisfying as well as personally threatening experiences (Claus and Bailey,
1980; Sellek, 1982). Concentrating on the stressful experience for a moment,
many nurses would readily agree that their experiences of stressful episodes
can also be more complex than the examples we have quoted. Third-year
SRN individual stress protocols recorded by Bailey (1982b) show that this is
indeed the case.

Senior student protocol no. 1

Factors which I found stressful:

> I think I feel most stress in situations that are out of my control, i.e. when
> people are dying and whatever you do does not alleviate their suffering.
> When you cannot get your professional colleagues to do what you think
> they ought to do, and when you cannot get supplies and hospital
> backing for your patients to help fulfil their needs. It is not very nice
> when you have an old lady admitted as an emergency and there is no
> nightdress to be had in the corridor. Differences in professional status
> can also be stressful. One week you can be working on nights and in
> charge – trusted with the lives of patients – the next week you can be
> back in school with a learner nurse status. Also it can be stressful on the
> wards – one day in charge – the next in the sluice.

We can usefully analyse this protocol against the CPT model of stress and
coping. Here we can infer the nurse seems to be saying that there is a lack of

external coping resources present in the situations she describes. It is also evident that effective coping for her can depend on a network of support systems such as colleagues (Kaplan *et al.* 1977; Baldwin, 1983). Stress may occur when support or collective coping are not readily available (Bailey, 1982a, 1984, 1985, 1986). We would conclude that sometimes the relationship between demanding situations, and the lack of available coping resources gives the nurse the impression she has no control over these circumstances and this is when she experiences most stress (Bailey *et al.*, 1983; Clarke, 1984).

Senior student nurse protocol no. 2

Factors which I found stressful:

> In my first and second years of nursing this was: changing wards and getting used to a new routine and getting used to new senior members of staff, not knowing patients well enough, and their conditions. Coping with distressed relatives. A patient I nursed died very suddenly of a rup-tured aorta. It was within a few hours of his reaching hospital. His wife was very distressed and hysterical. I found this very upsetting and could not cope with it.

> Being left in charge of a ward, and the doctor asking me for something, or about something, I did not know.

> Seeing patients suffer pain due to inadequate pain control in terminal illness.

> Facing exams in the school of nursing.

> Being told I am unable to go to the standard of SRN, and I should go down to SEN training.

> Waiting for exam results.

> Bad organization with off-duty, so you have to work ten days in a row.

We can see how this protocol is more complex and implies a more intricate and dynamic view of stress which the CPT view of stress and coping is better conceptualized to analyse than other models of stress. There are many diffe-rent situations appraised as stressful. Some of these are directly concerned with patient care, others involving relatives, professional relationships with doctors, the school of nursing and the nursing administration. There is also some suggestion of these circumstances being appraised and the nurse feeling uncertain about what to do, until she gets used to the coping routines of the ward and the condition of patients. Put another way, her appraisal suggests that getting to know what is expected of her may help to reduce the situations regarded as stressful (Berger and Luckman, 1968; Clarke, 1984; Bailey, 1985). Indeed there is considerable evidence that when behaviour, appearance, manner, or custom is outside the range of what a nurse is used to encountering it will arouse stress – particularly anxiety. (Kramer, 1974) This often leads to a demand for change in the behaviour of the person whose expectations are violated (Goffman, 1963).

Senior student nurse protocol no. 3

Factors I found stressful:

> The pressures all around add up to constant pressure of one sort or another. There is the pressure of Blocks – the pressure of sitting and passing exams. The pressure to behave correctly and keep up a neat appearance (I am not saying this is a bad thing) and set an example.

> The actual pressure of starting a new ward every three months, and of getting on with staff and the ward sister.

> Constantly learning – often by mistakes – and then teaching others.

> The work load is usually heavy so you are physically tired as well as being mentally drained because of the learning required and the need to think all of the time. The stress of being put through a teaching session during ward report, although very interesting and essential, leaves you red-faced and tired.

> The ward assessments (there are four) are something else to be revised for, and they invariably cause a sleepless night before they are taken on the day. The responsibility is enormous – you get home thinking 'have I done everything I should have'; 'have I told staff going on duty all I should have during report'; 'have I given the right drugs'; 'have I forgotten to tell the doctor anything'. Although highly unlikely that you have not done everything, you doubt yourself.

> On top of this you have to teach others, and must learn your facts correctly before you teach others anything.

> There is the actual stress of work itself; the patient dying and his relatives; sudden emergency situations, e.g. cardiac arrests, respiratory arrests, shock, collapse, epileptic fits, etc.

> I have assessed the stress that I found, and I find I coped well at the time, perhaps because of the crisis; but I soon 'go to pieces' after it is over. There are good points about the job as well.

> It is very rewarding and varied. At the end of each ward allocation you

receive a ward report, and hard as you try, it may not be as good as you hoped for – disappointment.

On top of all this especially the unsocial working hours – I had only one weekend off whilst on the wards in the whole of my first year.

Night duty is another great strain on the emotions, especially when you are married.

There are long spells of duty which makes it difficult to try and live a life outside of the hospital.

Being a married older student I find it very tiring to look after a husband, look after a house and garden, and work at a tiring job, and then start studying.

The pay is certainly no incentive.

To cope it means an understanding husband and family (sorry, can't see you this weekend I'm working) and late nights when there is studying to be done. I am sure at some stage everyone feels like giving up, but to go and do what?

Sometimes when I have been particularly abused at work I feel like wearing a sticker saying 'I am a person, not a machine'.

   This nurse points out that for her the pressures or demands are appraised as having a cumulative effect on her functioning. The stress experienced is mainly physical and mental fatigue, and features of disorganization and lack of certainty which are characterized by self-doubt. Specific situations similar to the other protocols are mentioned. She noted that she coped well with these at the time and suffered later. The effort of doing this seems to have a disruptive influence on her family life and at times exhausts her. Interestingly, she noted that some aspects of nursing are rewarding. In the interpretation of this stress protocol we may infer that the nurse appraised many demands of nursing as being stressful but also indicated good and rewarding or satisfying aspects of the job (see also Bailey, 1982b, 1985, 1986; Sellek, 1982).

We have included these senior student nurse stress protocols just as they were recorded. To shorten them would give a misleading impression of how each nurse viewed stress and what, if anything, they did about it. Interestingly, they have a number of important issues in common. First, these nurses observe the vast range of situations or circumstances which they regard as stress-inducing. Second, the reader may notice that the sources of threat, stress and coping are very much inter-dependent. In practical nursing this means being aware of the overlapping relationship between sources of threat for nurses, the forms of stress they may experience and the coping which might be adopted to deal with it. Fortunately, the CPT model of stress and coping we have discussed is in many ways robust enough for us to analyse and begin to interpret the complex psychological processes related to stress described by nurses. Although this is as yet a qualitative analysis, it should in no way discourage us from attempts at measuring quantitatively those emotions or physical complaints within nurses which are assumed to be indicators of stress or coping. The important point for nurses is to recognize when they are appraising any event as threatening, if it is experienced as stressful or not, and what, if any, coping resources may be required to alleviate their difficulties. Does this mean nurses should simply keep a personal record of their particular problems associated with nursing, a kind of threat, stress and coping diary? We believe this is an important tactic for nurses in training for a number of reasons. In the first instance, learner nurses may wish to consider if and how their sources of threat, stress and coping change over time, coupled with their ward allocations and school or college education. A second and more active approach might be for nurses to initiate coping strategies which can either regulate their stress levels (Luthe, 1965) or defuse the threat appraisal (Meichenbaum, 1976) or increase their clinical and personal skills. This approach can lead to mastery over stress-inducing threatening situations and more personal control by the nurse over her own psychobiological functioning. The attractive consequences for nurses in overcoming debilitating levels of stress in training might be to facilitate the development of 'self-coherence' (Antonovsky, 1979). We interpret this to mean a personal belief in one's own individual resources and professional abilities. Nurse motivation and competence may also be increased as a result (White, 1959).

Status of individual reports

We view these individual reports by nurses to have at least a three-fold appeal. First, they clearly demonstrate the rich diversity of situations and circumstances which nurses regard as threatening to them and the kinds of stress they experienced. Second, it is evident that a deeper understanding of the nurse can be achieved by investigation of the individual case (see also Shapiro, 1974; Bailey, 1986). Third, and not the least important, the individual stress protocols and cameos suggest environmental threat and the experienced stress related to coping efforts by the individual may proceed from a simple appraisal to increasingly complex psychological processes. We may not be able to test these directly, but by critical application of reasonable inference in each case, we may gain deeper insights into the individual nurse. Another attraction of this approach to stress comes from interpreting such reports against the cognitive–phenomenological–transactional (CPT) model of stress and coping. Application of the model helps us to make good clinical sense of what constitutes a threat to nurses carrying out the sometimes hazardous and initially shocking demands of nursing (Kramer, 1974).

The individual reports and protocols however, also illustrate the need for a coherent conceptual and theoretical basis for interpreting and proffering plausible explanations of stress whether they be of a qualitative or quantitative kind. More systematic study employing the CPT model of stress and coping needs to be carried out with individuals and groups of nurses. Undoubtedly its greatest virtue lies in the way in which the CPT analysis may begin to account for the great composite of data reflecting individual differences in stress experienced by individual nurses, and what is significantly threatening to them and their well-being (Claus and Bailey, 1980). Of equal interest and importance is to discover if the CPT model we have discussed may account for groups of nurses who report stress and different forms of coping under varying occupational demands. For instance, similar situations may concern many nurses but each appraises them in different ways which can affect their stress level, the form it takes or the coping employed. Again, it may be that there are specific circumstances (e.g. patient death and dying) which are not only of concern to most nurses but are appraised in similar ways which give rise to similar reports of stress amongst particular groups of nurses. Lazarus and Cohen (1977) have already noted both individual and group research is necessary for our further knowledge of stress and coping. The analysis of these data by the CPT views of stress and coping are also, therefore, compatible for groups of nurses (Folkman and Lazarus, 1980). However, as we shall observe, most studies of stress involving groups of nurses have tended to employ the simplistic cause–effect models we criticized in the opening section concerned with concepts and models of stress. We now turn to an examination of some of the studies relating to groups of nurses as opposed to individuals, the first of which is strictly speaking not a research paper.

3.3 GROUPS OF NURSES AND STUDIES OF NURSES IN TRAINING

Stress associated with nurses in training

Sheahan's work

Sheahan (1979) in a clinical and non-research based paper suggests that stress amongst nurses is caused by boredom, frustration and lack of security. Unfortunately Sheahan's conceptual framework in this paper is far from logical. He not only fails to use concepts from within the stress literature but he uses interpretations based upon psychiatric insights. Sheahan's work highlights a fairly common problem within the discussion of stress in nursing, i.e. lack of good conceptual frameworks for discussing and analysing stress.

There has also been an increase in the amount of carefully conducted empirical studies of stress amongst learner nurses, their education, and the stress they may experience during the course of their occupation and training (Birch, 1978, 1979; Parkes, 1980a, 1980b; Sellek, 1982). These studies have done much to overcome the criticisms made by Cang (1979), Clarke (1976), Gott (1981), Orr (1979) and Smith (1979) regarding the poor standard of nursing research. A critical evaluation of some of the more instructive studies of stress amongst nurses in the UK and USA shows that progress has been made, but substantial problems of statistical analyses, methods of investigation, research design, interpretation and conceptualization remain. Particularly enlightening efforts have been made to investigate stress that may be associated with becoming a nurse. One principal concern has been to focus on the relationship between anxiety and nurse education.

Birch's study

ANXIETY AND NURSE EDUCATION

Birch (1978) researched anxiety and stressful situations in a sample of 207 nurses in training from four schools of nursing in the North of England. He subsequently published some of these results in a paper entitled 'The anxious learners' (Birch, 1979). The central interest of his work was to consider anxiety connected with clinical situations and its possible relationship to curricula planned by tutorial staff in periods of block study. The IPAT Anxiety Scale was used (Cattel and Scheier, 1963) and the Situations Checklist at intermittent periods in the learner's education. The situations checklist was drawn up in collaboration with a group of nurses. The IPAT Anxiety Scale was administered during the introductory block for pupil and student nurses, and thereafter at 8, 16 and 24 months. The situation checklist was administered at 8 months and 24 months for all learners.

Birch found that many of the nurses in the study reported unacceptably high levels of anxiety. Pupils were noted to have higher levels of anxiety than students 'throughout their entire training'. Birch (1979) noted these differences to be significantly different at the $p < 0.05$ level of significance. Some of the scores also suggested that some nurses had levels of anxiety indicative of poor adjustment and indicative of psychological morbidity. It should be of great concern that so many of the participants in Birch's study scored such high levels of anxiety (sten scores of 6 +).

Anxiety levels however fell between the initial testing and subsequent assessment periods at 8 and 16 months. Interestingly, they rose again when tested at 24 months of their training. We note that Birch (1979, p. 18) attributes this rise to the fact that 'they were facing final examinations at the time'. This confirms the results from other studies that anxiety often arises due to the demands of examinations (see Brown, 1938; Mechanic, 1962; Melcer *et al.*, 1973; Sarason, 1980).

ANXIETY AND STRESSFUL SITUATIONS

The rank order of anxiety-inducing situations changed somewhat between the two periods of assessment. Nursing the patient in pain was considered the highest rank in the first administration of the questionnaire. This, however, had dropped to rank 6 on the second administration of the checklist at 24 months. Progress tests in blocks of study became less stress-inducing, these being ranked 3 on the first occasion and 6 on the second rank ordering at 24 months. Many of the ranks only changed slightly and remained similar to the initial period of testing. 'Being shown up on the ward in front of patients and other staff', 'Dealing with patients with cancer', 'Care of the terminally ill', 'Care of the dying', and 'Dealing with bereaved relatives', all seemed to concern nurses in this study much the same at 24 months as they did earlier in their training at 8 months testing. With the exception of 'Understaffing' being the highest ranking concern, 'Dealing with cardiac arrest', (Rank 10), 'Dealing with sputum' (Rank 11), and 'Dealing with children with incurable disease' (Rank 9) at 24 months, most other situations had similar positions on the same rank orders on the first and second administration of the stress-inducing situation checklist. Put another way, the *same* kinds of situations bothered nurses both earlier and later in their training. However, we would point out that no indication was given if these situations induced

(i)   the same intensity of stress; and
(ii) if they occurred more or less frequently or about the same at the different periods they were tested in training.

Clearly then, some situations changed and others did not in terms of their perceived stressfulness. Birch (1979) made the passing point that anxiety levels changed with the passage of time. We also suggest that the ranking of stressful situations may or may not change over time (Bailey, 1985). Moreover, Birch (1979) concluded that:

1. preparation of nurse learners was carried out inadequately;
2. stress was inevitable in nurse learners; and
3. stress was *not* minimized by training.

Birch's (1978) thesis usefully identified a set of situations which was common to many nurses and regarded as being potentially very stressful; that was dealing with death and dying. Considered within the CPT model of stress and coping this category of demands on nurses may also be subject to similar appraisals by nurses, and these remain to be researched for their anxiety-inducing or coping characteristics. Nonetheless the work by Birch (1979) at the very least confirmed that nurses in training do experience high anxiety, and have particular concerns over clinical situations at different points in their education.

Ward stress

The concern for groups of nurses has been pursued by Parkes (1980a, b) who investigated the relationships between student nurses' stress and the wards they were allocated to as part of their training. A total of 101 first-year female student nurses from two general hospitals participated in this study from the Barnet Area Schools of Nursing. They were allocated to one of four ward combinations for their first ward, and rotated on subsequent ward allocations. The allocations in Parkes' (1980a) study involved a total of 15 wards: 7 surgical and 8 medical. After the initial introductory 8-week block in school, student nurses' ward allocations were made. The first ward allocation lasted 11 weeks and was followed by a second ward allocation of 13 weeks' duration.

A number of questionnaires were used to investigate personality, work environment–climate, work satisfaction and the nurses' own emotional well-being. The main measures were Eysenck's Personality Inventory (EPI), The Middlesex Health Questionnaire, the General Health Questionnaire, The Work Satisfaction Scale and The Work Environment Scale. Short-term sickness absence was also recorded. The students were assessed on four different occasions. Their first assessment was completed prior to their ward placement – during the last week of their introductory course in the school of nursing. Follow-up assessments were carried out at the mid-point of each ward allocation.

The majority of the students in her study were stable extroverts – 43% fell into this category. Only 25% would be expected to be selected by random selection procedures. Two points need to be made about this finding. First, Parkes' findings are at variance with Birch (1978) who found the nurses in his study had poor adjustment. However, different questionnaires were used in the studies and are not directly comparable. Second, the tendency to extroversion in student nurses is now fairly well established (Lewis and Cooper, 1976; Crown and Crisp, 1979; Lewis, 1980; Bailey, 1983, 1985). Yet, personality profiles alone tell us little about the stress *experienced* by nurses. Parkes' (1980a, b) other measures and follow-up studies on the different wards did shed some light on ward stress.

Medical and surgical wards

Follow-up assessments on medical and surgical wards did show a significant difference in psychological distress. This was particularly noticeable for anxiety and depression. Students reported significantly more anxiety ($p <$ 0.05 level) and depression ($p < 0.01$ level) on medical wards than on surgical wards. Work satisfaction was also significantly different, with satisfaction scores consistently lower on medical wards when compared with surgical wards ($p < 0.05$ level). Interestingly though, no difference was observed in the periods of short-term sickness records.

As a group, these students reflected a tendency to more anxiety and depression on medical wards. We feel it is worth commenting though, that all levels of stress were not highly significant, e.g. there were no significant differences on medical and surgical wards – just somatic symptoms. Parkes does not publish the data on phobic, obsessional or hysteria dimensions of The Middlesex Health Questionnaire. Yet the results may be a helpful guide for those nurses concerned with appropriate ward-placement experience for nurses. For instance, should the majority of nurses be placed on surgical wards before medical allocation? No predictions of this kind were made or intended by the Parkes (1980a) paper, but it does suggest an area for future applied stress research with nurses. Also, if medical wards were more stressful than surgical, why was there no difference in sickness absence?

Perhaps this can be accounted for in the higher stress profiles reported by students from their medical placements. We might argue that medical-ward experience takes more out of the nurse or that surgical-ward experience does not make demands on the nurse which are appraised as threatening compared with medical wards. This may leave the nurse more free to use the available coping resources to meet difficulties which might arise. These group results are valuable for they suggest that as well as individual differences in nurses, some similarity can be claimed for groups of nurses and stress related to specific ward demands, and the type of nursing involved in practising nursing care (Bailey, 1985).

Yet studies like these, albeit not their intention, fail to identify those nurses who find surgical and medical wards equally demanding. Nor indeed can they reveal the nurse who has a tendency for greater stress and discomfort in medical wards as opposed to surgical ward nursing. The recorded individual stress protocols of third-year student nurses confirm this possibility (Bailey, 1982b). However there was general support for Parkes' (1980a, p. 116), conclusion that:

> differences between the nursing tasks involved, or the ward environment more generally, give rise to the higher levels of anxiety and depression and lower work satisfaction in medical wards.

Why should this be so? We have seen how neither the tasks themselves, nor the situations necessarily contain inherent stressors. We have argued that it is essentially the way the nurse appraises the demands made on her which matters and this is consistent with Lazarus' thinking and research programme on stress and coping. However, the question may also be asked why appraisals in medical wards, seem if anything, to induce more stress than surgical ward nursing? Clarke (1983) has made the useful point that simplistic models of stress overlook the importance of socially determined norms of behaviour which the nurse has to learn. In its broadest terms we may refer to this as the 'culture of nursing'. This is important for broadening our perspective on understanding ward stress in particular and stress amongst nurses in general. With respect to ward stress, the surgical ward seems to conform more to the behaviour implied in the medical model of care (i.e. admission, diagnosis, treatment, cure . . . discharge, and in a very short time), than does the medical ward where cure may not be the outcome.

In medical wards the model of care seems to be less clear and the behaviour expected more ambiguous and involving closer personal relationships. Clarke (1983) also noted that 'where the prevailing ideology is the medical model I presume students would experience less conflict. . .'. We can take this insight and match it to Berger and Luckman's (1968) observation that people learn what is expected of them and that they are constructing 'social reality'. Thus those realities which are more congruent with what the nurse has learned about what nurses do, and are, are likely to be less stressful than her appraisal of environmental demands which are incongruent with her expectations. If we accept this view then medical wards are not simply more stressful than surgical wards because of the appraisal made by nurses, but rather because the appraisals of the ward environment are somehow incongruent with the behavioural expectations of the nurse. This does not preclude the role of cognitive processes in stress and coping. Rather it seems to suggest that nurse appraisals of demands must by definition be made within a given ward culture which is either congruent or incongruent with the expectations of the nurse (Bailey, 1985). When incongruity arises there may be a 'misfit' between the nurse and the immediate situation. It is this that can give rise to stress. However, as Goffman (1963, p. 12) has noted we do not become aware of the norms that operate in any environment until they are infringed, or as he puts it 'until an active question arises as to whether or not they will be fulfilled'. Clearly there is a need to consider closely the congruence–incongruence between the nurses, type of ward and cognitive appraisal processes of stress and coping. We can infer this theme again in Parkes' comparisons of student nurses' experiences of anxiety, work satisfaction and sickness absence, and male and female wards.

The work environment

Further light is shed on the intricacies of ward stressors by the student nurse responses to the Work Environment Scale. The 'social climate' or prevailing cultures of the medical and surgical wards were somewhat similar. For example Parkes' (1980a) student nurses did not differ markedly in their perceptions of the degree of control senior staff had over their work. However, this area and 'work pressure' were given the highest scores. In other words they were more demanding than other aspects of the work environment. There were some significant differences as well. Support from peers was greater for the surgical wards, compared with medical wards. Indeed, support from senior staff was greater for surgical wards. On these wards student nurses also felt more involved in their job, had more autonomy, and were encouraged to experience a variety of nursing tasks. This seemed to be confirmed by the higher task orientation and innovation of surgical wards compared to medical wards. However, the extent to which nurses knew what to do (role clarity) was also greater, but not statistically significant, for surgical compared to medical wards. We can concur with Parkes (1980a) that the work environment scales showed a more favourable picture for the surgical wards than the medical ones. Interestingly though, in most respects, the Work Environment Scale profiles for male and female wards were notably similar. This was closest for task orientation–organization of work on the ward, high work pressure, and control by senior staff. Innovation and change seemed slightly lower but the same for male and female wards. Role clarity, indicating behavioural expectations of the student nurse, were remarkably the same for male and female wards. However, more autonomy was observed for female wards, and greater peer cohesion on male wards compared to female wards. These results suggest that our arguments in favour of ward cultures should also consider autonomy as an important variable in ward stress.

Type of ward and nursing the different sexes

The Work Environment Scale (WES) profiles for male and female wards consistently reflected the strikingly similar shape of the work environment profiles for the different-sex wards. Anxiety in particular was higher for female student nurses working on medical and male wards compared with female surgial wards. However, other indicators of stress such as somatic complaints and depression were significantly different for male and female wards. Concerning medical versus surgical ward, depression was significantly higher for surgical-ward experience of student nurses. The work satisfaction was significantly higher for student nurses' experience of surgical wards and nursing male patients, though work satisfaction was recorded as still being high for medical-ward allocation and nursing male and female patients.

MALE AND FEMALE WARDS

Here Parkes (1980b) found three results of further interest:

1. Anxiety as measured by the General Health Questionnaire and Middlesex Health Questionnaire (MHQ) was higher for students in male wards,

but only the MHQ showed a significantly greater level of anxiety for male wards compared with female wards. All of the other sub-scales on these questionnaires showed no substantial differences between male and female wards.

2. Student nurses reported more work satisfaction on male wards despite their *higher* level of anxiety compared with female wards.
3. No differences were recorded for sickness absence between the students allocated to male or female wards.

In our view these results have important implications for a deeper understanding of clinical nursing. The combination of high anxiety and high job satisfaction in particular helps to dispense with at least two myths of occupational stress. First, high anxiety does not necessarily predict low job satisfaction (though this may be the case for some nurses). Secondly, and conversely, high job satisfaction does not mean nurses will report low anxiety. Other studies provide additional support for the association of high anxiety with high job satisfaction. Similar results have been found in related occupational groups such as doctors and dentists (Burke, 1976; Mallinger, 1978; McCue, 1982; Bailey, 1985, 1986).

Clearly, the relationship between job satisfaction and stress is not a simple one. The ward sister who finds that nurses on the ward complain of various kinds of stress should not instantly infer they are not getting much satisfaction out of their job. Equally, for those nurses who do not show any of the signs of anxiety, it cannot be assumed they are satisfied with their jobs. Unfortunately, they may simply not be interested in their job and invest less of themselves into it (Bailey, 1985). One consequence of such circumstances we might conclude, is that there are nurses with low job satisfaction and low anxiety. Further, we can speculate and argue that where this is evident we might expect more sickness absence reported compared with those nurses who had higher job satisfaction and stress levels. Perhaps the combination to avoid for nurses is high stress and low job satisfaction. Whatever the circumstances, it would seem to be premature to draw conclusions about nurses' job satisfaction from their anxiety levels alone, or indeed to infer estimates of job satisfaction from anxiety reports. What we can, and should emphasize though, is the finding that many nurses experience unacceptable levels of anxiety (Birch, 1979; Bailey, 1985, 1986) but still find their job satisfying. In other words anxiety and depression may be some of the price the student nurse pays for becoming a nurse, but this may be offset by the satisfactions of the job (Claus and Bailey, 1980; Sellek, 1982).

Where these change over time, as anxiety did in Birch's (1978, 1979) research, this may be related to 'the rites of passage' and 'learning the ropes', and adjusting to the demands of nursing (Kramer, 1974) or learning improved coping (Bailey, 1985). In Clarke's (1983) view and Berger and Luckman's (1968), the student nurse, in learning of the social expectations of the ward, may alter her anxiety level and her job-satisfaction. Familiarity with what is expected (Goffman, 1979) is likely to increase with time, and such familiarity may reduce uncertainty of expected professional behaviour. If this is the case and we would argue that it is, then the nurse is probably learning to appraise the situations arising in the wards as less threatening or deciding she has the coping skills necessary to tolerate or change the circumstances. The course of time for many nurses is likely to alter their appraisal of threat, or loss, or their perception of challenge to their nursing competence. The good nurse in this sense then becomes someone who can cope effectively with the cognitive appraisals of the demands she regards as being upon her at any given moment. Simply assuming that it is the job, the nurse, or the stresses of nursing, just does not take into account the complexity of nurse–environmental relationships. These considerations clearly alert us to not uncritically rely on unwarranted assumptions about anxiety and job-satisfaction amongst student nurses.

INTERPRETATION AND IMPLICATIONS FOR CLINICAL NURSING

Why should there be greater work satisfaction on male wards for student nurses than female wards? Parkes (1980a, b) argues this is because of the common-sense explanation that male patients are more appreciative and by contrast, less demanding than female patients. In other words male patients are more popular to nurse than female patients (Stockwell, 1972). Another interpretation for the popularity of male over female patients might be that although females may have been equally appreciative, nurses prefer appreciation or compliments from male patients because of interpersonal attraction between the sexes (Huston and Levinger, 1978).

Perhaps this is even more evident when we remember that this finding was particularly striking on the male surgical wards where patients were younger on average than male medical patients. Parkes' interpretation may be open to question but her results are consistent with Moos' (1976) claim that differences in social atmosphere are related to peer cohesion. This view was strongly supported in the comparison of male and female wards.

We might be tempted to conclude these results support the practice of allocating female nurses to male wards. Conversely, it might be said male nurses should be allocated to female wards, but this hypothesis was never tested in Parkes' study which was based on an all-female sample of nurses in training. Furthermore, this is hardly a practical proposal. On the one hand, nursing is still predominantly a female profession, and is likely to be for the foreseeable future (Claus and Bailey, 1980). On the other hand, the nurse has a responsibility to provide nursing to patients without discrimination, irrespective of sex. Another problem that is pointed out by Parkes' (1980a, b) work is this: How are nurses under the present regulations and arrangements for nurse education and nursing practice to develop the skills and tolerance to deal with threats in the nursing environment which may lead to interfering levels of disabling stress? Surely, when the ideal allocation for each nurse cannot be made, there needs to be a back-up facility such as individual coping or counselling services (Annandale-Steiner 1979a, b; Hugill, 1979; Bailey 1981, 1982a, 1984, 1985, 1986). These benefit nurses in training and facilitate their coping efforts both to overcome, and to achieve personal control over different aspects of ward stress. We would claim it is as important – perhaps more important – for the nurse to develop her own coping resources than trying to arrange the ward environment to suit individual nurses.

Stress management and counselling facilities would encourage the nurse to develop her personal and professional expertise. It may be more stressful initially for the nurse on certain wards but it is impracticable to fit every nurse to wards or wards to nurses as a matter of nursing policy (Bailey *et al.*, 1983). If this were the case, some wards would never have nurses allocated to them.

We would make one further observation. If we look at the questionnaire data published by Parkes (see 1980a, b) and look for similarities of data and profiling rather than differences, some interesting possibilities immediately emerge. For instance, the student nurses' reports of psychological distress and work satisfaction are generally in the same direction, and there is no difference in sickness absence. This is consistent for the medical–surgical ward, and male–female ward analysis. Moreover, the remarkable similarity of the questionnaires' reports and the profile data, suggests that there is a common set of circumstances which nurses appraise as more threatening than others. Here again the notion of degree of threat from occupational demands of nursing by type of ward, or more properly ward climate, is connected both to the kinds of nursing demands and the appraisals made which lead to more or less stress. So that we might say, not only is appraisal in Lazarus' (1966, 1976, 1981) terms a highly individual phenomenon, it is also reasonable to suggest that under certain conditions common appraisals may be made. We would go further and claim this is likely to be reflected both in what we learn to regard as potentially dangerous, or hazardous, and also in societal taboos such as the tradition in the West at least, of avoiding discussion or confrontations about handicap, death and dying, and other stigmatized topics (Goffman, 1979; Whitfield, 1979; Jacobs, 1980). Put another way, the student nurse, like qualified nurses and indeed the population in general, as well as having their own individual ways of appraising environmental demands, have a culturally shared set of demands which are appraised as threatening to them. Also what is found threatening can be learned from one's professional peers (Allen, 1980; Clarke 1984). The evidence we have reviewed here is amenable to this interpretation. Simply being a student nurse, does not 'immunize' the nurse from some of the common threats inherent to the demands of becoming a nurse and practising nursing.

3.4 SUMMARY

We have considered the issue of stress amongst nurses in training. Personal examples show that stress is often a highly individual phenomenon. Moreover, we have demonstrated that stress for nurses in training can often be highly complex. But we have argued that the cognitive–psychological–transactional (CPT) model of stress and coping can account for these diverse complications. Considering the problem of stress more closely, we have found that the appraisal of stress depends on commonly shared cultures and the relationship it has between nurses in training and specific environmental demands. Particularly relevant here is the difference in social climate or ward cultures and levels of stress reported by nurses in training. We can conclude by saying that type of ward and the nursing demands of the same or opposite sex are significant variables in the study of stress amongst nurses. We also can claim the implications for clinical nursing suggest limitations in trying to fit the nurse to any particular ward climate culture. Stress management and counselling facilities are advocated as a progressive and productive development for nurses in training who wish to develop more competence in managing stress and coping with the often shocking demands of nursing (Kramer, 1974; Bailey, 1985, 1986).

REFERENCES

Allen, H. (1980) *The Ward Sister*, Heinemann, London.

Annandale-Steiner, D. (1979a) Unhappiness is the nurse who expected more, *Nursing Mirror* (November 29), 34–6.

Annandale-Steiner, D. (1979b) The nurse counsellor's role at Guy's. *Nursing Mirror* (August 13), 45–9.

Antonovsky, A. (1979) *Health, Stress and Coping*, Jossey-Bass, San Francisco.

Bailey, R. (1981) Counselling services for nurses – a forgotten responsibility. *Journal British Institute of Mental Handicap*, **9**, 45–7.

Bailey, R. (1982a) Counselling services for nurses. *Journal of British Association for Counselling*, B. A. C. Publications no. 39, 25–39.

Bailey, R. (1982b) *Senior Student Nurse Stress and Coping Profiles*. Dept. Records, Psychology Department, Manor House, Aylesbury.

Bailey, R. (1983) *Stress and Coping with the Demands of Caring*. Seminar at School of Nursing and School of Medicine, University of California, San Francisco.

Bailey, R. (1984) Autogenic regulation training and sickness absence amongst nurses in general training. *Journal of Advanced Nursing*, **9**, 581–8.

Bailey, R. (1985) *Autogenic Regulation Training (ART), Sickness Absence,*

Personal Problems, Time and The Emotional–Physical Stress of Student Nurses in General Training. PhD Thesis, University of Hull.

Bailey, R. (1986) *Coping with Stress in Caring*. Blackwell Scientific Publications, Oxford.

Bailey, J., Bailey, R. and Chiriboga, D. (1983) *Conceptual, Methodological and Research Issues in the Study of Stress*. Doctoral Seminars. School of Nursing and School of Medicine, University of California, San Francisco.

Berger, P. L. and Luckman, T. (1968) *The Social Construction of Reality*. Penguin, Harmondsworth.

Birch, J. (1978) *Anxiety in Nurse Education*. PhD Thesis. University of Newcastle.

Birch, J. (1979) The anxious learners. *Nursing Mirror* (February 8), 17–24.

Baldwin, D. (1983) *How Nurses Cope Successfully with Stress*. A Stanford Nursing Department Study, Stanford University Hospital, Stanford, CA.

Brown, C. (1938) Emotional reactions before examinations. *International Journal of Psychology*, **3** (5), 27–31.

Burke, R. J. (1976) Occupational stress and job satisfaction. *Journal of Social Psychology*, **100**, 235–44.

Cang, S. (1979) (Editorial). Nursing research: Problems of aim, method and content. *Journal of Advanced Nursing*, 453–8.

Cattel, R. and Scheier, I. (1963) *The IPAT Anxiety Scale*. The Institute of Personality and Ability Testing. Champaign, IL.

Clarke, M. (1976) A degree of nursing. *Nursing Mirror* (May 20), 60–61.

Clarke, M. (1983) Personal communication. Director of Nursing Studies, Institute of Nursing Studies, Hull University.

Clarke, M. (1984) Stress and Coping. Constructs for nursing. *J. Adv. Nursing*, **9**, 3–14.

Clarke, M. and Montague, S. (1980) Introduction. *Nursing*, 418–21.

Claus, K. and Bailey, J. (1980) *Living with Stress and Promoting Well-Being: A Handbook*. C. V. Mosby, St. Louis, MO.

Crown, S. and Crisp, A. H. (1979) *Manual of the Crown-Crisp Experiential Index*, Hodder and Stoughton, London.

Dosett, S. (1978) Nursing staff in high dependency areas. *Nursing Times*, (May 25), 886–9.

Folkman, S. and Lazarus, R. S. (1980) An analysis of coping in a middle-aged community sample. *Journal of Health and Social Behaviour*, **21**, 219–39.

Goffman, E. (1963) *Relations in Public*. Pelican, London.

Goffman, E. (1979) *Stigma: Notes on the Management of Spoilt Identity*, Prentice-Hall, Inglewood Cliffs, N.J.

Gott, M. (1981) A creative climate. *Nursing Mirror*, **2**, 44 and 47.

Hawkins, K. (1979) We need looking after too. *Nursing Mirror*, 1979

Hay, D. and Oken, D. (1972) The psychological stresses of intensive care unit nursing. *Journal Psychosomatic Medicine*, **34**, 109–18.

Haynes, G. (1978) The problem of stress. *Nursing Times* (May 4), 753–54.

Hugill, J. (1979) Nurse counselling. *Nursing Mirror* (April 10), 58–61.

Huston, T. L. and Levinger, G. (1978) Interpersonal attraction and relationship. *Annual Review of Psychology,* **29**, 115–56.

Jacobs, R. (1980) Personal communication, Stoke Mandeville Hospital, Bucks.

Kaplan, B. H., Cassel, J. C. and Gore, S. (1977) Social support and health. *Medical Care,* **15**, 47–58.

Kramer, M. (1974) *Reality Shock: Why Nurses Leave Nursing.* C. V. Mosby, St. Louis, MO.

Lazarus, R. (1966) *Psychological Stress and the Coping Process.* McGraw-Hill, New York, N.Y.

Lazarus, R. (1976) *Patterns of Adjustment.* McGraw-Hill, New York, N.Y.

Lazarus, R. (1981) The stress and coping paradigm, in *Theoretical Bases for Psychopathology* (eds C. Eisdorfer, D. Cohen, A. Kleinman and P. Maxim), Spectrum, New York, N.Y.

Lazarus, R. and Cohen, J. (1977) Environmental stress, in *Human Behavior and Environment: Advances in Theory and Research,* **2** (eds I. Altman and J. Wolhill), Plenum, New York, N.Y.

Lazarus, R. and Launier, R. (1978) Stress-related transactions between person and environment, in *Perspectives in Interactional Psychology* (eds L. Dervin and M. Lewis), Plenum, New York, N.Y., pp. 287–327.

Lewis, B. R. (1980) Personality profiles for qualified nurses: Possible implications for recruitment and selection of trainee nurses. *International Journal Nursing Studies,* **51**, 221–34.

Lewis, B. R. and Cooper, C. L. (1976) Personality measurement among nurses: A review. *International Journal Nursing Studies,* **13**, 209–29.

Luthe, W. (1965) *Autogenic Training,* Grune and Stratton, New York, N.Y.

McCue, J. (1982) The effect of stress on physicians and their medical practice. *New England Journal of Medicine,* **306**, 456–63.

Mallinger, M. (1978) Stress and success in dentistry. *Journal of Occupational Medicine,* **20**, 549–53.

Marshall, J. (1980) Stress amongst nurses, in *White Collar and Professional Stress* (Eds. C. Cooper and J. Marshall), J. Wiley, London.

Mechanic, D. (1962) *Students under Stress.* Free Press of Glencoe, New York, N.Y.

Meichenbaum, D. (1976) A self-instructional approach to stress management: A proposal for stress innoculation training, in *Stress and Anxiety in Modern Life* (eds C. Speilberger and I. Sarason), Winston, New York, N.Y.

Melcer, E., Kovacevic T., Strowanovic, L. and Duclovic, R. (1973) Test anxiety and its features. *Analytics,* **5**, 71–80.

Moos, R. (1976) *The Human Context: Environmental Determinants of Behavior.* J. Wiley, New York.

Orr, J. (1979) Nursing and the process of scientific inquiry. *Journal of Advanced Nursing*, **4**, 603–10.

Parkes, K. (1980a) Occupational stress among student nurses – 1. A comparison of medical and surgical wards. Occasional Papers. *Nursing Times*, **76** (25), 113–16.

Parkes, K. (1980b) Occupational stress among student nurses – 2. A comparison of male and female wards. Occasional Papers. *Nursing Times*, **76** (26), 117–19.

Sarason, I. (1972) Experimental approaches to test anxiety: Attention and the uses of information, in *Current Trends in Theory and Research*, (ed. C. Speilberger), Academic Press, New York, N.Y.

Sarason, I. (1980) *Test Anxiety: Theory, Research and Applications*. Lawrence Erlbaum Ass., London.

Sellek, T. (1982) Satisfying and anxiety–creating incidents for nursing students. *Nursing Times* (December 1), 137–40.

Shapiro, M. B. (1974) Intensive assessment of the single case: an inductive–deductive approach, in *The Psychological Assessment of Mental and Physical Handicaps* (ed. P. Mittler), Tavistock/Methuen, London, pp. 645–65.

Sheahan, J. (1979) Mental distress at work. *Nursing Mirror* (January 25), 16–19.

Smith, J. (1979) Is the nursing profession really research-based? *Journal of Advanced Nursing*, **4**, 319–25.

Stockwell, F. (1972) *The Unpopular Patient*. RCN Publications, London.

Thomson, J. (1983) Call sister–stress in the A & E Department. *Nursing Times* (August 3), 23–7.

White, R. (1959) Motivation reconsidered: The concept of competence. *Psychological Review*, **66** (5), 297–333.

Whitfield, S. (1979) *A Descriptive Study of Student Nurses' Ward Experiences With Dying Patients and Their Attitudes Towards Them*. MSc Thesis, University of Manchester.

CHAPTER FOUR

Stress, death and dying

In me thou seest the twilight of such day
As after sunset fadeth in the west,
Which by-and-by black night doth take away,
Death's second self, that seals up all in rest.

Shakespeare – *Sonnets*, LXXIII

4.1 INTERNATIONAL STUDIES

Nurses seem to experience considerable stress – particularly anxiety, depressed affect and guilt when dealing with death and dying (Folta, 1965; Glaserand Strauss, 1966, 1968; Gow and Williams, 1977; Birch 1978, 1979; Jones, 1978; Whitfield, 1979; Claus and Bailey, 1980; Bailey, 1982, 1985). As Sudnow (1967) has noted, many nurses actually try to avoid the corpse. Last offices may also be conducted in an impersonal way – referring to the corpse as a number or depersonalized object. However, this may be a necessary coping strategy. Glaser and Strauss (1966) have pointed out that distancing oneself from the dead patient may serve as a protective shield: a shield which permits the nurse to carry on with her duties.

We see a more complex picture of death and dying as a source of stress presented by Denton and Wisenbaker (1977), Giezhals (1976) and Shusterman and Sechrest (1973). The Shusterman and Sechrest (1973) study used a questionnaire concerned with six areas of attitudes towards death. These were:

1. Fear of death of self
2. Fear of death of others
3. Fear of dying of self
4. Fear of dying of others
5. Satisfaction with standard of nursing care
6. Self-confidence in own ability to care for dying patients

The investigators circulated 188 Registered Nurses in the surgical and medical wards of a general hospital. Perhaps not surprisingly only 50% of the intended sample completed the questionnaire. Put another way, half the sample refused to take part in the study. This may have been because of the threatening nature of the subject – particularly for the refusing group. Indeed those who replied reported little anxiety about death. Could it be that the nurses who coped best with death replied and those for whom death was a considerable anxiety did not? The other data in this study suggested that the nurses' ability to care for the dying was not related to anxiety. However, their self-confidence was rated as low. Their satisfaction with the nursing profession's standards of care for the dying was also recorded as being very low. We note that the age of respondent did seem a significant variable. Older nurses were apparently less anxious and more accepting of the standardized procedures for nursing the dying patient. Shusterman and Sechrest (1973) suggest self-selection procedures may have been operating in the sample response. We have interpreted this view to mean that those who coped better with death and dying participated in the study, whereas those who did not refused.

The researchers in this study also made the point that more attention should be spent on refining measures of response to death and dying. However, a substantially important aspect of this study must surely be the finding that age was significantly related to fear of dying. We would emphasize it is not clear though whether age *per se* alleviates fear of death and dying. Perhaps it is the length of time a nurse has contact with death and the dying, which matters most. For instance, Giezhals' (1976) work with ICU nurses and Occupational Therapists provides supplementary evidence for this view. Those ICU nurses and OTs who had their only contact with death and dying during student training, scored higher on her death anxiety scale than those who had greater contact with death and dying. However, this study also found that those of the sample who had had no previous contact with death or dying returned a low death anxiety score. Giezhals (1976) attributes the result to self-selection. We see the interpretation of these results as puzzling.

We suggest an alternative argument. Self-selection might be better understood in terms of relative differences in coping effectiveness. We can go further and speculate that self-selection can be understood within the paradigm of person–environment fit (Van Harrison, 1975; Caplan and Killilea, 1976). Such a conceptualization should make it possible to match environmental circumstances (e.g. death and dying) with the personal characteristics of individual nurses. The self-selection hypothesis in relation to research participation seems an impoverished inference to make – especially when it tells us nothing about the psychological dimensions along which self-selection – if at all – operates.

In an earlier American study, Folta (1965) covered a sample of 426 qualified and unqualified nurses. Three scales were used in the study. Their main concern was to evaluate:

1. Perceived dimensions of death
2. Sacred and secular views of death
3. Anxiety about death

The sample of nurses was taken from three hospitals. Folta (1965) found that most nurses expressed anxiety over death. However, many also viewed death as a natural event. Indeed some nurses in this study had positive perceptions of death. There are criticisms which can be made about this study. For instance, Folta (1965) did not enlist a control group or make distinctions between unqualified and qualified nurses' responses. Yet, allowing for these methodological limitations, the finding that some nurses see death in positive terms questions the assumption that death is a stressful event for nurses. Clearly, it does not follow that experience of death of a patient is necessarily always stressful to the nurse. This may not, of course, be the case for the nurses' experience of the dying patient (Glaser and Strauss, 1966, 1968). We would agree with the observation that in caring for the dying patient, the nurse is inevitably engaged in a close human relationship. It is at such times that 'human relationships are dangerous' (Bailey 1985; Parkes 1972).

Overcoming some of the methodological difficulties in the Folta work, Gow and Williams (1977) replicated and elaborated their study. Gow and Williams (1977) provided a more complex profile of the nurses' attitudes towards death. Their main aim was to compare the attitudes of 235 qualified nurses' attitudes towards death. This was done in three different areas of nursing:

1. The acute general hospital
2. Units for the chronically sick
3. Community care

Data from these were then related to the nurses' experience with death and dying patients. Analysis was also made of various demographic characteristics. The results of Gow and Williams' (1977) study was factor analysed and showed attitudes toward death and dying seemed to be largely influenced by (a) experience and (b) personal attributes. In other words, in this study, the type of nursing *per se* was not regarded as the central feature in attitudes towards death and dying. If this is the case, then type of nursing is not a strong predictor of 'type of nurse'.

Additional factors may be involved. To be sure, as Gow and Williams' (1977) investigation discovered, the older the nurse, the more positive her attitudes were towards the dying patient and death. This view also confirms the earlier study by Shusterman and Sechrest (1973).

A study which argues a more complex and critical relationship between the nurses' experience of death and death anxiety has been conducted by Denton and Wisenbaker (1977). They explored the assumption that greater contact with death would result in reduced levels of death anxiety. These authors collated medical data over three years and this was the basis for their study. The records of 76 baccalaureate nursing and graduate students provide the basis for this analysis. Death anxiety was measured using Templer's (1970) Death Anxiety Scale.

The results of their study seemed to reject their hypothesis that there is an inverse relationship between contact with death and death anxiety. In other words more contact with death did not lead to lower experienced death anxiety. Indeed, comparisons of the graduate nurses (more experienced) with the student nurses (less experienced) showed that the graduate nurses were more anxious about death than the students. One reason for this might be that student nurses in America are supernumerary to the staffing requirements for patient care. A consequence of this circumstance might be that they did not have to engage in situations which exposed them to death and dying as much as the graduate students.

The Denton and Wisenbaker (1977) study also points out that nursing staff's death anxiety may be tapping a more complex multi-dimensional concept. It is too simplistic to assume that death of a patient either does or does not lead to experienced anxiety by nurses. Indeed, in their analysis of their data they found three dimensions which may influence death anxiety. These were:

1. Death of a friend or relative
2. 'Experience' of violent death
3. Subjective near-death experience

These dimensions were related to the scores on the Templer Scale of Death Anxiety (1970).

Being associated with a violent or subjective death but not a close death (friend or relative) was significantly correlated with lower death anxiety. So it would seem that aspects such as the degree of personal relationships with others are important elements of death anxiety. Indeed, as Denton and Wisenbaker (1977) indicate, controlling for age and work experience did not change the feelings nurses expressed within these different dimensions of death anxiety.

Their study suggests that association with death and education does not necessarily result in reported lower anxiety. The Denton and Wisenbaker (1977) conclusion is contrary to those of Giezhals (1976) and Shusterman and Sechrest (1973). These differences however, may only be apparent when we take into consideration the multi-faceted possibilities of the phenomenon regarded as 'death anxiety' amongst nurses.

4.2 BRITISH STUDIES

Few British studies have addressed themselves to the specific study of the nurses' feelings in relationship to death and dying. However, Birch in his study of anxiety in the education of nurse learners makes an important contribution. He found that 6 out of 10 situations regarded as stressful (anxiety-provoking) were connected with death, dying and bereavement, and Jones (1978, p. 366) in his research arguing for a comprehensive counselling service for nurses, found that 80% of 50 student nurses irrespective of training year, were 'functioning under stress'. This study went on to record that 80% of the sample indicated anxiety over clinical situations, some of which were connected with death and dying. But this study can be criticized on similar grounds to Folta (1965) who did not control for different years of training. Indeed as Jones (1978, p. 361) noted, nearly 20% of the sample felt that the given clinical situations 'caused no anxiety at all'. Jones (1978) went on to highlight that this grouping could be divided into second- and third-year student nurses. Therefore it would seem a reasonable inference to claim that the 80% of students responding were predominantly from the first year of training. It should be mentioned, however, that Jones' (1978) questionnaire which was designed to estimate need for counselling, had other clinical situation questions included in it alongside those concerned with death, dying and last offices. In this respect it cannot be said to be a specific study of nurses' anxiety in relationship to death and dying.

Whitfield's study

The only substantial study of this kind in Britain has been carried out by Whitfield. Her thesis reported a descriptive study of student nurses' ward experiences with dying patients and their attitudes towards them (Whitfield, 1979). A total of 26 third-year student nurses from two different hospitals, and three different months during 1977 were involved in the project. School A provided 11 student nurses in February 1977, School B provided 10 third-year student nurses in May 1977, and another 5 third-year students during September 1977. Attitudes of these student nurses were measured using the Attitudes Questionnaire developed in the United States by Yeaworth *et al.* (1974), the 'Questionnaire for Understanding the Dying Patient and His Family' (Whitfield, 1979, p. 97). A questionnaire was also developed by Whitfield to investigate the students' ward experiences with the terminally ill, their religious beliefs and their feelings about death and dying. The research tools were piloted with two small groups of third-year students (no numbers are reported for the pilot study). Amendments were made to the American questionnaire. These were mainly concerned with wording of different questions. Whitfield (1979) decided to use only Part 1 of this questionnaire. This measured attitudes towards death and dying.

Procedure

The procedure for administering the questionnaires was simple and convenient. They were completed whilst the student nurses were in the School of Nursing. The researcher remained present to clarify any points arising from the questions. Discussion was also then focused on the death which had made the most impact on them. The discussion was then terminated and the students thanked for participating, and completing the questionnaires. The period allocated for the procedure was approximately one hour, and was included as a normal study period in the School of Nursing. Perhaps this is one reason why Whitfield (1979) had a 100% participation rate in her study.

Conclusions

From the analysis of her data Whitfield (1979) reached a number of conclusions.

First, the student nurses found it difficult to communicate with those patients who did not know they were dying (see also Glaser and Strauss, 1966, 1968). Insufficient discussion and guidance were given on this problem in the ward.

Second, the student nurses thought they needed to know more about the patients' psychological needs and these were not discussed enough, although the physical needs of the patients were usually met. Opinions were split about the spiritual needs of the dying patient. Whitfield (1979) suggests one explanation for this was confusion over the role the hospital chaplain had for providing spiritual care, alongside the nurse's responsibility for giving such care. We suggest that there was considerable role ambiguity in this area of nursing the dying (Kahn et al., 1964). However, no measures of role ambiguity were taken, and this can only be speculation on the part of the present authors.

Thirdly, nurses experienced difficulty in helping the family. This was attributed to not having sufficient information on how much the relatives knew about the patients' condition. Lack of experience in dealing with bereaved relatives also added to the difficulties experienced by the nurses.

Fourthly, a conclusion suggested by Whitfield (1979) concerned nurses' feelings toward the terminally ill. They appeared to 'become emotionally involved with the patients of their own age, or whom they had got to know over a period of time' (Whitfield, 1979, p. 195). Some had mixed feelings when a patient died. These feelings included anger, guilt and depression. Other students reported having a fear of their own death. A number also had difficulty in controlling their emotional involvement with the dying patient. Sixteen students said they had difficulty in coping with their feelings. This amounted to 61.5% of the total sample. Additionally, 17 students (65.3%) were confronted with Last Offices within the first six months of their training. However, here most nurses (17 or 65.3%) said they were given enough help to deal with this experience.

Examining the student nurses' views about patients in different age categories Whitfield (1979) found that 16/26 or 61.5% of the sample felt most difficulty in dealing with young adults. This was followed by the middle aged (11), children (9) babies (1) and the elderly (1). These figures suggest more than one category of significant difficulty for the student nurses in this study. Perhaps as Whitfield (1979) has suggested the young adults were the highest category of concern because the student nurses identified themselves more with this age group. In doing so they may have sensed their own vulnerability and mortality (Barton, 1977). However, by selecting more than one age group as the most difficult death it may have also depended on the way the patient died (Whitfield, 1979) that influenced how the particular nurse felt about it.

Evaluated within a framework of stress and coping, such as that of Lazarus (1966, 1976, 1981), we might say it was the way in which the nurse 'saw' or appraised the way a patient died which influenced how she felt about their death. Interestingly, Whitfield (1979), Gow and Williams (1977) and Shusterman and Sechrest (1973) found some nurses perceived the death of a patient in a positive way. Perhaps this may as these authors suggest be related to age or experience. These variables are of course, not necessarily the same thing, and are discussed in some detail later. Moreover, rather than age or experience being an explanation as such, it could be more productive to assess the changes in nurses' cognitive appraisals which may take place with age and experience, death, and the nursing of dying patients.

The descriptive study conducted by Whitfield (1979) does present a rich, grounded-research approach (Glaser and Strauss, 1968) to the study of student nurses' attitudes towards nursing dying patients and their feelings towards their death. Whitfield suggested there should be more research into the needs of relatives of dying patients. She argued this 'is necessary in order to provide information to improve the support they are given' (Whitfield, 1979, p. 197). We also need to know more about the opinions nurses have about the procedure of Last Offices. Finally, Whitfield (1979) suggests a larger scale study of student nurses should be carried out to 'find out whether or not the experiences and problems of the nurses in the sample are typical of the general population of third year student nurses' (Whitfield, 1979, p. 197).

For the moment however we may cautiously agree with Whitfield's (1979) general conclusions that the findings of her study . . . 'have shown that *some* nurses do have difficulties in caring for the dying' (Whitfield, 1979, p. 197). [italics added]

The most general finding in the studies of response to death and dying is that nurses can experience a mixture of feelings. These may include positive and negative experiences. Positive experiences may be those such as relief that the nurse has done the best for the patient or that they died peacefully. Negative experiences may be connected with the emotions of anger, anxiety, guilt and depression. Thus a wide range of feelings may be experienced by nurses caring for the dying patient and their response to death (Folta, 1965; Denton and Wisenbaker, 1977; Gow and Williams, 1977; Hooper, 1979; Luckman, 1979; Whitfield, 1979). Some evidence suggests that older nurses have more positive attitudes towards the dying (Shusterman and Sechrest, 1973). Other studies have inferred that it is experience with death and dying which is more important than age of the nurse. In these studies, 'more experience' has been considered to be related to fewer reports of stressful experiences with death and nursing dying patients (Gow and Williams, 1977; Whitfield, 1979). However, this hypothesis has also been rejected, for the Death Anxiety score may depend on the degree of relationship the nurse has had with the dying or dead patient (Denton and Wisenbaker, 1977). Additionally, much may depend on the age group of the patient (Shusterman and Sechrest, 1973; Whitfield, 1979), the way they died (Whitfield, 1979) and personal attributes of the nurse (Gow and Williams, 1977). A number of substantial issues are raised by these studies which deserve further discussion. We shall now examine them in greater detail. They are: age and experience, and the relationship between dying patients, their death and death anxiety.

Age and experience

The studies we have considered here argue that age and experience may be important variables in the nurses' feelings towards death and dying. Yet, although providing an insight into variables associated with nurses' response to death and dying, this deserves further critical comment. For instance, are age and experience the same thing? We would propose they are not. Age is a variable easily defined, experience is not. Take those studies purporting to have found that age is a central issue in nurses' feelings in relationship to death and dying (Shusterman and Sechrest, 1973): age *per se* may not have been a significant variable in the study. Rather age may have simply represented experience. Moreover, this need not have represented experience acquired in nursing. Indeed, as Hooper (1979) discovered, previous contact with old and frail people, prior to nursing, helped the student nurses in their study involving geriatric patients. Those investigators who argue that experience is a central factor in determining whether stress is experienced, or some satisfaction in nursing the dying (e.g. Whitfield, 1979) may be meaning different things when they refer to experience. For instance, Gow and Williams (1977) seem to use the term experience interchangeably with age.

Whitfield (1979) avoids this confusion. She appears to equate experience with the amount of previous contact with patients. However, this is not made explicit anywhere in her work. There are additional problems. How is experience to be measured – if at all? And if it is feasible, what experiences are to be considered as being relevant to the study of nurses' feelings and their attitudes towards death and dying patients? Perhaps the nurses' self-reports adopted in many of the studies are useful ways to proceed. They seem as helpful as any other ways of investigating the experience of the individual or groups of nurses (Lazarus, 1976; Bailey, 1985). We must concede however we can never have direct access to experience. We should be content with aiming to refine measures which provide self-reported experience as the method of enquiry.

McKay (1980) has presented an excellent critical review of self-report measures, and their use in psychological research, and concludes that many of the measures are highly reliable and valid. Inclusion of self-report scales and interview material is therefore justifiable in many of these researches, and indeed this is true of stress research in general. However, it must be acknowledged that experience may never be operationalized as a construct. In the event, we then can say that studies of the self-report kind, if not combined with other objective, or unobtrusive measures (Webb *et al.*, 1972) are inferential knowledge. By this is meant knowledge which is dependent on the kinds of inference that can be made about any group of data. Indeed, in one sense, all knowledge can be said to be inferential. But, with un-operationalized terms such as 'experience', the range of inferences, and therefore interpretations of the data are arguably potentially greater than working within the stricter parameters of operationalized frames of enquiry. This may not be any bad thing. Perhaps it is even desirable. For just as the failure to operationalize terms of enquiry results in wider possibilities, operationalizing research entirely severely circumscribes interpretation of the data generated by research.

These issues are raised here not to enter the debate about the preference for one or other approach to research. Rather, we have presented them to illustrate some of the complex problems raised by the studies of nurses' stress and their relationship to death and dying.

The relationship between death, dying and death anxiety amongst nurses

We see a further difficulty – studies of death and dying do not always distinguish one from the other. Yet, this seems an essential distinction if we are to examine any differences, or similarities between the two conditions and their possible associations with stress amongst nurses. Perhaps the Denton and Wisenbaker (1977, p. 64) investigation, more than others reviewed here, argues this point most forcibly: these researchers also argue that their findings 'suggest a need for examining the *conditions* under which death "experience" – death anxiety are related either positively or negatively' [italics added]. Summarizing, we may conclude that the death of a patient in itself is not necessarily associated with high death anxiety. Moreover, it seems important to investigate aspects of dying (e.g behavioural expressions, vocalizations, etc.) which may be associated with death anxiety amongst nurses or, indeed, its absence. To support these lines of enquiry, Denton and Wisenbaker's (1977) breakdown into sub-groups of their general conclusions suggests an even more complex set of relationships which can exist amongst nurses' experiences of death and death anxiety. Indeed as they intriguingly illustrate the assumption that nurses' 'experience' with death and dying is inversely related to death anxiety, is only partially supported by their study. Clearly, the relationship between contact with death, dying and the nurses' death anxiety is a complex matter and deserves further research along the lines suggested by Denton and Wisenbaker (1977) in their provocative paper.

One further point of considerable relevance concerns the recent development of death awareness training in nursing, and death and death anxiety workshops (Bailey, 1985).

We wonder from the complexity of the relationships between contact with death and dying and nurse anxiety and other feelings, whether the simple inauguration of death awareness training and death and dying workshops (a) reduces death anxiety amongst nurses or (b) increases sensitivity to death anxiety amongst nurses. Implications from our present review of studies suggests a cautious reservation. It is this: The 'dealing with death' packages for many nurses may be a premature pursuit and indeed for some, a knowledge which has consequences contrary to the apparently desirable goal of reducing death anxiety. Indeed, perhaps the fundamental assumption that death and dying are morbid, terrible, and terrifying, requires to be questioned, and further distinctions between these and other phenomena such as the nurses' appraisal of these circumstances. Whatever the future holds, studies to date have helped to indicate the complexity that may exist rather than a simplistic choice between direct or inverse relationships, on nurses' attitudes or feelings about death and the dying patient.

4.3 SUMMARY

In this chapter we have considered the problem of nurse stress in relationship to death and the dying patient. Death and dying has been highlighted as particularly demanding to nurses in training and qualified nurses. Various sources of stress have been highlighted including the nurses' knowledge of death and dying, contact with death, fear of her own mortality and the degree of kinship and emotional involvement with dying patients. Age and experience have also been seen as significant variables in the stress experienced by nurses nursing the dying and their reports of death anxiety. However, we also noted nurses do not always find nursing the dying patient or their contact with death stressful. Much may also depend on the way the patient dies and the cultural values we assign to the importance of death in our society. We also expressed our reservations about the contribution death and dying workshops play in helping nurses to alleviate the fear, anxiety, guilt and depression often associated with nursing the dying and contact with death.

REFERENCES

Bailey, R. (1982) Senior Student Nurse Stress and Coping Profiles, Dept. Records. Psychology Department, Manor House, Aylesbury.

Bailey, R. (1984) Autogenic regulation training and sickness absence amongst nurses in general training. *Journal of Advanced Nursing*, **9**, 581–8.

Bailey, R. (1985) *Autogenic Regulation Training (ART), Sickness Absence, Personal Problems, Time and the Emotional–Physical Stress of Student Nurses in General Training*. PhD Thesis, University of Hull.

Barton, D. (1977) The caregiver, in *Dying and Death, A Clinical Guide for Caregivers* (ed. D. Barton), Williams, Baltimore, MD.

Birch, J. (1978) *Anxiety in Nurse Education*. PhD Thesis, University of Newcastle.

Birch, J. (1979) The anxious learners. *Nursing Mirror* (February 8), 17–24.

Caplan, G. and Killilea, M. (1976) *Support Systems and Mutual Help*. Grune and Stratton, New York, N.Y.

Claus, K. and Bailey, J. (1980) *Living with Stress and Promoting Well-Being: A Handbook*, C. V. Mosby, St. Louis, MO.

Denton, J. A. and Wisenbaker, V. (1977) Death experience and death anxiety amongst nurses and nursing students. *Nursing Research*, **26**, 61–4.

Folta, J. R. (1965) The Perception of death. *Nursing Research*, **14**, 232–5.

Giezhals, J. S. (1976) Attitudes toward death and dying: A study of occupational therapists and nurses. *Journal of Thematology*, **3**, 243–69.

Glaser, B. and Strauss, A. (1966) *Awareness of Dying*. Weidenfield and Nicholson, London.

Glaser, B. and Strauss, A. (1968) *Time for Dying*. Aldine, IL.

Gow, C. M. and Williams, J. A. (1977) Nurses' attitudes toward death and dying: A causal interpretation. *Social Science and Medicine*, **11** (3), 191–8.

Hooper, J. (1979) *An Exploratory Study of Student and Pupil Nurses' Attitudes Towards, and Expectation of, Nursing Geriatric Patients in Hospital*. MSc Thesis, University of Surrey.

Jones, D. (1978) The need for a comprehensive counselling service for nursing students. *Journal of Advanced Nursing*, **3**, 359–68.

Kahn, R., Wolfe, D. M., Quinn, R. P., Snoek, J. D. and Rosenthal, R. A. (1964) *Occupational Stress: Studies in Role Conflict and Ambiguity*. J. Wiley, New York, N.Y.

Lazarus, R. (1966) *Psychological Stress and the Coping Process*. McGraw-Hill, New York, N.Y.

Lazarus, R. (1976) *Patterns of Adjustment*. McGraw-Hill, New York, N.Y.

Lazarus, R. (1981) The stress and coping paradigm, in *Theoretical Bases for Psychopathology*, (eds C. Eisdorfer, D. Cohen, A Kleinman and P. Maxim), Spectrum, New York, N.Y.

Luckman, D. (1979) The nurse who asked why. *Nursing,* **148** (14), 18–19.

McKay, C. J. (1980) The measurement of mood and psychophysiological activity using self-report techniques, in *Techniques in Psychophysiology,* (eds I. Martin and P. H. Venables), J. Wiley, New York, N.Y., pp. 501–61.

Parkes, C. M. (1972), Determinants of outcome following bereavement. *Omega,* **6**, 303–23.

Shusterman, L. R. and Sechrest, L. (1973) Attitudes of registered nurses toward death in a general hospital. *Psychiatry in Medicine,* **4** (4), 411–26.

Sudnow, D. (1967) *Passing On: The Social Organization of Dying.* Prentice-Hall, N.J.

Templer, D. I. (1970) The construction and validation of a death anxiety scale. *Journal of General Psychology,* **82**, 165–77.

Van Harrison, R. (1975) Job Stress and Worker Health: Person–Environment Misfit. Paper presented at 103rd Annual Meeting of American Public Health Association 1–2.

Webb, E. J. Campbell, D. T., Schwartz, R. D. and Sechrest, L. (1972) *Unobtrusive Measures: Non-reactive Measures in the Social Sciences.* Rond McNally, Chicago.

Whitfield, S. (1979) *A Descriptive Study of Student Nurses' Ward Experiences with Dying Patients and Their Attitudes Towards Them.* MSc Thesis, University of Manchester.

Yeaworth, R. C., Kapp, F. T. and Winget, C. (1974) Attitudes of nursing students toward the dying patient. *Nursing Research,* **23** (1), 20–4.

CHAPTER FIVE

Nurses and the intensive care unit: A special case

5.1 INTRODUCTION

There is now a large body of evidence to show that working in the intensive care unit (ICU) seems to be particularly stressful for many nurses (Vreeland and Ellis, 1969; Michaels, 1971; Gentry *et al.*, 1972; Hay and Oken, 1972; Cassem and Hackett, 1975; Jacobson, 1978; Huckaby and Jagla, 1979; Steffen, 1980). A classical, descriptive study by Hay and Oken (1972, p. 110) portrays the often excessive and insistent complex demands made on the ICU nurse.

As part of her daily routine, the nurse must reassure and comfort the man who is dying of cancer; she must calm the awakening disturbed 'overdose' patient; she must bathe the genitalia of the helpless and comatose; she must wipe away the bloody stool of the gastrointestinal bleeder; she must comfort the anguished young wife who knows her husband is dying. It is hard to imagine any other situation that involves such intimacy with the frightening, repulsive and forbidden ... But there is more; there is something uncanny about the picture the patients present. Many are neither alive nor dead. Most have 'tubes in every orifice'. Their sounds and actions (or inaction) are almost non-human. Bodily areas and organs, ordinarily unseen, are openly exposed or deformed by bandages. All of this directly challenges the definition of being human, one's most fundamental sense of ego identity, for nurse as well as patient. Though consciously the nurse quickly learns to accept this surrealism, she is unremittingly exposed to these multiple threats to the stability of her body boundaries, her sense of self, and her feelings of humanity and reality ... To all this is added a repetitive contact with death. And if exposure to death is merely frequent, that to dying is constant. The ICU nurse thus quickly becomes adept at identifying the signs and symptoms that foretell a downhill trend for her patient. This becomes an awesome burden of the nurse who has been caring for the patient and must continue to do so, knowing his outcome.

This continuous combination of diverse and potentially highly threatening demands, Hay and Oken (1972) suggest, culminates in an inexorable work load for the nurse engaged in ICU nursing. Complicating these demands even further they noted there were frequent breakdowns in communications between nurses and doctors (Hay and Oken, 1972; Huckaby and Jagla, 1979; Steffen, 1980). The nurses' attempts at coping with these demands seem to come from banding together (Kaplan *et al.*, 1977) and supporting each other; becoming a special club who can perform 'beyond the call of duty'. Here, however, we might say that doing this may well increase the expectations the nurse working in intensive care has of herself. In our terms, a high demand culture awaits the nurse who wishes to practice ICU nursing. If this is so, then their coping efforts are merely palliation or ultimately exhausting attempts to deal with the continuous catena of demands emanating from caring for patients in the ICU. Other apparently bizarre palliative coping efforts include singing, joking and talking loudly with an apparent sense of gaiety. We would argue this is a nurses' way of trying to cope with the knowledge that their caring responses will frequently have little or no influence on patient outcomes.

Predicting that the patient will die is hardly comforting, and we would also claim it is antagonistic to many of the precepts of nursing which assume patient responsiveness to treatment. We might also ask what other options are there open to the ICU nurse when Hay and Oken (1972, p. 112) summarize her plight as having 'no place to hide'? We have already suggested one possibility – altering the appraisal system or more generally the frame of reference within which nurses view their role in ICU. For instance ICU nurses could be encouraged to view ICU nursing as similar to hospice nursing. Here the assumption of the nurse's role is explicitly palliative. Making the palliation role the basis of caring, rather than attempts to save life at all costs, seems a controversial proposal. However, this might be associated with not only a reduction in experienced stress problems but also a change in the source of these problems. Thus the problems of those demands which are appraised as threatening could be reconstrued in a way which transformed their meaning.

However, within the present culture of ICU nursing (see Hay and Oken, 1972; Huckaby and Jagla, 1979; Steffen, 1980; Anderson *et al.*, 1981) the nurse's role expectations seem to be incongruent with the reality of the ICU demands. Much of what the ICU nurse appears to do is palliative nursing care. In Watzlawick *et al.*'s (1974) terms, there can be no solution to the threatening demands or losses associated with a patient's death and the subsequent stress unless the nurse's frame of reference is changed. Changed to what? For instance, as mentioned above it may be worthwhile advocating that the ICU nurse views (frames) her role as a palliative one. Doing this may not defuse all of the threatening demands made on her. However, it would arguably change the appraisals made about what is expected of *her* (e.g. the recovery of the patient) and draw it into closer congruence with what may be the real outcome of ICU nursing (i.e. the patient's death).

Later empirical studies have confirmed many of the observations made by Hay and Oken (1972). In a study of 46 registered nurses Huckaby and Jagla (1979) confirmed that patient care and communication between colleagues were of major concern to nurses, as shown by the rank order of responses. Closely following this were demands connected with the ICU environment such as noise level, equipment and its failure, the physical environment and risk of physical injury to the nurse. Perhaps a little surprisingly, requiring a sound knowledge base, although a source of stress to the ICU nurse, came lowest in the rankings of stressful factors of the ICU for the nurses in the Huckaby and Jagla (1979) research. However, this finding is consistent with Steffen's (1980) later and more comprehensive study of ICU nurses. From the nurse's point of view, perhaps we can say that, although she has a substantial knowledge base, this is still regarded as being insufficient to deal with the demands intrinsic to ICU nursing. This is hardly surprising if we accept the earlier arguments we have made regarding knowledge and coping effectiveness among nurses.

Interestingly, Huckaby and Jagla (1979) interpreted their results against Lefcourt's locus of control theory (Lefcourt, 1976, 1981) and Janis' (1958) view that knowledge reduces stress. Before proceeding, we believe it merits comment that Lefcourt did not introduce the notion of locus of control in psychology. This honour rightly belongs to Julian Rotter (1954, 1966, 1975). However, Lefcourt has done much to develop Rotter's ideas, both at a conceptual and research level (see e.g. Lefcourt, 1976, 1981). Briefly, Rotter developed the notion that people lie along a continuum between an internal and an external locus of control. In its simplest form, an 'internal' individual is oriented to believe that control over reinforcement is due largely to their own actions. Conversely, an externally oriented individual believes that reinforcement is not controlled by themselves but by other people – particularly those regarded as important and powerful (Rotter, 1954, 1966; Lefcourt, 1976).

Internal–External Locus of Control Scales have been developed to measure these dimensions, and have generated much useful discussion amongst psychologists (Mirels, 1971; Strickland, 1978; Lefcourt, 1981). The arguments and research for and against these scales are not elaborated any further here. The main purpose is to mention the assumptions behind the Locus of Control construct in psychology. We may now consider Huckaby and Jagla's (1979) interpretation of their data against this background knowledge.

Discussing the patient care and interpersonal communication categories these investigators suggest both can be understood by interpreting them within locus of control theory. On patient care Huckaby and Jagla (1979, p. 24) reported:

> ... the patient care category presents the ICU nurse with threatening situations that are controlled externally rather than internally and are therefore more difficult to direct and control. For instance, the death of a patient and the amount of physical work cannot be controlled by the nurse through either learning or experience and were, therefore, rated as more stressful.

A similar interpretation was made of the second highest ranking category of sources of stress – interpersonal communications. Here, Huckaby and Jagla (1979) claimed communications between staff members, and between staff and other departments were rated low on stressfulness. Compared with this communications between the staff and nursing office, and between staff and physicians were rated very highly stressful. Viewing these data along the external dimension of locus of control, they further suggested:

> The physicians and persons in the nursing office are seen as superiors who have dominance over the nurse. Situations involving them are externally controlled and therefore perceived as highly stressful.

Regarding the environmental category, they proposed this category may have been rated on an intermediate position because there was little the ICU nurse could do to alter external events. However they also suggest the more the nurse becomes familiar with a stressful situation the more control she experiences over the situation and the less stressful the situation is perceived. This seems a very plausible interpretation. However we would also consider a converse point. Many nurses engaged in the ICU may become sensitized to perceiving very frequently lack of control in the way they experience situations arising in the course of their work. Consequently such sensitization may induce more stress not less. Having an insufficient knowledge base was interpreted against Janis' (1958) early work which suggested surgical patients may recover more quickly if provided with information and permitted to carry out the 'work of worrying'. We can see how Huckaby and Jagla (1979) paralleled this finding with ICU nurses. We must regard these convincing considerations with some caution. A number of other points must be made here. First, Janis (1958) questioned the efficacy of giving information to *all* groups of patients. Second, in a more recent seminar Borkovec (1983) questions whether worrying is of any real help to individuals trying to overcome stress.

Borkovec (1983) distinguished the work of worrying from problem-solving, a more potentially adaptive form of coping. The relevance for the Huckaby and Jagla (1979) study can only be speculative. But we might cautiously suggest that giving knowledge can also increase stress for some ICU nurses. One reason for this may be that knowledge heightens the awareness of ICU nurses to the gravity of the patient's condition, a consequence of this being a sharpening of the ICU nurse's perception of the demands made on her. In a psychoanalytically focused study Gunther (1977) calls this 'the burden of rehabilitation' (see also Hay and Oken, 1972). Finally, a compound question which is of interest to us, but unfortunately was not pursued in the Huckaby and Jagla (1979) study is, 'which groups of nurses did not identify the need for more knowledge and why?'. Despite these criticisms of interpretation, for the ICU nurses in the Huckaby and Jagla (1979) study at least, insufficient knowledge was regarded as a substantial concern.

Theoretical and other issues

Some other points need to be made about Huckaby and Jagla's (1979) interpretation of locus of control theory, its relationship to the study and the stressful situations questionnaire.

First, locus of control theory is based on the belief the individual has about the control they have or do not have in ensuring reinforcement for their actions (Rotter, 1954, 1966; Lefcourt, 1976). In principle, it is irrelevant whether events in the external environment which are reinforcing are objectively under the individual's control or not. This brings us to the second point. Huckaby and Jagla (1979) seem to assign lack of control over events in the ICU, such as patient care, and interpersonal communication difficulties as being due to 'threatening situations that are controlled externally rather than internally . . .'. In doing so they then infer backwards suggesting this is how events in the ICU are perceived. This is an intriguing possibility and obviously worth further investigation. However, it is noticeable to us that there is some confusion in their understanding of locus of control and its background.

Clearly, it is difficult to say from the study data alone whether or not the ICU nurses regarded the patient care, interpersonal communications, and the ICU categories of stress, as being outside their control.

It is not unreasonable to speculate on these matters, but no measures were taken to establish the locus of control orientation in the ICU nurses of this study.

This study does raise another issue. Even though external events may be largely uncontrollable and perceived as such, and supposing ICU nurses do perceive them in that way, stress need not necessarily be reported. It is conceivable that given these circumstances, the nurse who has no need, or a low need for internal control, would not report any concern over externally-controlled events. Similarly, the nurse who has no need or a low need for external control would not be concerned either. Seen in this way, it is the need for control by the individual nurse rather than the actual control of reinforcement which influences perception of stress (Shipley, 1981). We appreciate that these speculations are more properly criticisms of the assumptions of the locus of control construct, and research which uses locus of control measures. However, we have mentioned them here to highlight the complex nature of locus of control theory, and its possibilities of interpretation within research using locus of control measures and stress (Rotter, 1954, 1966, 1975; Lefcourt, 1976, 1981; Strickland, 1977; Wallston *et al.*, 1978).

A final point we would like to make concerns the significance that work load and amount of physical work had in the study. Huckaby and Jagla (1979) found this received the highest stress score from the ICU nurses. Accordingly, they allocated this to rank 1 in their rank-ordering of components of stressful factors. But what does work load signify? Is it a discrete category of its own? Role load studies by Kahn *et al.* (1964) would tend to support this view. However, Kahn and his co-workers adopted a role-based model of stress–strain in their studies of foremen, and not a locus of control framework like Huckaby and Jagla (1979). Moreover, it may be argued that we might easily expect work load to be the highest ranked source of stress – particularly since it is a catch-all category encompassing all others. For instance, death of a patient, communication problems between staff and death of a patient, communication problems between staff and nursing office, and physicians, meeting the needs of the family, and the other components of stress mentioned by Huckaby and Jagla (1979) are all arguably elements of work load. Thus, whereas work load is a useful general indicator of sources of stress for the ICU nurse, we may argue that rather than being a component of stress, it may be considered to be a summary of all the other components in the questionnaire. Indeed, we would suggest this is the way in which ICU nurses may have responded to the questionnaire. These speculations do not detract from the great concern over work load ICU nurses showed in this and other studies (see e.g. Hay and Oken, 1972; Cassem and Hackett, 1975; Steffen, 1980). Clearly work load is a considerable source of stress for ICU nurses. It is for this reason we urge closer attention should be paid to the elements of work load and how it might be better managed to cut down unnecessary stress. An analysis of demographic variables of age, level of nursing education, and years of experience of general nursing showed they were not significantly related to the stress factor score. However, there was a significantly small inverse correlation ($r = 0.35$, $p < 0.05$) between years of experience on the ICU and the stress factor score. Huckaby and Jagla (1979, p. 25) interpret this finding to mean that 'the nurse who works longer on the ICU has acquired knowledge and proficiency in regard to functioning in the ICU'. They further concluded that 'the new nurse does not have that knowledge or mastery of skills and, therefore her stress level is higher'. These views were claimed to be consistent with Janis' (1958) theory that knowledge of events decreases anxiety.

We say this common-sense view, elegant though it may be, requires further examination. In the first instance, it is clear from the data that the correlation coefficient is quite small. Second, no mention is made about how many ICU nurses constituted this sub-group of the sample. Third, Huckaby and Jagla (1979) apparently attribute the length of ICU nursing experience as having causal significance in the lower stress of these nurses. It is equally plausible to argue that because nurses have a lower stress level they stay longer in ICU nursing. No causal mechanisms were actually identified in this study. This seems to be an error made in the use of correlational studies in general and has recently been cogently criticized by Clarke (1978). Fourthly, no reference is made about the variance in the nurses' estimates of stress. Did some nurses, for example, report substantial stress scores and also have longer periods of service on the ICU unit?

A fifth consideration is that, whereas knowledge may reduce some forms of stress such as anxiety, it may not be applicable to others such as anger or depression. Sixth, even if knowledge reduces reported or perceived stress, experience may not. Knowledge and experience seem to be used inter-changeably by Huckaby and Jagla (1979). We would argue that there is a case for arguing they are not the same thing. Nor indeed should they be treated as such, for a nurse may come to the ICU with knowledge but not experience (Lathlean *et al.*, 1986). Alternatively, it is at least possible for a nurse to gain experience but not knowledge. This seems to be rhetorical – inherent to the sequence of events. If this is the case, then we might argue that important distinctions about knowledge prior to experience on the ICU, and kinds of acquired knowledge linked with experience whilst engaged in ICU nursing need to be made, if we are to understand more fully what Huckaby and Jagla (1979) mean when they claim stress is reduced by knowledge and experience of the ICU. These points can also be made of Anderson and Basteyns' (1981) Milwaukee replication project involving a larger sample (182) of full-time registered nurses in critical care nursing. They investigated 17 different hospitals with ICUs and came to empirical and theoretical conclusions similar to Huckaby and Jagla (1979).

Implications for nurses

Our critical reservations apart, Huckaby and Jagla (1979) have some useful observations and recommendations to make for nurses in the ICU. They suggest introducing orientation programmes and more supervised practice for nurses' in-service education on the ICU. They note more should also be made of seminars and curriculum development to incorporate some of the items on the ranked components of stress scale such as coping with death and dying (see also Birch, 1978; Whitfield, 1979). Nursing administrators' atten-tion should be drawn to the importance of in-service training and tackle the problem of work load. Huckaby and Jagla (1979) persuasively note that increasing manpower on the ICU is not enough, but this should also be supported by more education and experiential learning (see also Borzak, 1981). To begin to deal with problems of interpersonal communication, these authors recommend regular meetings between staff and the appointment of a clinical nurse specialist liaison consultant to facilitate more agreeable communications. Huckaby and Jagla (1979, p. 25) propose this will all lead to reduced stress by decreasing the ICU staff's feelings of loss of control concerning their 'work situation and environment, such as staffing and workload'. Whether this would be the outcome of such changes is debatable. However, we would expect that these changes, if introduced, would be the subject of future research. Indeed this is what the authors suggest. It is an area of research which arguably requires urgent but systematic investigation. Before this though, it would follow from some of the reservations made about locus of control theory, its measurement and its implications for nurses employed in ICU nursing, that important clarifications need to be made by Huckaby and Jagla (1979) to avoid further confusion in this crucial area of stress and coping in nursing.

5.2 1800 ICU NURSES TELL THEIR STORY

A larger-scale sample totalling 1794 ICU nurses was conducted more recently by Steffen (1980). This study confirmed some of Huckaby and Jagla's (1979) views and concurs with the findings of Anderson and Basteyns (1981). The categories of sources of stress were similar. However, Steffen found additional categories, slightly different rankings, and also evaluated satisfactions, emanating from ICU nursing as well as sources of stress.

Like the Huckaby and Jagla (1979) and Anderson and Basteyns (1981) investigations, Steffen (1980) researched the perceived (appraised) stressors of the ICU designated by the nurses in the sample. Steffen (1980) also considered perceived–appraised sources of satisfaction and initial attractors to ICU nursing in the same way. A 'free-response' format was used in the study as opposed to a forced-choice checklist.

The study questionnaire

Steffen (1980, p. 41) reports that the study questionnaire was developed by 'a panel of experts, including intensive care nurses, a psychologist, a nursing educator and a research specialist . . .'. The final questionnaire comprised of two parts. Part 1 asked forced-response questions on demographic data, and initial attractors to ICU nursing. Part 2 involved asking free-response questions of sources of stress and satisfaction in ICU nursing. No further details of the questionnaire are published in Steffen's paper.

Sample

The main sample was based on a regional and national survey. The regional survey was selected from the nine-county San Francisco Bay Area of California. Eighty-nine ICUs from 74 hospitals agreed to participate in the regional study. A 60% return rate of completed questionnaires was reported by Steffen (1980). For the regional survey this meant 1238 ICU nurses completed and returned their questionnaires. We could find no account of the total number of questionnaires sent out. However, we estimate this to be approximately 2063 on the present figures. The American Association of Critical Care Nurses (AACCN) requested to be included in the study to enlarge the scope for a national survey.

Analysis

These data were analysed separately and then combined to give national and regional statistics for attractors, and sources of satisfactions and stress for nurses and ICU nursing. The data were allocated similar to Huckaby and Jagla (1979) and rank-ordered for attractors, satisfactions and sources of stress. The attractors had 10 ranked categories, satisfactions 6 and sources of stress 7 each for the regional, national and combined survey analyses.

Initial attractors of the ICU

The initial attractors were ranked. The combined surveys showed that intellectual challenge (rank 1), opportunities for learning (rank 2), low patient/nurse ratios (rank 3), proficient use of skills (rank 4), variety and excitement (rank 5), were in the upper 50% of ranked attractors to the ICU. Other reasons were (rank 6) learning to handle emergencies (rank 7), being a member of an effective team (rank 8) and recognition and respect (rank 9) were all regarded as being of less importance as attractors to ICU nursing. Interestingly pay differential was the least important attractor to ICU nursing (rank 10). These rankings were not always consistent between the regional and national surveys. For instance, opportunities for learning was the highest attractor for the regional sample and low patient/nurse ratios for the national survey. Whereas intellectual challenge was rank 1 for the combined survey it was rank 2 for the separate regional and national surveys.

Perceived satisfactions and sources of stress

The perceived satisfactions and sources of stress were allocated using the category formulation method. Briefly, this method involves allocating free-responses to appropriate global categories until all of the free-responses have been used (Steffen, 1980). A point not made explicit in the Steffen (1980, p. 41) paper however, is the way in which each survey was ranked. We would infer from her study that the total number of responses was added together for each main category in satisfactions and sources of stress. This was done by a panel of two ICU nurses and a research specialist in order 'to objectify the responses and gain group consensus'. The rankings were therefore relative frequencies of response in any given category converted into percentages and then rank-ordered by the research panel of judges in the Steffen (1980) study.

Sources of satisfactions of the ICU nurses

The nurses in the regional and national surveys gave a wide range of individual responses. There were nine sub-categories of response for direct patient care, five for interpersonal relationships, four for acquisition of knowledge, five for performance and use of skills, four for the ICU environment, and two for reward systems.

The combined surveys showed that most satisfactions for the ICU nurse came from giving direct patient care. This was followed by interpersonal relationships, acquisition of knowledge, performance and use of skills. The ICU atmosphere and reward systems were seen as having less influence on the ICU nurses' sources of satisfaction. The regional and national survey rankings were at variance with the combined survey for several sources of satisfaction. Although these were the same, the rankings were different, the main differences being shown in rank 2 in the national survey as acquisition of knowledge. The regional and combined surveys ranked interpersonal relationships as their second greatest area of satisfaction. The regional and national surveys differed from the combined survey on rank 3. Here the regional survey showed performance and use of skills as the third greatest source of satisfaction. The national survey placed interpersonal relationships in this rank. Rank 4 – performance and use of skills – was consistent for the national and combined surveys but the regional survey allocated acquisition of knowledge to this rank. The other ranks (1, 5 and 6) – nature of direct patient care (1), ICU environment (5), reward systems (6) – were the same for the regional, national and combined survey data.

Perceived sources of stress

The perceived sources of stress by the ICU nurses were ranked in closer agreement than the sources of satisfaction. All of the ranks were in agreement with the exception of the regional survey where management of the unit was ranked highest as a source of stress and interpersonal conflicts second. The remaining survey information showed that interpersonal conflicts in the ICU were of the greatest concern to nurses. This was followed by management of the unit, nature of direct patient care, inadequate knowledge and skills, physical work environment, life events and lack of administrative rewards.

The sources of stress rankings generated an extra category compared with sources of satisfaction. However, it is interesting to note that the main sources of satisfaction were very similar to the sources of stress with only some variation in the ranks assigned to each. Unlike the Huckaby and Jagla (1979) study, Steffen's (1980) data showed that ICU nurses did find the inability to meet patients' and families' psychological needs a source of stress (see also Hay and Oken, 1972; Anderson and Basteyns, 1981). This was incorporated in the patient care category. Huckaby and Jagla's study suggests this source of potential stress was less demanding – placing the psychological needs of the patient at rank 13 in the order of priority. However, they placed the psychological needs of the family at rank 5 out of the 16 ranks cited for components of stress. From our preferred cognitive perspective we would suggest that the psychological needs of the family were of considerably more concern for the ICU nurses in the Huckaby and Jagla (1980) study.

Discussion and concluding remarks

The Steffen (1980) surveys seem to confirm the view that the exacting demands of ICU nursing can be attractive to nurses, and contrary to the popular view the satisfactions of the job, may also count for many as sources of stress in the ICU. The sources of attraction and satisfaction data help us to gain a broader appreciation of how nurses perceive the demands of ICU nursing. In part, Steffen (1980) also confirms the data (but not the theoretical interpretation) of Huckaby and Jagla (1979). We consider this argument to have some force, particularly since their evidence is based on a greater sample of ICU nurses. Moreover, regarding sources of satisfaction and stress, these appear to be associated with the same categories of demands made on ICU nurses. Steffen (1980) does not comment on this observation. But we would suggest Steffen (1980) has reported an important finding in this study. It is suggested that the same source or demands of ICU nursing which are appraised as satisfying can also be sources of stress. In other words we can claim the main sources of stress and satisfaction are largely identical for ICU nurses, but depend largely on how nurses appraise or frame the 'reality' (Berger and Luckman, 1968) of ICU nursing. Further, and by implication, it also highlights the significant mediating role cognitive evaluation has on nurses' perception of the demands of ICU nursing.

We however have a number of reservations about the Steffen (1980) surveys and comparisons with the earlier research of Huckaby and Jagla

(1979). First, the Steffen (1980) study can be said to be two separate surveys, the regional survey being conducted during autumn 1977, and the national survey in the winter of 1978. This is not necessarily to suggest seasonal variations affected perceptions, though this may have been a minor factor. Rather the criticism here is the length of time between data collection for the two surveys. It is possible however this makes the study more convincing – since despite the 15 months or so interval, similar rankings were found in the two surveys. A problem is raised here though. For although the permitted listing of perceived sources of satisfaction were the same for the regional and national surveys, this was not the case for the perceived sources of stress. In the regional survey, ICU nurse respondents were permitted to list as many as three 'stressors' (Steffen, 1980, p. 49). In the national survey, ICU nurse respondents were permitted to list as many as fifteen 'stressors'. It may be argued that being permitted to list more stressors (15 as opposed to 3) in the national survey data makes it a different survey from the regional survey of perceived stressors. It is doubtful if the two surveys are comparable on these grounds. If this is the case, and taking into consideration the gap between the data collection for the two surveys, it is also doubtful if we can simply combine the data from the two surveys and rank them as if they were, (a) from the same population, (b) assessed at similar times, and (c) based on the same response opportunities for ICU nurses completing the questionnaires.

Comparison between the Steffen (1980) and Huckaby and Jagla (1979) investigations is even less plausible than this when we consider that a different method of establishing the scores for ranking into categories was adopted. ICU nurses in the latter study estimated their perceived stress on a Likert scale which was then converted from the raw score into ranked data and categorized into the four main categories:

1. Patient Care
2. Interpersonal communication
3. Environmental
4. Knowledge base

Although similar categories were used by Steffen (1980) and allocated by judges similar to Huckaby and Jagla (1979), Susan Steffen's ranking was derived according to frequencies of responses converted to percentages and then ranked. Comparisons therefore seem questionable on the method of calculating ranks in these studies. However, this does not detract from the substantially important finding that, even though different approaches were used to collate and analyse the data in these studies, we have a greater understanding of the common sources of perceived stress in ICU nursing which was identified. And in the Steffen (1980) surveys, the claim may be extended that common sources of perceived satisfaction and stress were also established, as well as sources of attraction to ICU nursing.

Implications for ICU nurses

Steffen (1980) highlights the fact that ICU nurses in her study liked providing patient care. In doing so she emphasizes making direct patient care more rewarding to the ICU nurse. In connection with interpersonal communication difficulties between nurse–nurse, nurse–physician and nurse–supervisor as sources of stress, Steffen (1980) urges that methods for dealing with these 'people problems' need to be explored and solutions found. This may be through the setting up of consultative counselling or other ICU nurse support systems.

Another concern was the interpersonal conflicts between nurses, physicians and supervisors. Steffen (1980, p. 57) makes the plea by ICU nurses for more rewarding and positive feedback with its potential benefit in alleviating interpersonal conflicts amongst staffs, and goes further and endorses our view that the perception of the ICU nurse 'is crucial to any understanding of nursing stress'. Regarding coping, Steffen (1980) notes that stressful experiences may be turned into more satisfying ones with changes in perception of ICU nursing demands, in other words, by altered appraisals. Again, this is consistent with our own remarks about reframing. She also proposed enlarging the ICU nurses' awareness and extending the range of behaviours which may reduce sources of perceived stress. Steffen (1980, p. 57) makes the very plausible assumption that with such changes, the ICU nurse 'who previously felt powerless, *could* then actively control and influence a given situation'.

These are changes which are, in part, the topic of current research on coping by Steffen and Bailey and their associates based at the School of Nursing, University of California. But will altered perceptions or cognitive appraisal facilitate a sense of greater power and control over potentially stressful situations arising in the ICU? Arguably, the demands of the ICU may become more tolerable and less threatening but not necessarily have any direct influence on the source of threat such as the dying patient. The question of significance and personal control seems a central and complex issue in the study of stress and coping. It is something which we will return to again when we consider coping with stress in nursing and stress theory.

5.3 SUMMARY

Nurses working in the ICU have many diverse demands made on them which are reported as being stressful. Generally speaking, excessive work load has been, and continues to be of great concern to nurses engaged in ICU nursing. However, other elements of the role demands made on ICU nurses are important to consider in any examination of work load in the ICU. We have found that poor interpersonal communication between nurses and nurses, and nurses and doctors can increase role conflict and stress. Also patient care and the knowledge base of nurses in the ICU are further demands which all add to the work load of the ICU nurse. Of particular interest are the data which showed the role demands in the ICU which lead to stress can also be sources of satisfaction to nurses. Moreover, we found that the 'life and death' demands of the ICU may be some of the paradoxical reasons why nurses are attracted to practise ICU nursing in the first instance. However, we also pointed out that some of the conclusions reached by the larger survey studies of ICU nurses cannot always be confidently compared because of limitations in their research methodologies.

It was also argued that the ICU nurse's perception of the control over demands made on her in the ICU environment can influence whether or not she experiences stress. We have concluded this to be a significant and central concern in the study of ICU nursing and stress amongst nurses. However we have found that one particular study assuming a locus of control interpretation of stressful events in the ICU has failed to adopt appropriate measures to validate its theoretical position. Nevertheless, these criticisms do not detract from the clear conclusion that ICU nursing makes very exacting demands on nurses. Not the least of these is the acknowledged difficulty ICU nurses have in dealing with worried or bereaved relatives. And although nurses may be attracted and satisfied by many of the demands of ICU nursing, it inevitably is a continuing source of considerable stress. Working in the ICU perhaps should be made more rewarding for nurses. Yet we cannot avoid the inescapable conclusion that they need to be cared for and supported in their role performance as ICU nurses. Their often misunderstood attempts to cope with the stress of ICU nursing such as singing, joking, and laughing, are all signs of the battle of life against death.

REFERENCES

Anderson, C. A. and Basteyns, M. (1981) Stress and the critical care nurse reaffirmed, *Journal of Nursing Administration*, (1981).

Berger, P. L. and Luckman, T. (1968) *The Social Construction of Reality*. Penguin, London.

Birch, J. (1978) *Anxiety in Nurse Education*. PhD Thesis, University of Newcastle.

Borkovec, T. (1983) Treatment of General Tension States. Seminar. University of Oxford, Department of Psychiatry, Oxford.

Borzak, L. (1981) *Field Study: A Sourcebook for Experiential Learning*. Jossey-Bass, San Francisco, CA.

Cassem, N. and Hackett, T. (1975) Stress on the nurse and therapist in the intensive care unit and the coronary care unit. *Heart and Lung*, **4**, 252–9.

Clarke, A. D. B. (1978) Predicting human development: Problems, evidence, implications. *Bulletin of the The British Psychological Society*, **31**, 249–59.

Gentry, W. E., Forster, S. and Frǫehling, S. (1972) Psychologic responses to and situational stress in intensive and non-intensive nursing. *Heart and Lung*, **1**, 793–6.

Gunther, M. (1977) The threatened staff: A psychoanalytic contribution to medical psychology. *Journal Comprehensive Psychiatry*, **18** (4), 385–97.

Hay, D. and Oken, D. (1972) The psychological stresses of intensive care unit nursing. *Journal Psychosomatic Medicine*, **34**, 109–18.

Huckaby, L. M. D. and Jagla, B. (1979) Nurses' stress factors in the intensive care unit. *Journal of Nursing Administration*, **9**, 21–6.

Jacobson, B. (1978) Stressful situations for neonatal intensive care nurses. *American Journal Maternity Child Nursing*, **3**, 144–50.

Janis, I. (1958) *Psychological Stress*. J. Wiley, New York, N.Y.

Kahn, R., Wolfe, D. M., Quinn, R. P., Snoek, J. D. and Rosenthal, R. A. (1964) *Occupational Stress: Studies in Role Conflict and Ambiguity*. J. Wiley, New York, N.Y.

Kaplan, B. H., Cassel, J. C. and Gore, S. (1977) Social support and health. *Medical Care*, **15**, 47–58.

Lathlean, J., Miss, G. and Radley F. (1986) Post registration development schemes evaluation, in *The NERU Report 4*, Department of Nursing Studies King's College, London.

Lefcourt, H. (1976) *Locus of Control: Current Trends in Theory and Research*. Lawrence Erlbaum Associates, N.J.

Lefcourt, H. (1981) *Research with the Locus of Control Construct – Assessment 6*. Academic Press, New York, N.Y.

Michaels, D. (1971) Too much in need of support to give any? *American Journal of Nursing*, **71** (10), 1932–5.

Mirels, H. (1971) Dimensions of internal versus external control. *Journal of Consulting and Clinical Psychology*, **34**, 226–8.

Rotter, J. (1954) *Social Learning and Clinical Psychology*. Prentice-Hall, Englewood Cliffs, N.J.

Rotter, J. (1966) Generalized expectancies for internal versus external control of reinforcement. *Psychological Monographs*, **80** (609).

Rotter, J. (1975) Some problems and misconceptions related to the construct of internal versus external control of reinforcement. *Journal of Consulting and Clinical Psychology*, **43** (1), 56–7.

Shipley, P. (1981) Personal Communication. Department of Occupational Psychology, Birkbeck College, University of London.

Steffen, S. (1980) Perception of stress: 1800 nurses tell their stories, in *Living with Stress and Promoting Well-Being: A Handbook for Nurses*, (eds K. Claus and J. Bailey), C. V. Mosby, St. Louis, MO.

Strickland, B. (1977) Internal–external control of reinforcement, in *Persona-*

lity Variables in Social Behavior (ed. T. Blass), Lawrence Erlbaum Associates, N.J.

Strickland, B. (1978) Internal–external expectancies and health-related behaviors. *Journal of Consulting and Clinical Psychology*, **46** (6), 1192–212.

Vreeland, R. and Ellis, G. L. (1969) Stresses on the nurse in an intensive care unit. *Journal of American Medical Association*, **208**, 332–4.

Wallston, B., Wallston, K., Kaplan, G. and Maides, S. (1978) Locus of control in health: A review of the literature. *Health Education Monographs*, **6** (2), 107–17.

Watzlawick, P., Weakland, J. H. and Fisch, R. (1974) *Changes: Principles of Problem Formation and Problem Resolution*.

Whitfield, S. (1979) *A Descriptive Study of Student Nurses' Ward Experiences with Dying Patients and Their Attitudes Towards Them*. MSc Thesis, University of Manchester.

CHAPTER SIX

Stress control

Soul and body, as it seems to me, are affected
sympathetically by one another;

Aristotle, De Anima

6.1 STRESS AND THE NEED FOR CONTROL

Nursing tasks and role expectations of nurses are often unpredictable. As
Briggs (1972 para., 253, 80b) noted:

> Both nurses and midwives have to deal with situations and reactions
> which are individual, often unexpected, sometimes sudden and catas-
> trophic, and which require a far from routine response.

The emergency admission from a road traffic accident; the cardiac arrest; or
the sudden realization that a patient is dying (Whitfield, 1979) are all instances
which testify to this fact. These are all situations which call for a great deal of
composure and personal control on behalf of the nurse (Bailey, 1981, 1986a).
Personal control and competent composure can originate from successful
past experience (Mahoney, 1974), competence (Antonovsky, 1979), and
motivation (White, 1959). It is our view that the relationship between these
areas can be enhanced or diminished depending on the kinds of coping
adopted by nurses and patients to control their own stress.

Direct coping

Direct coping or problem-solving coping as it is sometimes called (Folkman
and Lazarus, 1980) can be utilized by the nurse in many nurse–patient
contacts. Giving an injection for instance, may relieve patient pain and at the
same time reduce nurse anxiety. Such a direct action might also help to calm
the patient because the nurse acted on the patient's complaints about pain. So
direct coping in this case would lead to reduction of reported physical pain in
the patient and feelings associated with such discomfort. Put another way, the
nurse would have employed her professional competence directly to cope
with the patient's distress. Where the nurse can employ nursing skills in this
way, she keeps the situation literally under control, and her own reactions to
the nursing demands made on her at any particular time. Other forms of

direct coping may be adopted by the nurse such as giving instructions to the patient on exercise, diet, and helping to turn patients who have, or are susceptible to bedsores. Yet as Briggs (1972) implies many of the demands made on nurses require the nurse to be sufficiently composed to carry out the professional skills learned in the school or training ward, but rarely practised.

Moreover, we would point out that direct coping may not be possible with many patients. That is to say, many patients may not respond to medical treatment or general nursing care (see for example Stone *et al.*, 1980). It is not reasonable or practically possible for nurses to cope directly with all of the demands and outcomes connected with patient care. We would argue this is the case despite adequate nursing skills and knowledge. Personal control by the nurse may be seriously impaired where the nurse appraises the patient's health problem as one which she is directly responsible for but cannot influence in the direction of recovery or rehabilitation (Bailey, 1985). Whitfield's (1979) research clearly shows how the nurse's inability to deal with her own feelings when caring for the dying may be so stressful that it interferes with nursing practice and performance. In these instances, direct coping may be rendered impossible because of the degree of threat it poses to nurses caring for terminally ill patients. Such threat may be sufficient to induce stress-related problems in nurses such as anxiety, depression, panic, tension headaches, hypertension and diarrhoea (Colligan *et al.*, 1977; Phillipson, 1978; Marshall, 1980; Parkes, 1980a, b; Ansell, 1981).

The use of palliative coping

In the many instances where direct coping is not possible, the nurse may look for other ways of reducing the amount of impact experienced due to any particular threat. This view, we feel holds for both qualified and unqualified nursing staff. The field studies we reviewed showed pupil, student, charge nurses, sisters, and Directors of Nursing all reporting considerable stress problems associated with their experience of nursing (see for example Arndt and Laeger, 1970a, b; Sobol, 1978; Redfern, 1978; Birch, 1979; Parkes, 1980a, b). Nurses who have insufficient coping resources to directly influence the kinds of threats raised for them by the demands of nursing may adopt palliative coping to deal with their problems. Palliative coping by definition is at best a temporary and limited method of coping with experienced stress. In other words, it is a 'stop-gap' measure to deal with upsetting emotions. Palliative coping doesn't actually help the nurse bring into play her professional skills and deployment of competence. Our understanding of palliative coping suggests it may even provide a maladaptive form of coping which interferes with the quality of nursing care and have damaging consequences for the nurse's own health and career. We would cite the studies on nurse smoking, alcohol consumption, late arrival for work and sickness absence as instances of palliative coping (Hillier, 1973; Cormack, 1973, 1981; Redfern, 1978, Clarke and Hussey, 1979; Hillier, 1981; Jacobson, 1981.)

The high attrition rate in nursing may also be connected with an over-reliance by nurses on palliative forms of coping. In the short-time, these are only likely to bring temporary relief and the illusion of controlling stress. The possible long-term effects may add to the increasing numbers of nurses leaving the profession from the 'burn-out' syndrome (Cherniss, 1980; Edelwich and Brodsky, 1980; Ansell, 1981; Bailey, 1986a, 1987a). Although definitions of burn-out vary, Cherniss (1980, p. 16) points out that the features are the same; burn-out is apparent when the caring professions begin 'To fail, wear out, or become exhausted by making excessive demands on their energy, strength or resources'. We would suggest that ineffectual coping increases the vulnerability of the nurse to burn-out. Obviously this may not be the sole reason for nurses leaving nursing. However, it is not unreasonable to suppose that many nurses do leave the profession because of an impoverished range of coping strategies for controlling their own levels of experienced stress. Put in personal control terms, nurses who leave nursing reluctantly, have not been shown, nor acquired, sufficient coping skills to reduce to individually manageable proportions the degree of threatening demands imposed by their work.

Controlling stress by indirect coping

One way of achieving more personal control, composure, and reduced stress in nursing, is for nurses to influence their own emotional and physical reactions to the many situations in nursing they anticipate or experience as threatening. To do this means taking an indirect approach to coping (see Lazarus, 1966, 1976, 1981; Lazarus and Launier, 1978). Psychologically speaking, indirect coping often entails the practice of physical or intrapsychic procedures to reduce threats that interfere with emotions, well-being and physical comfort. Working on herself, the nurse can reduce the degree the threat posed by external or indeed internal circumstances may have on her psychological health and performance. A number of stress control strategies are required which will assist the nurse, and which she may invoke:

1. When preparing for an anticipated highly threatening work period
2. When unexpected threatening events occur
3. To increase her personal control over such events so that stress may be avoided in the future

What then, can nurses do themselves to increase personal control over stress by indirect coping?

Stress-control techniques

A number of specific techniques have been developed by psychologists to increase indirect coping and enhance personal control over stress. Their main principle is the development of control over the involuntary sympathetic nervous system through the influence of the central nervous system and extending to the somatic functioning of the body (Schwartz, 1978). These techniques come under the broad title of mental training. Much mental training involves the practitioners talking to themselves internally and allowing these thoughts to act on the body and the mind (Luthe, 1965; Schultz and Luthe, 1969; Rosa, 1976). Other approaches have been concerned with allowing thoughts that are held about threatening situations to be corrected or altered. The outcomes of mental training when applied systematically have shown that behaviour and emotions can be changed (Meichenbaum, 1979; Zastrow, 1979). People can learn to let their body and mind relax together in a natural way. We believe that this is connected with the rest principle inherent in each human organism (Sinclair, 1981). Mental training and its related methods help to bring it about.

Walter Hess was probably the first person to experimentally demonstrate an organism's natural response to relaxation. This was done with infrahuman species. Hess (1957) used cats as experimental subjects. Stimulating the hypothalamus, Hess found it could produce what he termed 'trophotropic activity – a 'restful and restorative response'. Thus, the hypothalamus regarded as an important mechanism governing stress and the fight–flight response was also capable of producing processes leading to restorative equilibrium in the organism. The implications for health care, nurses and patients could be clinically important if similar activity could be produced in humans. Could it be that the hypothalamus – the stress alarm centre – would also produce restorative activity in people? In other words, could the stress alarm centre also have the function of being a healing centre as well? Later research and clinical work by Luthe (1965), Schultz and Luthe (1969), Lindemann (1974) and Rosa (1976), seems to uphold the view that this naturally restorative response is present in the human species. It can be invoked by the practice of mental training methods. Practitioners of mental training report varying degrees of relaxation and an increase in their general well-being as a result of regular training. The psychological name now given to these comfortable states and the feelings they engender in students of mental training is The Relaxation Response (Benson, 1980).

There are many ways of achieving the relaxation response which may give the nurse and patient more personal control over stress in nursing and aid recovery. Five methods in popular use are:

1. Progressive Relaxation (PR)
2. Relaxation with Desensitization (RD)

3. Cultivating Assertiveness
4. Autogenic Regulation Training (ART)
5. Stress-Inoculation Training (SIT)

1. *Progressive Relaxation (PR)*

Practising Progressive Relaxation (PR) techniques involves tensing and relaxing different sets of muscles in the body (Jacobson, 1934, 1938). It is carried out systematically – hence progressive relaxation (Bailey, 1986b). Attention is also brought to the practice of breathing awareness. Relaxation training proceeds through each successive step until the practitioner begins to report feelings of relaxation, comfort, calm, rest, peacefulness and other indicators that the relaxation response is present (Benson, 1980).

Physiological signs of rest accompanying the relaxation response are often reflected in lower respiration rate, galvanic skin response (GSR), heart rate and blood pressure (Benson *et al.*, 1974; Bloomfield *et al.*, 1976).

During PR practice, any reported discomfort is a signal which should generally be taken to terminate the relaxation session. Where this happens, it is often useful to return to a previous part of the procedure which was pleasant, and terminate relaxation training for the day at that point. It has been found to be clinically helpful too, for the practitioner to end each session in a comfortable state rather than attempting to 'race ahead' and cover all of the training exercises within a fixed time period. Our common sense backed up by research on psychological individual differences of humans tells us that each person may relax at their own particular rate. In our view, this suggests that just as we learn to achieve various goals in our lives, we can learn to relax. And although nurses and patients may learn to relax at their own tempo, the basic technique for PR and the conditions for carrying out progressive relaxation procedures should be the same for all practitioners of this method of stress control.

THE METHOD

General requirements
PR training should be conducted at least twice per day – once in the morning, and at night immediately on retiring to bed. Afternoon sessions can be substituted for the morning session or added on to make three sessions of PR per day. However, not all stress problems requiring relaxation need sessions three times each day. Another point here is although the patient might have time for several sessions each day, the nurse may not (Bailey, 1985, 1986a). No food should be consumed immediately prior to stress control practice periods.

Setting conditions

- Find a quiet spot where you are unlikely to be disturbed.
- Then decide upon a comfortable position to sit or lay down (a bed, couch, favourite chair, or any other position where your body is supported and not strained). Use cushions or blankets for support of muscles. Don't exert weight on muscles.
- Make sure the place in which you are to practise is not too hot or cold.
- Now loosen any restrictive clothing such as belts, bras, collars, headgear and shoes.
- Do a final check on your body. Make sure ankles, calves, thighs, pelvic region, back, hands, lower arms, upper arms, shoulders, neck and head are all supported by cushion, pillow or floor.
- Practise for a minimum of 10 minutes and a maximum of 20 minutes for each training period. Set this period as essential, and keep a clock at hand. Glance at it when you feel the practice period is over. Do not set an alarm as this will interfere with the development and effectiveness of progressive relaxation. Now practise the following relaxation–stress control procedure.

Progressive relaxation procedure

Step 1.   With each movement slowly count to five, hold the muscle stretch for about 5–10 seconds. Observe a steady and rhythmic inhalation and exhalation.

Step 2.   Direct your attention to both your feet, now bend your toes down away from your body. Feel the tension until it is 'tight' then slowly return the toes to their former position. As they travel to a natural stopping point, pause and feel the sensations of rest in your toes.

Step 3.   Carry out the same procedure for the feet, but this time stretch the feet upwards and toward the body. Again, slowly stretch to a count of five, hold for 5–10 seconds and gradually rest to stopping point. Feel the sensations and accept them.

Step 4.   Continue the procedure now at the level of the calf muscles. Carry out forward stretch – relax, and appreciate sensations of rest and relaxation.

Step 5.   Stretch – relax using the same procedure with the backward movement. Remember to bend to the point where the tension is tight. Hold and gradually let go. Relax and enjoy the sensations you are now feeling.

Step 6.   Now stiffen and tighten your thigh muscles. Relax them in the same way, gradually sensing the growing warmth and spreading relaxation in your body.

Step 7.   Move to your buttocks. Tense them until tight – then gradually relax them. Accept and appreciate the release of tension.

Step 8.   Now tense both of your fists and arms so tight they vibrate. Slowly release the tension, becoming aware of any warmth, heaviness, and general feeling of well-being.

Step 9.   Let your attention move to your neck and back muscles. Draw them in until they are bearably 'hard'. Then after a few seconds let go, allow this muscle group to find their own position of rest. Now relax and enjoy the release of tension in this area of your body.

Step 10. Next screw up all the muscles of the face; around the mouth, eyes, nose and forehead. Hold this position for 3–5 seconds and then allow all of your face muscles to return to their natural resting position. Feel the relaxation and any 'glow' from the aftermath of this exercise.

Step 11. Now link up all of the exercises you have done by tensing all of the groups of muscles together. Hold the tension then gradually release – allow the complete feeling of relaxation to permeate the whole of your body.

Step 12. Finally, imagine a pulsing ball of energy gradually and systematically travelling throughout all of the areas of your body you have relaxed. Feel how this energy ball – your life force – brings

Check that each part of your body is supported		
	Supported	
	Yes	No
Tick appropriate box:		
Head	☐	☐
Neck	☐	☐
Shoulders	☐	☐
Lower and upper arms	☐	☐
Hands	☐	☐
Back	☐	☐
Pelvic region	☐	☐
Thighs	☐	☐
Calves	☐	☐
Ankles and feet	☐	☐

Figure 6.1 Posture-relaxation checklist.

with it a sense of oneness and lightness in a state of comfortable calmness. Stay with this feeling of complete ease, and allow it to link up with all of your body so that you are now bathed in total relaxation. Your relaxation training session is now completed. Each session should be followed by a cancellation procedure.

Cancellation
Cancellation of progressive relaxation should be done by opening the eyes and making slow but deliberate movements of the body. No attempt should be made to tense and relax the muscles again. When the muscle tone has returned to your limbs, neck and face, you can stand up. After standing, take one or two deep breaths, then let your breathing carry on as it usually does. When the cancellation has been carried out, you can take up any task which requires your attention. Cancellation must be carried out in order to return to ready-alertness. Failure to cancel the relaxed state is not intrinsically a problem, but it may leave you feeling lethargic. If this happens, provided you do not have to carry out any tasks which demand close, clear attention, lack of cancellation presents no difficulty. But where you are likely to be preparing for a work period, it is unwise not to cancel the effects of the relaxation procedure. The only time cancellation can be usefully omitted is when practising progressive relaxation in bed shortly before going to sleep. Cancellation can be carried out naturally when you awaken next morning. This is easily done by opening your eyes, stretching and taking a few deep breaths. It is quite natural and largely mirrors what we do after a prolonged period of sleep whether or not we are practising stress control through relaxation training.

Relaxation with systematic desensitization
A system of combining progressive relaxation with systematic desensitization (see below) was developed by the American psychologist, Joseph Wolpe (1958, 1976). This system of stress control is helpful for dealing with specific stress reactions such as anxiety and phobias. Lazarus (1971) has shown the assumptions underlying this approach to stress control are both physiological and cognitive. People with specific stress reactions are sensitized to various situations or stimuli (Wolpe, 1958; Wolpe and Lazarus, 1966; Lazarus, 1976). The sensitization results in an increase in physiological arousal activity in the nervous system which is often coupled with a release of increased adrenaline, a stress hormone associated with different states of anxiety and reported fear (Wittkower and Warnes, 1977). Sensitization is also influenced by the way a person appraises situations or stimuli (Lazarus, 1966, 1976, 1981; Lazarus and Launier, 1978). For instance, a situation such as being asked to prepare a patient for surgery may increase physiological activity in the autonomic arousal system of the nurse. Thus the appraisal of

preparing someone for surgery for the first time is a stress-inducing threat which takes the form of increased adrenaline flow, and reported anxiety.

So physiological activity is triggered by the way a person views demands from the environment. For other nurses it could have been that preparing a patient for surgery induced a feeling of relief, thinking, perhaps, the patient would now receive corrective treatment. Therefore, thinking, or more properly cognition (Neisser, 1972) (which includes memory and associations as well as thinking) influences the presence or absence of experienced stress and different levels of physiological activity. The way the nurse 'sees' situations, what the nurse thinks about her work demands therefore, is important in two respects. First, changing the way a nurse thinks about the demands made upon her will change the threat potency of the nursing demands from her environment. Second, where stress-inducing threat is overcome, this should be seen in a transfer from the nurse having little personal control to a reported increase in personal control over previously stress-inducing threats. The nurse will be able to remain calm and composed in the face of situations or stimuli which she previously appraised as harmful, and consequently experienced anxiety, depression or fear. The same may be said for patients.

2. Relaxation with desensitization (RD)

CASE 1: A TYPICAL PROCEDURE

This approach to stress control is quite specific. The nurse or patient should have, as their goal, a state of relaxation and rational composure in the face of a previously disturbing or upsetting situation. Therefore, the first task for the nurse would be to identify and define precisely what it is that induces the threat and stress reaction. After this, the nurse should systematically practise progressive relaxation. This could be done using the typical procedure shown in the previous section, or some other procedure which permits the nurse to achieve a comfortable and relaxed state throughout the mind and body (Bailey, 1985, 1986a, 1986b). When the relaxation response can be achieved quite regularly and without great difficulty, the nurse or patient can then begin to desensitize themselves to the identified threatening situation.

Desensitization may be carried out in the imagination or in the presence of the threatening situation (Wolpe, 1958, 1976; Bakal, 1979), i.e. the conditions where and when the threat actually occurs. Many studies of systematic desensitization suggest that stress control can be effective in facing real situations by using imaginative desensitization (Lazarus, 1976). However, both procedures are often therapeutic. Selection of one or the other should depend on the nature of the threat, and the imaginative ability of the person to be desensitized. Before actually starting the desensitization sessions, the person wishing to exercise more control over stress should draw up a hierarchy of threatening situations, and their threat potency. This is a central component of systematic desensitization and should be constructed very carefully. If a nurse requires desensitization to any threat, e.g. panic attacks when asked to carry out Last Offices, a trained nurse counsellor or clinical psychologist should help her to draw up the panic hierarchy. Finally, the nurse should reach agreement with the nurse counsellor or clinical psychologist about what signs to use if psychological discomfort is experienced during the stress-control period. If nurses carry out desensitization programmes on themselves, care should be taken to ensure adequate systematic relaxation training has been established prior to attempts at desensitization (Bailey, 1986b). This is a general principle of stress control by desensitization. A desensitization protocol for use with a nurse's fear of blood, and satisfactory stress control over this threat illustrates the procedure.

Specific source of threat: The sight or thought of blood. Nurse's appraisal of this situation (anticipation – at the thought of it or when it occurs): *Oh no! Not again, I feel tense and queasy. I think I am going to faint.*

Preparation
The nurse was prepared for desensitization by attending a counselling clinic (Bailey, 1981). The clinic ran classes to show nurses how to practise progressive relaxation. The blood-phobic nurse practised progressive relaxation for four weeks until the relaxation response was established. During this time she was asked by the clinical psychologist to prepare a blood phobia hierarchy. Six situations of increasing threat were identified and marked for the degree of fear experienced. The blood phobia hierarchy could then be drawn up in the following way:

Blood Phobia Hierarchy

Threatening situations

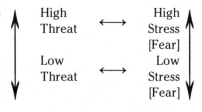

1. Blood seen on emergency admissions   High   High
2. Blood seen during theatre operations   Threat   ⟷   Stress
3. Blood seen on patients' dressings   [Fear]
4. Blood seen coming from a drip   Low   Low
5. Looking at bottles of blood   Threat   ⟷   Stress
6. The thought of blood   [Fear]

This threat–fear profile shows where the nurse's coping and personal control over 'blood' threat is manageable and breaks down: low threat induces little fear. In this case she can manage the threat of blood but with some discomfort. As the threats move up the threat hierarchy from the 'thought of blood' to 'blood seen on emergency admissions', there is an increase in experienced fear. At the high-fear point, this nurse found she panicked because of the unmanageable level of experienced fear. The blood-fear hierarchy must be completed before proceeding with combined relaxation–desensitization as a means of establishing and increasing stress control. Doing this provides a baseline measurement of the nurse's stress reaction to threat. Baseline measurements should be taken to assess the effects of any stress control interventions. We will say more about baseline measures later in this chapter (p. 155).

Practising stress control by combined relaxation and systematic desensitization

When the baseline measurement of the phobia hierarchy was complete and relaxation established, the nurse had adequately prepared for practising relaxation with systematic desensitization. Stress-control practice continued by combining the state of relaxation produced in progressive relaxation with gradual exposure to the threats listed by the nurse in the blood phobia hierarchy. The nurse was asked to prepare herself to deal with the threats connected with actual experience and thoughts of blood. The background to the reported fears was explained to her in the following way.

> We all have fears. Some are essential for our everyday survival such as fear of going without food, water or shelter for an unusually long period of time. But there are fears which are not helpful to our survival, such as fear of breathing, and of open or closed spaces. These fears may be so great that they interfere with our work and personal life. Most fears are learned. A person learns to fear things because they are seen as threatening. But just as we learn to fear things we find threatening, we can also learn to relax and be calm in the face of threats. When this is done, situations lose their threatening significance or 'threat potency'. Your fears can be changed in the same way. We are going to use a procedure called 'combined relaxation–systematic desensitization' to reduce the fear you experience from the threatening situations you have described.

The procedure was:

Step 1. The nurse practises progressive relaxation and establishes the relaxation response. This is indicated by physiological and psycho-logical measures showing a change of state. The practitioner may say, 'I'm relaxed, calm, at peace, I feel good' etc. Alternatively, they may be asked to press a button lighting a green light for 'relaxed state achieved'. A press button which produces a red light can be used when the practitioner wishes to 'stop the procedure'.

Step 2. Once the relaxed state is achieved, the least threatening situation on the hierarchy is presented (in this case, 'thought of blood'). The nurse is asked to think about the colour of blood, how blood is composed and its functions. Finally, in this instance, the nurse was told to imagine as clearly as possible how blood was central to the many tasks she carried out at work. In a matter of fact way, she was asked to imagine continuing her work despite any thoughts connected with blood. This part of the hierarchy was carried out for one week with the nurse indicating complete relaxation midway through the third session. This was the signal to continue up the hierarchy.

Step 3. Sessions continued for a period of eight weeks, five days per week, using the same approach. Relaxation was established, then she practised the ideas of seeing the items from the threat hierarchy and feeling calm.

Step 4. All of the threats on the hierarchy were submitted to this procedure. When the nurse continued to feel relaxed, and no longer saw the blood hierarchy as threatening, stress control training was terminated.

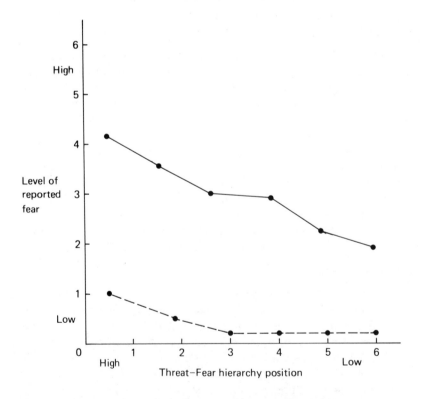

Figure 6.2 Effects of relaxation–desensitization for blood phobia.
Key: • —— •, baseline levels of reported fear; • ----- •, level of reported fear after practising stress control with systematic desensitization procedures.

The results were then recorded. Comparing them with the baseline measure, it can be seen how effective this stress control procedure has been with the nurse (Fig. 6.2). It can be seen only one threat remained which induced fear. This was the threat of seeing blood in emergency admissions. But now the intensity of the threat has come to the bottom of the threat hierarchy and it only induces a very low level of fear. Further practice sessions actually carried out during emergency admissions might ultimately remove this final threat.

CASE 2

A similar approach to removing an excessive fear of blood in a nurse has been reported in a case study by Max Rardin. This case characterized the problem experienced by the nurse as one of haemophobia, an incapacitating fear of blood. It was treated by a variation of the desensitization technique developed by Joseph Wolpe. A fear hierarchy and progressive relaxation was therefore the method of treatment.

The young woman in this case was an 18 year-old student nurse, in the first year of a nursing education programme. Rardin (1969, p. 125) reports the following history of events.

> The client indicated that she had been fearful of blood and generally squeamish for several years but her fears had not been a serious concern until she entered nursing – a career goal for her since childhood.

This case showed quite clearly the prominent threatening significance blood had for the student nurse. The particularly pressing concern for her proficiency as a nurse, and caring for patients, was her reaction to the threat of blood. It is evident in this case, that it impaired her personal control over a range of imagined and actual situations associated with blood, inducing a number of stressful reactions (Rardin, 1969, p. 125).

> Her reaction to blood and possible physical injury varied from moderate discomfort to dizziness and nausea depending on the topic and circumstances. The immediate concern was her reaction to the film shown in nursing classes which vividly depicted various medical conditions. On a number of occasions, she had to put her head down or leave the room. She felt she would faint or vomit if she continued to observe the film.

These reactions interfered so much with her watching films that the nursing faculty began to question her suitability for the profession.

At this point, the student nurse, with the encouragement of her nursing tutors, contacted a clinical psychologist about the possibility of controlling her fear of blood. Like the previous case study, a preparation and a practice period for stress control was adopted as the therapeutic strategy.

Preparation and practice

Step 1. The student nurse was given a detailed description of relaxation – desensitization and how it would be applied to her situation.
Step 2. Three sessions were then allocated to the practice of relaxation training.
Step 3. A fear hierarchy was constructed.

The fear hierarchy consisted of 16 items, involving increasing amounts of blood appearing due to injury, surgery and childbirth. Relaxation and vivid imagery established, she began to become desensitized to the fear hierarchy items. By the end of the nursing school term, 7 of 16 fear items indicated below had been successfully desensitized. These 7 items are asterisked.

- Bleeding from nose and mouth due to internal injury
- A sucking chest wound
- Seeing a blood sample drawn
- Blood foaming from mouth
- Waters breaking for childbirth
- Head emerging and effect on mother
- Blood flowing after birth
- Delivery of placenta
- Stitching after delivery
- Scraped elbow*
- A torn hangnail*
- Squeezing out one drop of blood*
- A cut in the sole of the foot*
- A compound fracture of the leg*
- Needle in the skin for a stitch*
- Gash in the arm with flowing blood*

The remaining threats in the fear hierarchy were desensitized by the nurse practising desensitization at home. Using a monologue prepared by the psychologist, she practised relaxation–desensitization five or six nights per week for a period of six weeks. This was found to be effective at home and generalized to actual events occurring at work (Rardin, 1969, p. 126).

At the end of 6 weeks she contacted the author and reported being able to imagine comfortably all of the items on the list and having visited the hospital maternity ward. She was late for the delivery but did see the cord being cut and the delivery of the placenta. At that point she felt mildly faint and left. She then requested that she be allowed to use smelling salts at her next birth observation since her dizziness was not accompanied by nausea. Because she attributed this faintness more to excitement than anxiety, she was given permission to use smelling salts with the condition that she should not force herself to observe if she felt highly anxious. She observed her next delivery successfully. The last session occurred after her return to (nursing) school and was primarily a review of events to complete the case history.

During this closing session (Rardin, 1969):

the student nurse reported having observed a complete delivery, successfully taken blood samples, and having her own blood sample taken. One year later she was a student nurse on an obstetric ward assisting in deliveries to the dabbing blood between vaginal stitches.

SUMMARY AND PROCEDURE FOR PRACTISING
RELAXATION–DESENSITIZATION

These two case studies serve to illustrate how a common incapacitating fear in nursing – haemophobia – can be brought under effective control. They also make the important point that baseline measures should be made before stress-control practices are initiated. More generally, it can be seen from the second study how the nurse may be educated to practise stress-control procedures on herself and reduce dependency on relaxation–desensitization sessions held in stress-control clinics. Promoting the management of stress by combined relaxation–desensitization, largely helps the practitioner to gain personal control over threatening situations by counter-conditioning (Wolpe and Lazarus, 1966). Whereas previously threats in the blood phobia hierarchy had conditioned the nurse to be sensitized or acutely anxious, pairing relaxation with each step in the hierarchy reconditioned the nurse to relax. This process has been called reciprocal inhibition (Wolpe, 1958). The relaxation response inhibits the physiological and psychological responses associated with fear, anxiety and other stress reactions. In this way the practitioner overcomes stress and gains control over significant demands in their internal or external environment.

PROCEDURE FOR PRACTISING RELAXATION WITH DESENSITIZATION

Step 1. Practise progressive relaxation. Establish the production of the relaxation response.

Step 2. Draw up a threat hierarchy and measure the stress response associated with each threat. Record these in written and graphic form.

Step 3. Begin systematic desensitization by relaxing and comparing first step on the threat hierarchy with relaxation state. Only progress up the threat hierarchy at the practitioner's pace. Where the practitioner indicates some discomfort or loss of relaxation at any item on the threat hierarchy, return to a lower level of threat where relaxation can be re-established. Always end stress-control sessions with the practitioner reporting a calm and composed state.

Step 4. Carry on practising the procedure until all the items on the threat hierarchy can be managed by the practitioner, and relax in their presence.

Step 5. Record any changes in threat–stress reactions during the stress control sessions.

Step 6. Terminate stress-control sessions when the stress reactions originally reported and measured (e.g. anxiety, fear, heart rate) have reached a comfortable level for the practitioner.

Step 7. Compare any changes in threat and reported stress reactions with the baseline measures taken prior to stress-control training.

Combining relaxation with systematic desensitization should permit the nurse or patient to practise stress control for a variety of specific problems. This form of stress control is best used where the threats to the nurse or patient are specific, identifiable, and for stress reactions such as panic–fear, anxiety and anger. Where a general and diffuse lack of well-being is evident across a wide range of nursing demands, a broader stress control practice such as meditation would seem more appropriate.

Cultivating assertiveness

Some of the situations nurses find themselves in will require an assertive response. Admittedly many situations are unpredictable (Briggs, 1972). Here nurses will need to keep their emotions in check and rely on practising relaxation, meditation, and systematic desensitization – especially in the presence of trying and gruesome events. But nurses also have to make plans and take courses of action to combat stress. In other words nurses are people who get things done. Stress-inoculation training should be of observable benefit in such circumstances. However, and more specifically, nurses have to meet, challenge and influence significant situations in their working environment. This calls for cultivating assertiveness: when a nurse needs to make it clear to a patient what is required; when a nurse thinks it is important for a superior to know her position and how she feels about it; when a nurse needs to refuse to do something that is against her beliefs, principles or outside the law, then it is important to avoid or manage stress assertively.

WHAT IS ASSERTIVENESS?

First of all being assertive is not being aggressive. Nor is it being passive. Perhaps nurses have been passive for too long and this position of apparent helplessness has caused them considerable stress, especially what Oswin has termed professional depression (Oswin, 1978). Being passive is saying 'kick-me, I don't count'. The 'you're OK – I'm not OK' position. Conversely, by being aggressive, we are saying 'I kick you – you don't count' (Bailey, 1988). The 'I'm OK, you're not OK' position. However by being assertive we express ourselves in a way that says, ' I count and you count too'. The parity position – I'm OK and you're OK too', (Harris, 1969). Managing stress through assertiveness means being able to influence significant events that are important to us but not railroading them through at the expense of someone else. Assertiveness is not about putdowns or being put down. It is a method of communicating that is characterized by being honest, direct and fair. Practising assertive skills in their communications has already proved to be of considerable benefit to nurses (Clark, 1978). It is a potent method that gets results, reduces anxiety and self-doubt and promotes influence and confidence in its practitioners.

PREPARING TO BE ASSERTIVE

The first thing we need to do in preparing for asssertiveness is to have the courage to carry it out. The American author Cora Harris put it this way:

> The bravest thing you can do when you are not brave is to profess courage and act accordingly. Why is it important to profess courage? The simplest answer is that by doing so we provide a basis for action. Assertiveness is about action. We suggest you go further than this and practice bolstering up your courage. Try this exercise; it has worked for many people who claimed they never had the courage to be assertive.

Six tactics to encourage assertiveness

Tactic 1. Describe the natural abilities and skills you have.
Begin each statement by saying . . . I am naturally gifted at/able to . . . and I am especially skilled at . . .
I am ....
....
....
....
....

Tactic 2. Specify the things that you do better than others.
Begin each statement by saying . . . I can do . . . better than others because . . .
I can ....
....
....
....
....

Tactic 3. Identify particular ways in which you have grown personally
              in the last six/twelve months.
Begin each statement by saying . . . I have made progress in these areas of my
life in the past six/twelve months. For example I have . . .
I have ....
....
....
For example I have ....
....
....
....

Tactic 4. State without compromise the most difficult things you have
              achieved in the past six/twelve months.
Begin each statement by saying . . . This last six months/year I have
achieved . . .
This last six months/year *I have achieved* ....
....
....
....
....

Tactic 5. Describe your most recent proudest moment.
Begin each statement by saying . . . My proudest moment was when
I . . .
My proudest moment was when I ....
....
....
....
....

Tactic 6. Specifically describe those aspects of yourself about which
              you would like to receive compliments.
Begin each statement by saying . . . I would like to be complimented on
my . . .
I would like to be complimented on my. ....
....
....
....
....

PUTTING COURAGE INTO PRACTICE

Nurses cannot be faulted on their courageousness. But they may be on
occasions prone to modesty. For assertiveness to be effective it is important

not to hide your light under a bushel. Take these six tactics and practise them with your colleagues, patients, and superiors. It is often helpful to develop this stage of assertiveness in an assertiveness-at-work group. It forms the basis for increasing self-confidence and managing stress more assertively (Bailey, 1988).

NON-VERBAL AND VERBAL BEHAVIOURS – THE KEYS TO ASSERTIVENESS

Non-verbal communications

Courage is a necessary but not a sufficient condition to manage stress more assertively. It is also important to practice and establish the range of identifiable non-verbal and verbal behaviours which makes for assertiveness instead of passive or aggressive behaviour (Table 6.1). First, check out where you fall on the range of non-verbal behaviours. Are you more aggressive or passive than you thought? If so, identify those assertive non-verbal behaviours and introduce them to your communications with those people with whom you have decided to be more assertive. Notice particularly your facial expression, the tone of voice, pitch, volume, timing, eye contact, posture and gestures you adopt. Keep rehearsing the non-verbal assertive behaviours until they become 'second nature' to you.

Table 6.1 Non-verbal behaviours associated with being aggressive, passive and assertive

	Aggressive	Passive	Assertive
Facial expression	Teeth clenched, frown, eyes staring, curled lip	Head hung down, eyes look up to others, lips quiver	Mouth relaxed firm, head level, eyes steady
Tone of voice	Loud, sharp threatening	Quiet, strained, child-like	Low-pitched, steady, modulated
Timing	Interrupts 'bulldozes'	Hesitates, quiet, waffles, long gaps	Puts own view concisely
Eye contact	Hard gaze, glaring	Avoids looking into others eyes	Direct gaze but not staring
Posture	Stoic stance, hands on hips, feet/legs stiff	Round-shouldered, slumped, chest down, head down	Upright balanced, facing squarely, suitable distance
Gesture	Poking/pointing, stabbing finger, banging fist, jaw-grinding, 'hand-cruncher', 'back-slapper'	Fidgety (hands/arms/legs), fiddling movements, e.g. crossing/uncrossing legs	Open flow of co-ordinated movements, relaxed, 'composed gesticulation'

Assertive verbal communications

It is essential to combine appropriate assertive verbal behaviours with assertive non-verbal behaviours when we are communicating. Why? Because, if not we run the risk of (1) confusing the receiver of the communication and (2) reducing the impact of our own communication. For instance, there we will have little influence on a situation if our non-verbal behaviour is passive but our verbal behaviour is clear, direct and assertive. Similarly, if we are indirect, unclear and 'woolly' in our verbal expression and assertive in our non-verbal behaviour we will still be ineffective. Nurses should aim to match assertive non-verbal behaviours with assertive verbal behaviours. Then we not only can become more confident, but also more competent, and influential in our communications with others (Bailey, 1988; Clark, 1978)

Two methods of assertive verbal communication that have produced good results are the (a) 'I, . . . THEN' method and (b) 'DESCRIBE EXPRESS, SPECIFY, CONSEQUENCES (DESC)' approach to developing effective assertiveness.

(a) 'I . . . THEN'

With 'I . . . then' we say clearly directly and honestly what we think and feel and then what we will do about any particular situation. For example, when a nurse is asked to treat a patient who is not in a critical condition or in some emergency she could say, 'I will first finish dressing Mr Noble, then I will attend to Mr Hawkins'. The 'I . . . then' method of being assertive involves first of all stating what you think/feel and following it by saying what you will do.

Now identify those situations where you want to use the 'I . . . then' method of asserting yourself. Remember to combine the 'I . . . then' verbal expression with appropriate assertive non-verbal behaviour and firmness and eveness of tone in your voice.

I . . . Then

I will use the 'I . . . then' method of asserting myself verbally when/if the following situations arise:

Situation 1
Brief Description ....
....
....
....
....

Use of 'I . . . Then' ....
....
....
....
....

Situation 2
Brief Description ....
....
....
....
....

Use of 'I . . . Then' ....
....
....
....
....

Situation 3
Brief Description ....
....
....
....
....

Use of 'I . . . Then' ....
....
....
....
....

(b) 'DESC'

Another practicable method is DESC. It has proved to be a useful and powerful addition to increasing the assertiveness of individuals and groups. Nurses in general and women in particular seem to increase the amount of influence they have on their surroundings at work and in their personal lives. Try it for yourself either in an assertiveness-at-work group or in your relationships with others. An example shows how DESC can be used and applied to real life situations: the day shift/night shift nightmare.

A charge nurse sister is angry at the way the shortage of staff in the unit for sick children has meant more nurses have to be 'shuttled round and

round' to meet the needs of patients. This has resulted in a very unsatisfactory situation. The nurses on the unit complain, dislike the sister, are
tired much of the time and anxious that the nightmare of suddenly
having to move from the night shift to the day shift and back again is
'ruining' their personal lives.

Here is how the sister used the DESC method to communicate *assertively*
to:
(i) the unit manager,
(ii) all of the nurses on the unit for sick children.

(i) Meeting with the unit manager

Describe   When I see my nurses having to cope with the extra demands
being made on them – especially extra shifts between the day and night time
staff.

Express   I feel livid, and realize we are just digging ourselves into a bigger
hole. I feel the staff are just getting worn out, are under-appreciated and are
simply expected to carry on.

Specify   Particularly on the third and fourth weekends of each month for an
extra twelve hours per week.

Consequences   I am no longer prepared to maintain this arrangement unless
either the staff are given a more predictable schedule or extra nurses are
found for the additional hours. If you are unable to do either of these things
we will lose more nurses from the unit. I think that would be most undesirable
and I believe we should avoid it at all costs. I want to sort out the work
schedule immediately and make arrangements to relieve the nurses within
the next month.

(ii) Meeting with the unit nurses

Describe   After our last staff meeting I realized just how much the extra
demands our current day and night shift schedule was having on our
performance at work and for some of our personal lives. I decided to inform
the unit manager of our position.

Express   I can also tell you what I told the unit manager. I said how angry I
was – seeing how much stress this arrangement for shifts was generating. I
said we were becoming worn out and not given sufficient recognition for the
work we do.

Specify   I made it clear when the shift problem was occurring – as you
described it to me. I emphasized the main difficulty was the third and fourth
weekends of each month and the extra twelve hours per week most of us had
to find to meet the needs of our patients.

Consequences   I pointed out I was no longer prepared to accept this arrangement. I believe carrying on in this way would end up with more staff leaving

and this would only put even more pressure on us all round. What I want for us is a dependable work schedule and less extra hours.

REHEARSE, PRACTICE AND APPLY

Much of what we have been saying about assertiveness is about practising, rehearsing and transferring it to important situations at work and in our personal lives. But unless we rehearse, practice and apply, we will only be assertive 'in our heads'. So don't underestimate the importance *of rehearsing, practising and applying* assertive behaviour. Use this exercise to get underway and into assertive action.

Describe   (to the person or persons the situation as *you* see it).
Start by saying: *When I* .... or simply, I ....
....
....
....
....

Express   (remember to put *your* expression in the first person – how *you* feel).
I Feel/think ....
....
....
....
....

Specify   (make *your* assertive expression specific and identifiable).
What I find particularly evident is ....
....
....
....
....

Consequences   (state the results as *you* or the group *you* represent sees them)
I believe what will happen is .... and/or *As a consequence I will/will not* ....
....
....
....
....

GETTING YOUR POINT OVER – USING 'THE BROKEN RECORD'

An efficient and effective way of asserting ourselves is to use the method colloquially called 'The Broken Record'. The main principle here is just as when a record gets stuck in a groove we hear the same piece of music or singing, so in assertiveness we keep repeating our position until the receiver of the communication acknowledges it in some way. On many occasions they will not only acknowledge it but will act on it and carry out our request. The broken record method can be employed in many situations in which nurses find themselves. Perhaps one of the most obvious is working with unpopular or 'difficult' patients (Stockwell, 1972). Study this example and then identify your own situations where you will practice the broken record method of asserting yourself.

Scenario. Patient refuses medicine/injection . . . trying to smokescreen and sidetrack nurse. May use ridicule to try and provoke anger or submissiveness and anxiety. The nurse uses the broken record to avoid falling into these two traps and gets her point over and the patient co-operates at the end of this potentially stressful episode.

Patient: No I'm not having that stuff . . . definitely not.

Nurse: I want you to take your medicine. It is the one prescribed and it is time to take it.

Patient: You're just trying to butter me up. You are like all the other nurses, bossy boots . . .

Nurse: I know you must think that, but it is time for your medicine and I want you to take it now.

Patient: I don't have to take it. Nobody else is having to take it just now.

Nurse: That is true; nobody has their medicine at exactly the same time. It is time for your medicine and I would like you to take it now, 'cos this is the right time for you to have it.

Patient: Why do I have to take it right now? Can't I have it later? I'd rather . . . You're just a young nurse; what do you know about my medicine? Are you sure it is the right one for me? I mean I'm not sure if . . .

Nurse: I am sure this is the right medicine and it is the right time for you to have it, I want you to take it now. It is the right one.

Patient: Well if you are sure then it's alright. I'll take it . . . You are sure aren't you?

Nurse: Yes I am sure.

Patient: Alright I'll take it. Thanks . . .

ACCENT ON ASSERTIVENESS

Clearly there are many ways we can manage stress by being more assertive. Cultivating assertiveness at work will do a great deal to alleviate unnecessary anxiety and aggression. By identifying the appropriate non-verbal and verbal behaviour associated with assertiveness nurses should be in a position to strengthen their communications with colleagues at work and patients receiving clinical nursing care. They are also likely to be less vulnerable in their personal lives. Avoiding the anxious pitfalls of submissive behaviour and aggressive actions makes it possible for nurses to have more influence over their own behaviour. However, and much more importantly, by identifying, rehearsing and practising assertiveness, nurses will be listened to and respected by those with whom they work. Assertiveness should not be seen as being in competition with the other stress management strategies we have covered in this book. In our view assertiveness is a powerful option for managing stress. The selection of any specific method for managing stress will depend on the circumstances, the purpose for which it is chosen and the goals we set out to achieve. We must first feel confident and relaxed enough before we can effectively practise communicating assertively. On other occasions we may want to use just one of the tension – reduction or stress-inoculation methods for managing stress. Nurses who have a wider range of stress management and assertive behaviours to call on will be much less at the mercy of the occupational demands made on them.

4. Autogenic regulation training (ART)

Autogenic Regulation Training (ART) was orginally devised by Dr Johannes Schultz, a Berlin neurologist, and later elaborated by Dr Wolfgang Luthe in Montreal. Schultz noticed his patients moved into a trophotropic or healing state when they practised giving covert verbal instructions to different parts of their body. Initially these were cognitive formulae designed to influence the involuntary nervous system. For example, practitioners of ART can regulate the flow of blood to their upper limbs by phrases such as 'my hands and arms are heavy and warm'. Reports of regulating heart rate, decreasing respiratory functioning, lowering blood pressure, and reducing muscle tension, have all been validated by research after practising ART (Luthe, 1965, 1973; Schultz and Luthe, 1969). Alpha waves – recorded by an electroencephalogram (EEG) – can also increase with the practice of autogenic regulation training. These brain waves are usually accompanied by reports of increased relaxation, peace, tranquillity, creativity and well-being.

ATTITUDE

Practising ART requires the nurse or patient to adopt a passive attitude towards stress-control training. This passive attitude means letting the body and the mind work together to reduce stress through more regulated and natural functioning. In more prosaic terms ART helps to 'flush-out' stress and prevent us from becoming 'glued-up' (Bailey, 1987a). A central assumption of autogenic regulation training is that the human organism is a natural self-regulating psychophysiological system. Each individual is thought to have a natural psychobiological balance which maintains the equilibrium of organ processes and functions of their body. In biological terms we know this equilibrium is called 'homeostasis'. But because stress relations are induced by cognitive appraisal (an appraisal that personal harm is anticipated) we believe it is more appropriate to refer to psychobiological homeostasis. One implication of this restated position is that just as the body learns to react to threatening situations by anxiety, anger and sadness, so too can it learn to be calm and composed. Conversely, where a person tries to hold back those feelings, they can also learn to relax and let them go. This can be done by carrying out a series of cognitive instructions using autogenic regulation training procedures. They may involve the nurse or patient covertly 'talking' to different parts of their body, and giving themselves cognitive instructions of heaviness, warmth, calm, peacefulness, composure and control. Each autogenic training assignment is graded, and should be tailored to the psychobiological progress of the practitioner. As progress with autogenic regulation training becomes evident, previously disturbing events will often lose their threatening significance and stress reactions become less intense. Bottled-up stress is often discharged from the body and can take many forms such as laughter, tears, shouting, and feeling of hotness, coldness, shivering, limb tremor and muscular spasms. These autogenic discharges flush out stress and lead to a more harmonious functioning of the whole individual. The underlying process is called autogenic neutralization (Luthe, 1973) or just simply neutralization.

BEGINNING ART

The techniques employed in autogenic regulation training have been developed to promote natural self-healing by the psychophysiological systems operating in each person. The main emphasis is on removing blocks to the self-regulating and restorative processes which give rise to the trophotropic state, and relaxation (Luthe, 1973).

After initial training in each autogenic regulation exercise and controlled practice of ART, nurses or patients can carry out ART assignments in their own privacy, and in their own time. A number of preparatory checks should however be made.

1. The practitioner of ART should have no medical condition preventing its practice.
2. The practitioner of ART should have the support of a clinical psychologist, physician or nurse counsellor qualified in ART.
3. Passive concentration should be explained as simply 'letting it happen' and that no conscious or deliberate concentrated attempt should be made by the practitioner to bring about the benefits associated with ART.
4. The basic ideas behind ART and its practice should be explained to the practitioner.

PRACTISING ART

We believe the nurse or patient practising ART should carry out the anti-stress training assignments first thing in the morning, midday or early evening, and immediately before retiring for the evening. Corresponding with this practice, three different positions can be adopted which encourage good results.

(a) The simple sitting posture
(b) The reclining armchair position
(c) The lying horizontal position

Procedure

Step 1. Regularly practise ART in a quiet place, e.g. bedroom, library, until the trophotropic state and relaxation is readily achieved. Thereafter the degree of noise or visual stimulation should not interfere with ART practice and its effects.
Step 2. Practise ART in the morning in the simple sitting posture.
Step 3. ART sessions at midday or early evening should be carried out in the reclining armchair position.
Step 4. The final ART session should be carried out in bed prior to sleep. This session should be conducted in the horizontal position. (Do not be concerned if you fall asleep during this session. You probably have entered the trophotropic state and can cancel the state when you wake in the morning by naturally stretching arms, legs and toes, and taking a deep breath of fresh air.)
Step 5. Repeat each exercise three times i.e. say to yourself the formula three times for each position at different times of the day.
Step 6. Cancel each session by:
    (i)   clenching the fists and briskly flexing the arms back towards the shoulders;
    (ii) taking a deep inhalation of air; and
    (iii) opening the eyes.

The autogenic regulation training session is then over. You can stand up and carry on in your usual way, after cancelling each exercise. Remember to cancel each ART session to avoid any 'sluggishness'. Cancelling also fulfils the function of toning up the muscles and bringing the individual's consciousness back into an alert attentiveness.

ART ASSIGNMENT SCHEDULE

The following schedule is a shortened version of ART which can be practised by nurses or patients who want to alleviate stress, gain more control over stress and facilitate recovery and healing processes.

Example: first ART exercise
Practise this exercise three times per day in sitting, reclining, and lying horizontal position.
1. Sit quietly, close your eyes.
2. Repeat three times silently to yourself:

My right arm is heavy (RAH)	Say this to yourself three times
My left arm is heavy (LAH)	" " " " " "
Both my arms are heavy (BAH)	" " " " " "
My right leg is heavy (RLH)	" " " " " "
My left leg is heavy (LLH)	" " " " " "
Both my legs are heavy (BLH)	" " " " " "
My arms and legs are heavy (ALH)	" " " " " "
I am calm and at peace (IACAP)	" " " " " "

Now cancel exercise by clenching fists, flexing arms to shoulders; take a deep breath and open your eyes.

CHANGES AND BENEFITS FROM ART

Each weekly ART exercise should be monitored for its therapeutic effects. The total autogenic regulation training period can also be assessed for its efficacy by the practitioner. This is usually best done in consultation with a supervising counsellor who is familiar with ART and the range of its possible effects. Early changes from practising ART often come through the practitioner's self-report and body movements. These reports can range from feelings of well-being to some initial discomfort associated with relief and the discharge of tension from the body (Schultz and Luthe, 1969; Luthe, 1973). These forms of tension release are termed 'autogenic discharges' (Bailey, 1985). Some typical observations reported by practitioners of ART are:

- heaviness
- warmth
- twitching
- happiness
- laughter
- elation
- relaxation
- tingling
- floating
- pain
- anxiety
- sadness
- tearfulness
- tension

The benefits of autogenic discharges may therefore be either pleasant or discomforting or some mixture of both. Discomforting discharges benefit the practitioner in that the brain and body work together to flush out the barriers to natural self-regulation, and psychomedical homeostasis. So, for instance, crying may precede laughter or anxiety. There is, however, no set sequence of autogenic discharges. Many people carrying out autogenic regulation training do not experience feelings of tension or any discomfort. In general, they report feelings of relaxation, peacefulness, physical and psychological well-being. We note a wide range of psychological, medical and physical benefits are reported in the literature (Luthe and Schultz, 1969). Practitioners of ART often claim an increase in their awareness of themselves and their reactions to their surroundings (Schultz and Luthe, 1969; Lindemann, 1974; Rosa, 1976).

A number of specific benefits have also been reported in the research literature. For instance asthmatic attacks and tension headaches occur less often (Rosa, 1976; Wittkower and Warnes, 1977; Schwartz, 1978). Also ART patients diagnosed as suffering from angina pectoris developed fewer myocardial infarctions as a group compared with patients relying on medication alone (Luthe and Blumberger, 1977). Other studies suggest ART practitioners become less depressed and anxious. Sleep patterns may also improve and may be accompanied by an increase in alertness during waking hours (Lindeman, 1974; Luthe and Blumberger, 1977; Bailey, 1987a).

Sickness absence may also be reduced significantly. Bailey (1984, 1986a) reported a longitudinal study involving an ART trained group (n = 25) and a comparison group (n = 20) of student nurses in general training. The group that received autogenic regulation training clearly had significantly fewer days off overall than the comparison group. Proportionally, no significant differences were found between the numbers reporting sick. But the interesting result here was that the ART group spent less time absent compared with the comparison group of student nurses – an indication that ART had played some mediating influence on those reporting sick and their recovery rate. Interestingly, fewer students in the ART group transferred to other forms of nurse training. And significantly more student nurses in the comparison group left the NHS altogether. An analysis of individual stress profiles however showed that whereas ART may be of considerable benefit as a strategy for preventing stress, some nurses only practised ART when they needed it most. We may presume from these data that ART is used when stress is experienced as being 'uncomfortable' and the nurse could no longer manage either using her own coping resources or by enlisting available social supports to reduce stress (such as colleagues, nurse tutor, counsellor, friends, family etc.) (Caplan and Killilea, 1976). There were of course a few student nurses in the ART-trained group who neither needed nor practised ART after their initial training period. This helps us to make another point about this study. Simply having a potent stress management strategy available may be sufficient for nurses to better control their stress level and the different forms it takes (Bailey 1982, 1985). We agree with Miller (1980) who observed that if we can 'stop the roller-coaster' we won't want to come off. In other words, if we know we can control stress through ART or any other method of managing stress, just knowing we can do it increases our perceived control over significant demands being made on us at any one time and in specific environments.

However, it should be clearly acknowledged that ART, like other stress-control techniques, is not a panacea for all psycho-medical ills. For instance, it may not work effectively with practitioners who cannot make the cognitive–behavioural link-up with the verbal formulae of autogenic regulation training. Additionally, those people who are repeatedly exposed to stress-inducing situations may find it difficult to maintain their psycho-biological equilibrium. A saturation effect may develop which has a major disrupting influence on the psychological functioning of the nurse or patient. Where this is excessive, psychiatric illness may appear. Autogenic regulation training should not be used in these cases unless in close collaboration with a clinical psychologist, qualified nurse, or psychiatrist. However, ART is an appropriate and efficacious method to practise with the softer psychological signs of stress such as anxiety, anger, phobias, hypertension, compulsive obsessions and mild depression. Insomnia, headaches, bronchial asthma, writer's cramp, and other somatic complaints also show considerable improvement during and after autogenic regulation training (Luthe and Schultz, 1969; Luthe and Blumberger, 1977). Perhaps the four strongest reasons for adopting ART are that it is at once:

1. A method for preventing, or at least minimizing, the threatening impact of demands in the individual's environment.
2. A method for intervening in undesirably high levels of stress and reducing them to manageable proportions.
3. A method that can be applied to a wide range of stress problems and potentially threatening situations.
4. A method which genuinely increases the amount of control we can have over stress and our own psychobiological functions.

Viewed from this perspective, autogenic regulation training seems to be a useful method which can be enlisted by nurses to deal with the many forms of stress they experience at work and for patients coping with the stress associated with physical illness (Moos, 1979; Stone *et al.*, 1980; Charlesworth *et al.*, 1981; Bailey, 1986a).

5. Stress-inoculation training (SIT): Cognition and altered appraisal

Another method of stress control involves adopting a comprehensive set of coping skills to deal with a wide range of stress-inducing situations. This approach has been developed by Meichenbaum (1979) and Novaco (1975). It is popularly termed stress-inoculation training (SIT). These coping skills involve the practitioner learning to modify their inner or private dialogue. The private dialogue that individuals have with themselves (i.e. what they say to themselves about situations, what they believe about the effects they have on them, and the memories of what threatens them and how they cope) influences whether or not they will experience some form of stress. In other words it is the cognitive appraisal each person makes of their environment that determines their physical, mental and emotional reactions to situations, and their feelings about the physiological activity taking place in their own body (Beck, 1972, 1976). For instance, a nurse may say to herself 'dying children make my adrenaline flow and I feel anxious at not being able to help. In fact, I feel helpless'. By adopting stress-inoculation training procedure, the nurse or patient can learn to alter their inner thoughts and appraisals of these situations and others which might be disturbing. Different stages of SIT show how changing the labels and thoughts about threatening situations can alter individual emotional reactions. Stress-inoculation training procedures can also be self-administered by patients after a period of coaching and training. Two beneficial consequences arise from these circumstances. One is patients become less dependent on nurses and the health-care system because they can gain personal control over their own levels of stress. The other is patients are likely to reduce the unreasonable demands they may make on the nurses' time.

STRESS-INOCULATION TRAINING PROCEDURES

The procedure for SIT usually involves four phases: (i) educational behaviour, (ii) rehearsal, (iii) application and (iv) self-reinforcement.

Phase 1 – education. During this phase, the causes of stress are explained in terms that the practitioner can understand rather than in scientific concepts. However, the explanation rests heavily on a theory of emotion put forward by Stanley Schachter, a research psychologist (Schachter and Singer, 1962). In simple terms, the theory is conveyed to the SIT student in the following way:

1. When we get sensations in our bodies, we try to make sense of them. In doing so we label our sensations to describe our states and moods, and general health.
2. It is these labels which give rise to whether or not we say we are anxious, depressed, angry, elated, bored, calm, cool or collected.

Although this theory has been subjected to criticism (see Meichenbaum, 1979), it is still useful to conceptualize directly how stress arises, and by implication, how it can be controlled, and overcome. Just as we learn to label our sensations which then give rise to our experience of emotion, it is explained to the student that relabelling sensations and how we think about them changes the emotions we experience. In turn this relabelling, and the change of the inner dialogue we have, should influence our physiological levels of arousal. One consequence of this relabelling of sensations in relation to different levels of physiological activity is a reduction in reported stress reactions. After the education phase, the student of SIT then rehearses the ideas learned.

Phase 2 – behaviour rehearsal. During behaviour rehearsal, the SIT student carries out the procedure of relabelling the different sensations she has identified as threatening. In clearly set-out instructions, the SIT student practises 'talking to herself' (himself, themselves) in a different way about situations which previously threatened her to the extent that they caused psychological and physical discomfort (Meichenbaum, 1979). This is an application of coping self-talk and often achieves three goals (Zastrow, 1979). First, it changes the perception and primary appraisal of the situation – usually resulting in a reduction in its threatening significance. Second, it allows the practitioner of stress control to take a less-stressful view of the sensations experienced in her own body (secondary appraisal). Third, when these sensations are relabelled, they usually result in the practitioner of stress-inoculation training reporting dramatic reductions in experienced stress (reappraisal).

Phase 3 – application. In this phase the person applies what they have learned about stress-inoculation training after a period of rehearsal using new thoughts and behaviours in previously stress-inducing situations. This is the period when the new-thinking and new-behaving should be put into practice (Bailey, 1987a). It is essential that Phase 3 is applied consistently and in the same way that it was practised during the rehearsal phase of stress-innoculation training. By doing this, we increase the likelihood of achieving successful stress control. Also it is easier and more systematic to identify where any improvements need to be made to enhance practical control over stress by individuals or groups. If all of the phases of stress-inoculation strategy are followed carefully, significant increases in stress control will follow.

Phase 4 – self-reinforcement. To make the new-thinking, new-behaving aspects of stress-inoculation training effective and lasting, it is important for practitioners to reward themselves in some way so as to reinforce and maintain their new-found control over stress. Failure to do so runs the risk of reducing the effects and the duration of effective stress control. Self-reinforcement can either be covert or overt. Saying to yourself 'I did well', 'I really did it that time', 'I do have control', are all examples of covert self-reinforcement. More overt forms may involve buying a gift for yourself, giving yourself a score out of say 100 for how well you applied the stress-inoculation strategy or just simply going out to your favourite restaurant. Self-reinforcement is a central part of the SIT programme and should not be omitted on the grounds of false modesty or worse still disbelief in the influence it has on establishing and increasing our cognitive and behavioural control over stress.

Internationally, many programmes of stress-inoculation instruction have been developed and tested with efficacious results (Meichenbaum, 1979). The schedule of training permits the individual to move from a position of learned helplessness (see e.g. Seligman, 1977; Abramson *et al.* 1978; Garber and Seligman, 1980) to one of acquired learned resourcefulness, renewed competence and progressive mastery over stress. In other words, the practitioner of stress-inoculation training develops more comprehensive appraisal and coping skills to control her own level of stress. This phased and systematic approach to stress control permit individuals and groups to:

1. Prepare for a threat that induces stress
2. Confront and deal with stress-inducing threats
3. Cope with feelings of inadequacy or being overwhelmed
4. Achieve self-reinforcing statements which lead to personal control over stress.

Using a stress-innoculation training format of this kind also allows the individual to estimate how much threat they are under and how well they are coping. This can be done in a fairly detailed way. For instance, the nurse or patient can estimate how much difficulty they have with different situations, and the feelings and thoughts they engender. They may also get a clear idea of how well they confront experienced stress and the effect this has both on themselves and the threatening situation. Finally, they should be able to assess whether their methods of coping are ones which promote personal control over threatening events and experienced stress.

A useful way of applying the SIT format is to measure the present reaction to threat, confrontation, feelings of being overwhelmed, and kind of self-statements, before carrying out any stress-control programme. This is a principle which can also be applied to the previously-mentioned methods of stress control. Doing this achieves three goals important for any stress control assessment and training. First, it will give nurses or patients 'a stress-control profile'. The profile would show both areas where they are doing well, and where they need help to establish or re-establish personal control over stress. Not all areas of the stress-control profile would therefore require a comprehensive scheme of stress-inoculation training. For example, a nurse may effectively prepare to meet a threat – such as being reprimanded by a superior in front of patients. She may also cope with feelings of embarrassment or anger, by being calm and polite without being servile. However, on the SIT assessment she may reveal being dissatisfied with the way she confronted such a situation. It is also possible she never congratulated herself on the dignified way in which she coped with the encounter. In such an instance, insufficient self-reinforcing statements leading to personal control would be evident. This example of a baseline assessment prior to SIT highlights the second goal. It informs the nurse or the patient which parts of their reactions to the situation have to be changed. In the example, the nurse could be taught to confront 'being shown up in front of patients' by ignoring the incident, asking to discuss the matter in private, suggesting it should be written down and discussed at a later date when she was not so busy, and relabelling her present view of how she confronted the incident. Relabelling could involve her saying to herself, 'this is below my dignity', 'I am handling this the right way, I am calm and in control', 'this is a matter which is of no importance to me', and other self-talk which would neutralize the threatening significance of the experienced situation. The activation of relabelling would also be followed by self-reinforcing statements such as, 'I didn't panic', 'staying cool was the right thing to do', 'I'm glad I reacted the way I did' 'I have control of the situation and myself', etc. These are all examples of self-statements which promote the nurse's personal control over potentially stressful threatening demands in nursing.

Evaluation
Once these aspects of SIT have been established, the goal – efficacy of the programme – can be evaluated.

In its simplest form, this can be done by going through each stage of the SIT programme with the nurse or the patient. The typical sequence involves checking once again the reactions to each stage of the programme. In the example we have given, we would check that the nurse still felt prepared to deal with the threat and cope with her feelings. But we would expect to see her use a different style of confrontation and look for self-reinforcing statements leading to an increase in her personal control. This change in style and relabelling would show up in the nurse's response to the phases outlined in the SIT programme. And where these therapeutic changes were noted, we should find a corresponding decrease in the forms of reported stress.

Stress-inoculation training would seem to have an important part to play in the future of the nursing profession. Its main contribution could be in helping nurses and their patients to maximize their personal control over threat, and enhancing their coping skills to combat disabling forms of stress such as acute anxiety, reactive depression and anger. Its main appeal lies in the nurse being able to adopt a varied range of appraisal and coping skills within and across different threatening situations. One slight drawback with SIT, however, is that initially at least, the SIT student must rely on a qualified clinical psychologist, nurse, or counsellor to coach them through the early training sessions. This only presents a minor problem though when compared with the time-consuming character of other forms of therapist-dependent therapies such as traditional psychoanalysis. For the most part, SIT, like the other methods of stress control detailed in this chapter, can be self-administered by the nurse or patient after a short period of supervised practice.

6.2 PRACTICAL CONSIDERATIONS AND SPECULATIONS FOR THE FUTURE OF STRESS CONTROL

The stress-control and self-regulation coping strategies covered in this chapter present a number of realistic options for nurses who wish to practise stress control for themselves and their patients. Training in stress control techniques could also be adopted by schools and colleges of nursing and incorporated into their educational curricula. Nursing management and district and regional health authorities should support and research the efficacy of stress control on patient health and nurse effectiveness. We have already shown how sickness absence can be reduced in student nurses through the availability of autogenic relaxation training. There are also further potential benefits to the management of nursing services. Nursing in general may also become more cost-effective from a management-administrative perspective by the practice of stress control methods. We would speculate further still and suggest that nurse tutors, and qualified ward and management nurses would also benefit from using some of the techniques in this chapter to avoid or reduce already disabling levels of stress amongst themselves and their patients. However, these areas should also be properly researched for their association with other financial and health-care variables rather than being introduced uncritically into nursing and health-care systems. At present though, we can have some clinical confidence in offering a range of stress-control techniques for use by nurses and patients which at least provide a coherent means of direct and indirect coping with threat, harm, loss, and the stress arising from significant demands in health-care environments. The detail of how nurses and patients might learn to use direct or indirect stress-control skills which lead to the more effective control of stress does not seem to us prohibitive. All the techniques we have considered here can be self-administered after an initial period of appropriate training.

6.3 SUMMARY

In this chapter we have argued that stress-control techniques can be used to better prepare nurses and patients for dealing with predictable threatening aspects of their environment. Unexpected or unpredictable sources of threat, common to nurses (Briggs, 1972), can also be defused through the regular practice of stress-control techniques. Other benefits might also stem from the very knowledge that nurses and patients have the means to control their levels of stress – even though they do not put them into practice. In other words, just knowing that we can exert some personal control over disturbing internal or external threats such as pain or anxiety is in itself enough to limit the impact of otherwise stress-producing events in our lives (Pervin, 1963; Glass and Singer, 1972; Bailey, 1982). Simply put, controlling stress may also help immunize the nurse and patient against helplessness (Seligman, 1977; Abramson *et al.*, 1979; Meichenbaum, 1979). In this respect, acquiring stress-control techniques and practising them are not to be confused as the same thing, although they both seem to be connected with achieving personal control over stress-inducing threats in the context of delivering health-care systems.

We conclude, therefore, that the availability of stress-control techniques can serve a number of important functions in maintaining and promoting human health.

REFERENCES

Abramson, L., Seligman, M. and Teasdale, J. (1978) Learned helplessness in humans: Critique and reformulation. *Journal of Abnormal Behaviour*, **87**, 49–74.

Ansell, E. (1981) Professional burn-out: Recognition and management. *Journal American Association of Nurse Anaesthetics*. **49**(2), 135–42.

Antonovsky, A. (1979) *Health, Stress and Coping*, Jossey-Bass, San Francisco.

Arndt, C. and Laeger, E. (1970a) Role strain in a diversified role set: The Director of Nursing Service, *Journal of Nursing Research*, **1**(19), 253–9.

Arndt, C. and Laeger, E. (1970b) Role strain in a diversified role set: The Director of Nursing Service, sources of stress. *Journal of Nursing Research*, **2**(19), 495–501.

Bailey, R. (1981). Counselling services for nurses – a forgotten responsibility. *Journal British Institute of Mental Handicap*, **9**, 45–7.

Bailey, R. (1982) Senior Student Nurse Stress and Coping Profiles. Dept. Records. Psychology Department, Manor House, Aylesbury.

Bailey, R. (1984) Autogenic regulation training and sickness absence amongst nurses in general training. *Journal of Advanced Nursing*, **9**, 581–8.

Bailey, R. (1985) *Autogenic Regulation Training (ART), Sickness Absence, Personal Problems, Time and The Emotional-Physical Stress of Student Nurses in General Training*. PhD Thesis. University of Hull.

Bailey, R. (1986a) *Coping with Stress in Caring*, (2nd edn), Blackwell Scientific Publications, Oxford.

Bailey, R. (1986b) *Systematic Relaxation*. Winslow Press, London.

Bailey, R. (1987a) *Masterstress*. (In preparation).

Bailey, R. (1987b) *Regulating Stress – A Self-Management Method for Controlling Sickness Absence.* Stress and the Public Services Conference, Loughborough.

Bailey, R. (1988) *Managing More Assertively. Training and Management Development Methods.* MCB University Press, Bradford.

Bakal, D. (1979) *Psychology and Medicine.* Tavistock Publications, London.

Beck, A. (1972) *Depression: Causes and Treatment.* International Universities Press, New York, N.Y.

Beck, A. (1976) *Cognitive Therapy and the Emotional Disorders.* International Universities Press, New York, N.Y.

Benson, H. (1980) *The Relaxation Response.* Fontana, London.

Benson, H., Marzetta, B. R. and Rosner, B. A. (1974) Decreased blood pressure associated with the regular elicitation of the relaxation response: A study of hypertensive subjects, in *Contemporary Problems in Cardiology, Stress and Heart* (ed. R. S. Eliot), Futura, Mt. Kisco, New York, N.Y.

Birch J. (1979) The anxious learner. *Nursing Mirror* (February 8), 17–24.

Bloomfield, H. H., Cain, M. P., Jaffe, T. and Kory, R. (1976) *TM: Discovering Inner Energy and Overcoming Stress.* George Allen and Unwin, London.

Briggs, A. (1972) Report of the Committee on Nursing. Cmnd. No. 5115, HMSO, London.

Caplan, G. and Killilea, M. (1976) *Support Systems and Mutual Help.* Grune and Stratton, New York, N.Y.

Charlesworth, E. A., Murphy, S. and Beutler, L. E. (1981) Stress management for nursing students. *Journal of Clinical Psychology,* **37**, 284–90.

Cherniss, C. (1980) *Staff Burn-Out: Job Stress in the Human Services.* Sage Publications, London.

Clark, C. C. (1978) *Assertive Skills for Nurses.* Contemporary Publishing, Wakefield, MA.

Clarke, S. and Hussey, D. G. (1979) Sickness amongst nursing staff at two hospitals. *Journal of Social and Occupational Medicine,* **29**, 126–30.

Colligan, M., Smith, M. and Horrel, J. (1977) Occupational incidence – rates of mental health disorder. *Journal of Human Stress,* **13**, 34–9.

Cormack, D. (1973) *Sickness and Absence Amongst Nursing Staffs in a Psychiatric Mental Deficiency Hospital Group.* Royal Dundee Liff Hospital, Dundee.

Edelwich, J. and Brodsky A. (1980) *Burn-Out: Stages of Disillusionment in the Helping Professions.* Human Sciences Press.

Folkman, S. and Lazarus, R. S. (1980) An analysis of coping in a middle-aged community sample. *Journal of Health and Social Behaviour,* **21**, 219–39.

Garber, J. and Seligman, M. E. P. (1980) *Human Helplessness: Theory and Applications.* Academic Press, New York, N.Y.

Glass D. C. and Singer, J. E. (1972) *Urban Stress: Experiments on Noise and Social Stressors*. Academic Press, New York, N.Y.

Goleman, D. (1976) Meditation helps break the stress spiral. *Psychology Today*, **V**. 82–6. 93.

Harris, T. (1969) *I'm OK – You're OK*. Harper and Row, New York, N.Y.

Hess, W. R. (1957) *The Functional Organization of the Diencephalon*. Grune and Stratton, New York, N.Y.

Hillier, S. (1973) Nurses' smoking habits. *Postgraduate Medical Journal*, 1981. **49**, 693–4.

Hillier, S. (1981) Stresses, strains and smoking. *Nursing Mirror* (February 12), 26–30.

Jacobson, E. (1934) *You Must Relax*. Whittley House, New York, N.Y.

Jacobson, E. (1938) *Progressive Relaxation*. University of Chicago Press, Chicago, IL.

Lazarus, R. (1966) *Psychological Stress and the Coping Process*. McGraw-Hill, New York, N.Y.

Lazarus, A. (1971) *Behavior Therapy and Beyond*. McGraw-Hill, New York, N.Y.

Lazarus, R. (1976) *Patterns of Adjustment*. McGraw-Hill, New York, N.Y.

Lazarus, R. (1981) The stress and coping paradigm, in *Theoretical Bases for Psychopathology* (eds C. Eisdorfer, D. Cohen, A. Kleinman and P. Maxim), Spectrum, New York, N.Y.

Lazarus, R. and Launier, R. (1978) Stress-related transactions between person and environment, in *Perspectives in Interactional Psychology* (eds L. Dervin and M. Lewis), Plenum, New York, N.Y., pp. 287–327.

Lindemann, H. (1974) *Relieve Tension the Autogenic Way*. Abelard-Schuman, London.

Luckman, D. (1979) The nurse who asked why. *Nursing*, **148**(14), 18–19.

Luthe, W. (1965) *Autogenic Training*. Grune and Stratton, New York, N.Y.

Luthe, W. (1973) *Autogenic Therapy: Treatment with Autogenic Neutralization*. Grune and Stratton, New York, N.Y.

Luthe, W. and Blumberger, S. (1977) Autogenic therapy, in *Psychosomatic Medicine: Its Clinical Applications*, (eds E. D. Wittkower and H. Warnes), Harper and Row, London.

Luthe, W. and Schultz, W. (1969) *Autogenic Therapy: Autogenic Methods*. Grune and Stratton, New York, N.Y.

Mahoney, M. (1974) *Cognition and Behavior Modification*, Ballinger, Massachusetts.

Marshall, J. (1980) Stress amongst nurses, in *White Collar and Professional Stress* (eds C. Cooper and J. Marshall), J. Wiley, London.

Meichenbaum, D. (1979) *Cognitive Behavior Modification*. Plenum, New York, N.Y.

Miller, S. M. (1980) Why having control reduces stress: If I can stop the roller coaster I don't want to get off, in *Human Helplessness: Theory and Applications*, (eds J. Garber and M. E. P. Seligman), Academic Press, New York, N.Y.

Moos, R. (1979) *The Human Context: Environmental Determinants of Behavior*. J. Wiley, New York, N.Y.

Neisser, U. (1972) *Cognitive Psychology*. Appleton-Century-Crofts, U. S.

Novaco, R. (1975) *Anger Control: The Development and Evaluation of an Experimental Treatment*, Heath, Lexington, MA.

Oswin, M. (1978) *Children Living in Long-Stay Hospital*. Spastics International, Lavenham Press, Suffolk.

Parkes, K. (1980a) Occupational stress among student nurses – 1. A comparison of medical and surgical wards. Occasional papers. *Nursing Times*, **76**(25), 113–16.

Parkes, K. (1980b) Occupational stress among student nurses – 2. A comparison of male and female wards. Occasional papers. *Nursing Times*, **76**(26) 117–19.

Pervin, L. (1963) The need to predict and control under conditions of threat. *Journal of Personality*, **31**, 570–85.

Phillipson, P. A. J. (1978) The reason learners go absent. *Nursing Mirror* (June 8), 12–15.

Rardin, M. (1969) Treatment of a phobia by partial self-desensitization. *Journal of Consulting and Clinical Psychology*, **33**, 125–6.

Redfern, S. (1978) Absence and wastage in trained nurses: A selective review of the literature. *Journal of Advanced Nursing*, **3**, 231–49.

Rosa, K. (1976) *Autogenic Training*. Victor Gollanz, London.

Schachter, S. and Singer, J. E. (1962) Cognitive, social and physiological determinants of emotional state. *Psychology Review*, **69**, 379–99.

Schultz, J. and Luthe, W. (1969) *Autogenic Training: A Psychophysiological Approach to Psychotherapy*. Grune and Stratton, New York, N.Y.

Schwartz, J. (1978) *Voluntary Controls*. E. P. Dutton, New York, N.Y.

Seligman, M. E. P. (1977) *Helplessness*. W. H. Freeman, San Francisco, CA.

Sinclair, J. D. (1981) *The Rest Principle: A Neurophysiological Theory of Behavior*. Lawrence Erlbaum Associates, N.J.

Sobol, E. (1978) Self-actualization. The baccalaureate nursing student's response to stress. *Nursing Research*, **27**(4) 238–44.

Stockwell, F. (1972) *The Unpopular Patient*, Croom Helm, London.

Stone, G., Cohen, F. and Adler, N. (1980) *Health Psychology – A Handbook*. Jossey-Bass, San Francisco, CA.

White, R. (1959) Motivation reconsidered: The concept of competence, *Psychological Review*, **66**(5), 297–333.

Whitfield, S. (1979) A Descriptive Study of Student Nurses' Ward Experiences with Dying Patients and Their Attitudes Towards Them. MSc Thesis, University of Manchester.

Wittkower, E. D. and Warnes, H. (1977) *Psychosomatic Medicine: Its Applications*. Grune and Stratton, New York, N.Y.

Wolpe, J. (1958) *Psychotherapy by Reciprocal Inhibition*. Stanford University Press, Stanford, CA.

Wolpe, J. (1976) *The Practice of Behaviour Therapy* (2nd edn), Pergamon Press, Oxford and New York.

Wolpe, J. and Lazarus, A. (1966) *Behaviour Therapy Techniques*. Pergamon Press, Oxford.

Wood, E. (1969) *Yoga*. Pelican, Penguin Books, Harmondsworth.

Zastrow, C. (1979) *Talk to Yourself: Using the Power of Self-Talk*. Spectrum Books, New York, N.Y.

PART THREE

PATIENTS – STRESS AND COPING

In general, books on stress and coping for the nursing profession focus either upon the stress considered to be inherent within the nursing role, or on stress and coping associated with the patient's role. However, we have chosen to include both aspects within this book. We have done this because the same theoretical considerations apply whether one is interested in nurses or patients.

We also believe that nurses should gain understanding of themselves from empathizing with patients and gain empathy with patients from understanding themselves. Nurses and patients are not two separate species subject to different pressures but are part of the same humanity. Not only that, but nurses may become patients and some patients may become nurses.

Finally, we believe that a major source of stress for nurses is their perception of the stress suffered by patients, and evidence for this was reported by Menzies (1961). Helping patients to cope is, therefore, a healthy method of coping for the nurse, helping to reduce his or her own stress by direct action, rather than through the use of mental defence mechanisms as described by Menzies (1961).

Reference

Menzies, I. (1961) *The Functioning of Social Systems as a Defence Against Anxiety*, Tavistock Press, London.

CHAPTER SEVEN

Hospital admission: coping and recovery

Research has shown that going into hospital may be perceived as a source of threat by many patients. For the majority who enter hospital for treatment, one major threat, that of perceiving that one is ill, is already being confronted. Having to go into hospital acquires a social meaning; it implies the presence of an illness too serious to be treated by the doctor in his office or within the patient's own home (Kornfield, 1979). On top of this, 'illness alters the patient's social role and his social relationships and hospitalisation dramatises this stage' (Coser, 1962).

Apart from the significance which hospital admission may have in terms of illness and the disruption to the social role and relationships, there are other dimensions of hospital admission which may be appraised as threatening. These include the strangeness of the environment, interference with normal daily activities, potential and actual control by others, depersonalisation, and the possibility of encountering unpleasant sights and sounds.

Within the cognitive–phenomenological–transactional (CPT) view of stress and coping we emphasize individual appraisal of threat and it would be wrong to suggest that every person under every circumstance finds hospital admission threatening. Informal evidence from talking to patients suggests that for some, going into hospital is a relief and a comfort. In particular people who normally live alone and are lonely have said that going into hospital gives them companionship and reassurance. Patients who have been waiting a long time for a hip-replacement operation, for example, have also said that they welcome going into hospital. Nonetheless, even for those who find it a relief to be admitted to hospital, there are certain critical events within the total experience of hospital which patients may appraise as particularly threatening (Wilson-Barnett and Carrigy, 1978). Becoming a patient in hospital means the patient must (Kornfield, 1979)

> face the reality of his own mortality. Man does not usually live with this anxiety in the forefront of his consciousness. It is hard to do otherwise in the hospital where one is surrounded by serious illness and death twenty-four hours a day. Certainly each patient deals with this situation in his own way but each must come to grips with it. The question is, how

does the hospital environment affect the individual patient in his struggle with this anxiety-provoking situation?

Before discussing the research in which the answer to this question has been studied, it is useful at this point to elaborate further the authors' theoretical position with regard to stress and coping.

Stress and emotions

Stress is considered to be a meta-concept: one which embraces several other concepts. It is concerned, by definition, with the appraisal of threat and coping with that threat. However, when considering individuals, their experience of threat is frequently in terms of felt emotion. For example, fear, anxiety, depression and anger are frequently experienced in the face of threat, even when the threat has not been recognized at a conscious level. In turn the emotions experienced may themselves be appraised as threatening and may enhance the perceived threat from a recognized source.

In terms of adaptation and coping any emotional response which occurs may interfere with behavioural or somatic coping. For example, high levels of anxiety have been shown by Ley and Spelman (1967) to interfere with the processes of acquiring, retaining and retrieval of medical information. Extreme fear may disrupt behaviour in animals, preventing them from making effective responses at all (Karsh, 1970). Tremor due to anxiety or anger may interfere with fine hand movement in humans, reducing performance levels in manual tasks. This relationship has been incorporated in the well known Yerkes–Dodson Law (1908).

This complex relationship between stress and emotion has been addressed within Lazarus's work on coping and its two functions which he designates as (1) the regulation of emotional responses and (2) the regulation of instrumental or behavioural aspects of transactions with the environment (Lazarus and Launier, 1978).

This issue has been raised at this point since it is crucial to the studies of patients' experience which will be discussed in this and subsequent chapters. In much of the research, it is the patient's emotional responses to the illness, the hospital environment, the treatment procedures etc. which have been described and measured and generally treated as operational indicators of stress. Stress has not been used as a theoretical framework in all of the studies. Instead the emotional responses have been used as theoretical constructs in their own right.

Patients' verbalized appraisals have also been explored in some studies, as well as the emotional responses. Questions have been asked about 'worries' and what instigated the worry, for example (Franklin, 1974).

Another important feature of the research into the experience of patients has been the use of measures of emotional states as an indicator of the effectiveness of an experimental intervention aimed at reducing stress, i.e. they have been used as outcome measures. Thus the relationship between stress and emotion is an important one in the understanding of the research studies in this field.

A further issue which should be discussed at this stage is the measurement of anxiety. In the pyschological literature anxiety has been conceptualized as a dimension of personality (trait anxiety) and as a short-term response to threat (state anxiety). Individuals who exhibit trait anxiety have a tendency to respond with anxiety and worry to circumstances under which average individuals would not respond in such a way. Such individuals are likely to see a much wider variety of circumstances as threatening than most of us, i.e. anxiety is characteristic of them. State anxiety occurring in an individual who is low or average on trait anxiety is indicative of an event appraised by them as 'threatening'. The distinction between state and trait anxiety can be measured by a scale devised by Spielberger (1979). The Mood Adjective Check List (MACL) of Lishman (1972) measures state anxiety and this has been used frequently in research, together with a measure of trait anxiety such as the neuroticism scale of the Eysenck Personality Inventory (EPI) (Eysenck and Eysenck, 1972).

The EPI can be used to identify those patients who are high on trait anxiety. This is useful since such patients are particularly likely to develop an adverse emotional state in illness due to their anxiety proneness. A state anxiety measure is useful to identify those incidents and objects within a hospital which are appraised as threatening by patients in general.

7.1 ADMISSION TO HOSPITAL

We now wish to turn to the research evidence concerning patients' responses to hospital admission. In a study by Wilson-Barnett and Carrigy (1978) which has been mentioned above, the authors monitored the emotional reactions of 202 medical patients in two hospitals, each afternoon from the day of admission until discharge. In particular, patients' anxiety and depression were monitored and any score significantly higher than the median on scales relating to these emotions was considered to indicate a reaction to events which were perceived by the patients as of great importance to them.

Scores higher than normal were found on the day of admission, on the day of a special test, and in one of the study hospitals at weekends. A significantly lower than average score on anxiety and depression was found on the day of discharge in one of the study hospitals but not the other.

In this study, the results showed that negative emotions were aroused amongst patients at the time of admission and several studies have examined this event in particular.

The admission procedure

One of the earliest such studies in the UK was by Franklin (1974). She carried out a survey of 160 male surgical patients admitted to one ward in each of four different hospitals. Patients were surveyed either on the day of admission or on the following day. The aim of this study was to attempt to relate patient anxiety on admission to the admission procedure, patient knowledge of the hospital environment, diagnosis, etc. and patient opinion of nursing care. Anxiety was measured by the Cattell IPAT questionnaire which uses a rather global measure of anxiety, obscuring differences between trait and state anxiety. One of the most significant findings of the study was the relatively high average level of patient anxiety in comparison with published norms for the population as a whole. One-fifth of the patients recorded an anxiety level which was greater than that of patients attending an adult guidance centre. Patients were also asked to state how worried they had been about coming into hospital and the results correlated well with the anxiety scores. From the point of view of the CPT model of stress and coping the reasons people gave for their worry or lack of it are interesting.

Firstly, the reasons for not worrying were given as:

- Being tired of being ill and wanting to get it over with
- Being not the sort of person who worries
- Their illness was not serious
- Confidence in the hospital or doctor
- Knowing what to expect

Reasons for worrying were given as:

- Not knowing what to expect
- Worry about the operation and its outcome
- Worries about the anaesthetic
- Worry about their families
- A general dislike of hospitals

A further important finding was that 50% of patients who had received less than 4 days' notice of their admission to hospital complained. Franklin recommends that at least 6 days' notice of admission is required to allow business and personal arrangements to be made. A large majority of patients had found the pre-admission booklet helpful. This contained information about the hospital.

There was a suggestion of an inverse relationship between the quality of nursing care as rated by the patients and patient anxiety. That is to say that the more satisfactory the nursing care was seen to be by patient, the lower the anxiety they reported.

This study and others suggest that the way in which a patient is admitted to hospital can affect the way in which the patient reacts to admission. In particular the person admitting the patient can carry out their role in such a way as to reduce the threat appraised by patients. This person is usually a member of nursing staff and several studies by nurses have investigated the effects of the style of approach during admission upon patients.

One study carried out by Wong (1979) failed to include any control group. She attempted to evaluate a personalized admission procedure. A patient welfare inventory was completed by patients at home before admission and again after the admission procedure. Physiological indicators of anxiety (temperature, pulse, respiration and blood pressure) were recorded during the admission procedure and two hours later. The patients' perception of the admitting nurse was also evaluated. An improvement in the physiological variables was found between the pre- and post-admission recordings and similarly on the patient welfare inventory. The admitting nurses were given a positive rating. According to Wong this showed the effectiveness of the personalized approach. In the absence of any data from a control group of patients this claim is unsubstantiated however.

A more rigorous (and earlier) study had been carried out by Anderson *et al.* (1965). In this study a control group of patients was admitted to hospital in the normal way whilst the intervention group was admitted using a patient-centred nursing-process approach. Patients were randomly assigned to the control or intervention condition. However, the study sample was small, comprising 22 patients admitted as medical emergencies and 22 women admitted to a large state mental institution. Indicators of the effectiveness of the admission procedure were the patients' behaviour as recorded by process recording, the systolic blood pressure and the pulse rate.

Each measure used showed the greater effectiveness of the patient-centred admission procedure, but the difference between the intervention group and the control was greater for the medical patients than for the group being admitted to the mental institution.

A more refined study in which the special attention given to the inter-vention group was controlled for was carried out by Elms and Leonard (1966). The total study population comprised 75 patients admitted for elective gynaecological surgery. These were assigned to one of three groups. Group 1 was admitted by one of the researchers using an individualized approach in which an assessment of their individual needs was made. Group 2 was admitted in the normal way by the researcher and Group 3 was admitted as usual by a member of the hospital staff. The effectiveness of the individualized approach was shown by the lower average pulse and respiration rates of group one patients after admission. Patients were interviewed 'blind' by the other researcher about their knowledge and feelings. These subjective measures also demonstrated the effectiveness of the individual approach.

These studies are important for nursing since they point to the role which nursing can play in reducing in degree any threat perceived by the patient on being admitted to hospital. In particular, these studies suggest that it is attention to the emotional experience of the patient which is important and that whilst giving factual information is useful, the personal approach means identifying those patients who reveal greater than normal anxiety and encouraging them to express their anxiety so that the source can be identified and addressed on an individual basis. Unfortunately in spite of the evidence, admitting a patient to hospital is still frequently seen as a routine procedure.

Franklin (1974) suggests that

> The impression given . . . by the author's experience on the wards, was that nursing staff rarely recognise anxiety as an important problem and that therapeutic discussion directed at anxiety relief is nearly non-existent. Patients who were worried remarked either that they did not discuss their worries with anyone, or that these discussions were with relatives and never with hospital staff. It is likely that with a little encouragement patients would be prepared to discuss their problems openly and previous studies have shown that such discussion can be beneficial.

Franklin's study points to the conclusion that information alone is not sufficient to relieve anxiety. However it also supported the case that information is necessary since patients had found the hospital booklets helpful. Information which patients need comes under the following headings (Baderman *et al.*, 1973).

(a) Information about the admission procedure so that they can be safely settled in hospital with the minimum delay or embarrassment.
(b) Information about the domestic details of ward life so that there will be no doubts or surprises to unsettle them.
(c) They should be informed about the different kinds of staff and services available to help them.
(d) Information about how best to obtain information from and communicate with the hospital staff.

Information needs of patients

This perspective emphasizes the information required by the patient on admission, but a large volume of research dating from the early 1960s points to the patients' needs for information throughout their hospital stay and beyond. An example of such research is that by Cartwright and Anderson (1981) who found that 31% of in-patients were dissatisfied with the information which they received about the progress of their illness. Patients' dissatisfaction with information is the most commonly mentioned item in satisfaction studies (Locker and Dunt, 1978).

One of the problems of research to identify patient satisfaction/dissatisfaction is to ensure that patients are willing to express their dissatisfactions whilst in hospital, since they feel that this is to criticize the staff. So much of the research probably underestimates its extent. A study in which dissatisfaction with information was explored in a post-discharge interview was carried out in Sweden by Engström (1984). This showed high levels of expressed dissatisfaction after discharge in spite of the fact that patients and staff knew the purpose of the study during the hospital stay. The sample comprised 120 patients who had been in surgical, medical and neurological wards in a university hospital.

Results showed that:

- 51% were dissatisfied with information about their progress
- 49% were dissatisfied with information about what the physician did during the medical examination and why he did it
- 48% were dissatisfied with information about their medications
- 47% were dissatisfied with diagnostic information
- 39% were dissatisfied with information about the ward routine
- 34% claimed to have had no information about routines, departmental facilities and equipment.

Most of the information about which patients were dissatisfied comes into the category of medical information. All was of great importance to patient welfare.

A study carried out by a medical student in the UK (Reynolds, 1978) focused upon patients' need for information from the medical staff: 100 patients on four surgical wards were interviewed. Patients' diagnoses were diverse, ranging from haemorrhoids to carcinoma. Patients were included in the study only if they had undergone at least one investigation.

The conduct of medical ward rounds provoked heavy criticism. Patients disliked being excluded from the conversation and the incomprehensible medical jargon. They wished to know the results of investigations but frequently had not been told them. Whilst patients did not like to ask about these, doctors expected them to ask if they wanted to know (10% of the patients interviewed wished to know little or nothing). Only 18/100 patients knew the result of their chest X-ray and many of the others worried unnecessarily about the results. In general, the fear of the unknown was the major problem for these patients.

The problem with lack of information is that it leaves the patient in a state of uncertainty. From the point of view of stress and coping it leaves the patient feeling threatened but unable to identify the threat except in the most general terms and thus unable to identify coping strategies (Clarke, 1984). Patients may also fear something worse than the reality since they attribute motives of the presence of a very serious illness when medical staff are reluctant to give them information.

A recent study by Mishel (1984) was based on the premise that uncertainty and stress are very closely associated with one another.

Uncertainty was predicted to occur in association with four classes of events:

(a) discomfort, incapacitation and other symptoms of illness;
(b) management of special treatment procedures and their side effects;
(c) technical environments including relating with medical and other health-care providers;
(d) assessment of the future and reassessing independence.

Mishel claimed that uncertainty in these areas hampers the task of recognition and classification and a cognitive structure of events is not formed, limiting severely the ability both to appraise and to cope. A total of 100 medical patients participated in the study when they had been in hospital for a minimum of 3 days. They completed several scales on one occasion between days 3 and 5 after admission. The scales used were: the Mishel Uncertainty in Illness Scale; the Volicer Hospital Stress Rating Scale and a seriousness of illness rating scale (Threat of Serious Illness Scale).

Results showed a strong relationship between uncertainty and stress. This suggested that it was vagueness and lack of information about events that accounted for their evaluation as being stressful rather than the events themselves. The Threat of Serious Illness Scale was found to have a curvilinear relationship with the uncertainty scale. This was interpreted by the author as meaning that moderate to highly uncertain events allowed the perception that the illness was not as serious as the patients feared. However as the actual seriousness of the illness increased uncertainty could not be maintained and stress occurred.

Potentially this is an important study because it shows a rationale for the small number of patients who prefer not to receive information in hospital. It is worth reiterating an interpretation of the findings, i.e. uncertainty is strongly associated with stress when the uncertainty leads to fear or appraisal that the event is more threatening than it actually is in reality. However when the event is indeed severely threatening, uncertainty is the more reassuring state.

The relationship between stress and being in hospital has been explored by Volicer and co-researchers in a programme of research during the 1970s. Patients in hospital and members of the public not in hospital at the time were asked to rate and rank the degree of stress associated with items describing events or potential events in hospital. As a result a 49-item Hospital Stress Rating Scale (Volicer and Bohannon, 1975) has been produced which can be used to identify a 'stress' score for patients as in the Mishel (1984) study above.

There has been a fair amount of consensus about the 'stress rating' of the items on the scale and some are of great interest since they suggest that uncertainty, worry, loss and lack of information are potent sources of stress.

Items which score highly as stressors are:

	Rank
Thinking you may lose your sight	1
Thinking you might have cancer	2
Thinking you might lose a kidney or some other organ	3
Knowing you have a serious illness	4
Thinking you might lose your hearing	5
Not being told what your diagnosis is	6
Not knowing for sure what illness you have	7
Not getting pain medication when you need it	8
Not knowing the results of or reasons for your treatments	9

'Not having your questions answered by staff' was ranked 13 and 'Not knowing when to expect things will be done to you' was ranked 25.

From this scale it is possible to see how important information is to patients. It provides further evidence of the link between uncertainty and stress.

Wilson-Barnett (1976) carried out a study in which she identified patients' emotional responses to a number of frequently occurring events: 200 medical patients were interviewed using a checklist of items, and were allowed to make free responses. These were later coded as indicating positive or negative emotional reactions. Items giving a negative response most frequently were:

- Using the bed-pan
- Anticipating that a treatment or procedure is likely to be painful
- Seeing another patient who is very ill
- Leaving your usual work whilst in hospital
- Being away from the family
- Your own condition or illness.

Among the items most frequently eliciting a response classified as positive were:

- Talking to staff nurses
- Talking to student nurses
- Talking to your visitors

- Sister's round when she comes on duty
- Talking to your consultant
- Talking to your junior doctor

This suggests that the opportunity for interaction with staff was not only highly valued but was highly reassuring, confirming the view that this is an important component of nursing care.

Wilson-Barnett and Carrigy (1978) also carried out the study which has already been referred to, to monitor anxiety and depression scores during a hospital stay. They found that patients with diagnoses of neoplastic or infective illness or who were undiagnosed tended to have higher scores on anxiety and depression than other patients, strengthening the evidence for a relationship between seriousness of threat, uncertainty and stress. It will also be recalled that this study showed that anxiety levels tended to be high on the day of a special test, and it is to the impact on patients of special tests and procedures that we now turn.

Information and the experience of tests and treatment procedures

Several pieces of research have been carried out to evaluate the effect of giving patients information about tests and procedures before they are carried out. Wilson-Barnett (1978) herself carried out a study of this kind using a schedule of information about barium X-rays. Patients were assigned to a control or experimental group. The control group received interaction from the researcher of a non-informative kind for the length of time it took to give the planned information to the experimental patients. Measures of the effectiveness of the information were collected by a second individual who did not know which patients had received information and which interaction alone. The EPI (Eysenck Personality Inventory) was used on one occasion only to identify those patients exhibiting high trait anxiety. Monitoring of the patients' emotional reactions to the test was carried out by using the Mood Adjective Check List on four occasions.

Amongst those patients undergoing a barium meal the informed group showed lower anxiety than the control group immediately after the X-ray. However by far the more dramatic difference between the informed patients and the controls was shown after patients had undergone barium enema, the more disturbing of the two procedures. This supports the view that the more distressing the procedure is likely to be the more important is the giving of information.

A programme of research has been carried out by Johnson and co-workers to investigate the effectiveness of what she calls sensory information. This is information given to patients before a procedure, about the sensations they are likely to experience during the time the procedure is being carried out and afterwards. She has investigated this in relation to investigations, treatments and pre- and post-operative care. The work in relation to surgery will be discussed in Chapter 8, but a discussion of the work on procedures which medical patients may undergo is included here.

Nurses are taught to give patients information before a procedure is carried out but this is usually interpreted as an instruction to tell patients what the staff are going to do and the reasons for it. This has been called procedural information within the literature (see for example Newman 1984 and Mathews and Ridgeway, 1984). Procedural information is a description of the procedure from the staff's point of view, and can be contrasted with sensory information which is information presented from the point of view of the patients, preparing them for what they will experience during the procedure. Thus sensory information is carefully designed to meet the patients' needs.

Johnson (1973) tested the hypothesis that sensory information was more effective than procedural information in a laboratory study of the ischaemic pain brought about by an inflated blood pressure cuff around the upper arm. Male subjects were given either sensory information or procedural information before the procedure. The effect of the information was estimated by the use of an analogue scale to mark the degree of distress and unpleasant sensation experienced. Subjects who had received the sensory information consistently reported less distress than those subjects who had received procedural information.

Since that study Johnson has investigated the effectiveness of sensory information in real life settings and shown its usefulness before gastro-endoscopy, orthopaedic cast removal among children (in Britain we would term this the removal of plaster of Paris) and pelvic examination.

Results from this research have been convincing enough for a volume of the Conduct and Utilization of Nursing (CURN) (1981) project to be devoted to 'Distress reduction through sensory preparation' based on Johnson's work. In this book guidelines for translating research findings into nursing practice are given. Principles are listed for the development of sensory information protocols. These are shown in Table 7.1 and the guidelines indicated have been compiled from the many publications related to sensory information.

Johnson (1983) considers that sensory information is useful in influencing 'the structure of a cognitive map or image of the impending experience' which

> provides a structure for predicting and monitoring the unfamiliar experience ... As in any familiar situation, the individual relies on previously learned skills and techniques to conduct transactions with the environment. The map-like image provides a structure for processing the stimuli encountered and allows the individual to respond as if in a familiar environment.

Table 7.1   Guidelines for Development of Sensory Information Messages

1. Identify the steps of the procedure.*
2. List what you perceive would have a sensory effect on patients – whatever relates to seeing, touching, smelling, tasting, hearing.*
3. Ask present patients for their perceptions. For example: How did you feel during the procedure? What did the speculum feel like? What did the tube feel like? How did it feel when the doctor was poking on your back before he put the needle in? How did it feel when the needle penetrated your skin? How did it feel when you were placed in that position? Was the table cold?*
4. Select the typical sensory experiences described by 50 or 60% of the patients.*
5. Choose several words to describe the sensations.*
6. Use the patients' words.*
7. Hit the high points – the things that almost everybody perceives.*
8. Use the word 'pain' sparingly. Some procedures cause discomfort, but patients may not describe them as painful. Taking a cast off is not painful. The endoscopy patients did not describe the procedure as painful.*
9. Although the focus of the content is upon *sensations* that patients are likely to experience, the message should also include the procedural information that is usually given.
10. The message should be personalized by using personal pronouns.
11. The described sensations should be presented in the sequence that they will most likely be experienced.
12. When recording, a non-threatening voice should be used. A woman's voice was used in the original studies.
13. A tape should be approximately 6 or 7 minutes in length for adults. Tapes for children should be approximately 2½ minutes in length.
14. If tapes are to be used, it will be convenient to have several copies available. All tapes should be copied from an original to ensure consistency in presentation.
15. Use aids when feasible. For example, in the cast removal study, a recording of the sound of the saw was used. Printed and audiovisual materials may be appropriate.*

Cautions
1. Don't try to describe how severe the 'pain' might be or how much sensation might be felt.*
2. Don't think sensory information can substitute for procedural information or instruction in exercises, ambulation, relaxation, or other patient activities. Information about sensations complements other instruction.*
3. Don't describe sensations that patients only rarely associate with a procedure.*
4. Don't tell patients that the sensory information you are giving them is meant to reduce distress.*
5. Don't try to teach patients how to cope with the threatening event. You teach the sensory information, and that, in turn, will have the effect of helping them cope with the experience.*
6. Remember that the tape does not relieve the nurse of teaching responsibility. Reinforce teaching with personal contact and an opportunity for patients to ask questions and clarify misunderstandings.

From Distress Reduction Through Sensory Preparation, *CURN Project (1981) Grune and Stratton, New York, N.Y.*
*Cited with permission from How to Include Sensory Information in Your Patient Teaching, *RN (1977), 40, 53–4.*

She goes on to suggest that the use of the image may be reducing the amount of effort used in worrying and organizing new experiences into a meaningful context.

Giving information is a form of teaching patients and as such, different methods of presentation of the information may be used. A study in which a film-tape of information was used to inform patients about the procedure of passing a naso-gastric tube was reported by Pallidla *et al.* (1981).

The objective of the study was to evaluate the effectiveness of various types of information content in reducing the distress felt by patients having a naso-gastric tube passed. These authors argue that information reduces the threat of the procedure and increases patients' feelings of control. They also argue that correspondence of feelings experienced during the procedure with the information previously given increases the individual's feelings of the predictability of events.

In Pallidla's study, 50 patients were randomly assigned to one of four groups, each group receiving different information. Group 1 was given procedural information only; Group 2 was given procedural and sensory information; Group 3 was given procedural information and information about coping behaviour which would increase comfort and Group 4 was given all three types of information. Patients were also asked the extent to which they preferred to have personal control in new situations.

Visual analogue scales were used by the patients before, during and after the intubation to identify their experience of pain, discomfort and anxiety. The filmstrip used for Group 4 which combined all three types of information was associated with the lowest levels of experienced distress, pain and discomfort and anxiety. This suggests that a filmstrip is an acceptable and effective way of giving information to patients and that the more information a patient is given, the more effective it is likely to be.

In addition to a considerable literature on the effect of giving patients information in helping them to cope with experiences within hospital there is also evidence for the importance of social support in helping patients to cope with emotional reactions in particular (Wilson-Barnett and Fordham, 1982).

Nuckalls *et al.* (1972) found that a meaningful and close supportive relationship mediated the effect of stress.

A recent study which explored the importance of social support was carried out by Ahmadi (1985). A total of 100 medical patients in two similar units were studied. The Volicer Hospital Stress Rating Scale revealed high stress scores among the sample. These were higher for Black patients than for White, particularly on those items relating to the hospital environment and staff–patient interaction. Results did reveal a positive relationship between having supportive family and friends and overall satisfaction as well as lower stress scores. There was also a relationship between the supportiveness of other patients and lower levels of stress. However, the author cautiously suggests that this needs further research to identify the direction of causality, since it

could be that those with lower levels of stress are more pleasant in their interactions and thus attract more social support.

So far in this chapter we have concentrated upon the aspects of the hospital
environment which are associated with distress and negative emotional
response amongst patients, together with an account of some of the strategies
which staff can use to reduce the degree of threat appraised by patients or to
improve patients' ability to cope. Discussion has centred on the more psychosocial strategies since these are aspects to which staff are least likely to give
attention. It should be remembered, though, that pain is a powerful stressor,
as is infection. The best psycho-social strategies may be undermined if
unnecessary pain is caused during a procedure through poor technique, or if
infection is caused through carelessness with asepsis. Thus competence and
attention to detail in physical aspects of care cannot be neglected. In
particular, adequate pain relief is crucial to the prevention of distress and
adverse emotions (see McCaffery, 1979).

The primary aim in admitting a patient to hospital is to ensure recovery or
symptom relief. 'Failure to cope with illness is synonymous with a reduction
in all the potential contributions and co-operation for the recovery process'
(Wilson-Barnett and Fordham, 1982). Thus the aim of distress reduction is not
only humanitarian but also, by helping the patient to cope, ensures a speedy
recovery.

7.2 DISCHARGE FROM HOSPITAL AND RECOVERY

Throughout a patient's stay in hospital the goal is that of helping him or her
into a condition where they can return home. From a common sense point of
view it seems that this is what patients want too, above all else, and therefore,
discharge from hospital will be unproblematic.

However, this is not always the case and discharge from hospital may be
stressful. Wilson-Barnett and Carrigy (1978) in their monitoring of patients'
emotional reactions throughout the hospital stay found that patients were not
always delighted to be going home. Whilst in one of the study hospitals the
average anxiety and depression scores were low on the day of discharge, this
was not the case for the other hospital. Several patients experienced negative
reactions for a number of reasons. Examples were worry about the arrangements for the journey and worry about coping at home with little or no
assistance. Some felt the goal of the hospital admission in terms of treatment
or identification of their health problems had not been met. Many patients
were unhappy about the short notice of discharge.

That notice of discharge from hospital may be very short has been
confirmed in other studies. For example, Gay and Pitkeathley (1979) investigated 124 patients discharged from acute hospitals of whom 37% complained

that not enough warning of discharge had been given and that there was a lack of services following discharge. In Scotland, Buchanan (1979) investigated the length of notice of discharge given to patients over the age of 70 years. Among those discharged from medical wards (as opposed to wards for the care of the elderly) 36% had been given less than 3 days' notice of discharge. In Skeet's (1970) large-scale study of patients' coping at home after discharge from hospital, she found that 17% of her sample had had 3 days' warning of discharge, 34% had had 2 days' warning, and 37% had had notice of only 24 hours or less. Interviewers noted that some elderly patients were agitated by the short notice given. Similarly worrying results were reported by Roberts (1975). She found that of her sample of 164 patients, 20% had been informed of the discharge on the day it happened, 36% were warned 1 day before and 21% had been given 2 days' warning.

These findings are a cause for concern. From the point of view of stress and coping the return home after a period of hospitalization demands not only physical organization but psychological adjustment to a new situation. The patient needs time to get used to the idea and to develop coping strategies.

Few people are completely fit on discharge home. This is increasingly the case due to pressure on hospital beds and the fact that in the present day sending patients for convalescence is the exception rather than the rule.

How patients will cope on return home will depend upon many factors, among which are:

(a) personality factors and how well the illness and the period in hospital have been coped with;
(b) how well patients have been prepared for discharge;
(c) the degree of adjustment to loss and/or disability and the amount of relearning required for functional independence;
(d) support and help from family and friends, how appropriate are the arrangements for continuity of care and how well they work in practice.

Factors which may interfere with or facilitate a patient's recovery

The relationship between stress, coping and rehabilitation is still relatively under-researched. Nonetheless some relationships have been established. Additional stress to that arising from the illness, if it occurs during the illness or recovery period is likely to interfere with recovery (Mayou et al., 1978). Feelings of helplessness, uncertainty and depression have been shown to be associated with a poor physical recovery (Viney and Westbrook, 1982; Viney et al., 1985). A slower recovery has been shown among patients with a high score on trait depression (Cohen and Lazarus, 1983). It is likely also that those patients who respond to hospital admission with high anxiety will also respond to discharge in the same way although there is conflicting evidence about the effect this has on recovery (Cohen and Lazarus, 1983).

Factors which seem to be positively associated with recovery are a positive self image (Rutter, 1978), taking a positive and active role in rehabilitation (Naismith *et al.*, 1979; Cohen and Lazarus, 1983), and having an accurate perception of the prognosis (Rosillo and Fogel, 1970).

Preparation for discharge

It is a truism, only too infrequently followed through in practice, that preparation for discharge should begin when the patient is admitted to hospital. Whatever the practice, in theory the term 'discharge' (Armitage, 1981) should not be

> regarded as a single event when the patient leaves hospital but as a stage in patient care situated towards one end of a continuum which has both a period of preparation and from which there are consequences. Discharge cannot effectively be examined in isolation from what has gone before. If patient care is to be regarded as continuous between hospital and community, then it also cannot be separated from what follows after the event when the patient leaves hospital.

Armitage goes on to say that 'It is difficult for those involved in any one stage of patient care to see the whole of it'. This is borne out by a hospital staff nurse quoted in Gay and Pitkeathley (1979): 'Actually you only see the patient in bed – you don't think of them in their kitchen or driving or anything else'.

The person, of course, who experiences all stages is the patient and it is the patient (or family and friends) who must play the co-ordinating role in care when once they have said goodbye to the hospital and its 24-hour provision of care, since however good the services laid on in the community by statutory or voluntary authorities, they will fall short of a 24-hour service. There is evidence, moreover, that the services provided may well fall short of what is needed. Hockey (1966) found that district nurses spent surprisingly little time in the nursing care of patients; they frequently had insufficient information and had little contact with hospital nurses. In Hockey's study of 1968 she concluded that the majority of simple nursing and household tasks were being shouldered by the family and the patient.

In the light of this it is very important to use a perspective that it is the patient who will be the co-ordinator of care and indeed the person responsible for care on leaving hospital if continuity is to be ensured. Thus throughout the patients' stay in hospital they will need information and teaching about their illness, treatment and care. By this means they can play their full role in recovery on discharge, and can cope more effectively on discharge.

Areas of patient education which are important include the following:

- Details of medication
- Special diets
- Obtaining supplies of dressings, drugs etc.
- Behaviour changes for healthy living
- How to cope with a colostomy or ileostomy, for example
- Appliances and prostheses
- Advice on pain and its management
- Information on the effects of treatment

The importance of this is underlined by a report made to Ferguson (1961) in a study of discharge, that 10% of all admissions to hospital were due to patients' failure to cope at home through lack of understanding and adherence to medications. It follows that there is a real danger of readmission to hospital if a patient fails to cope at home due to lack of compliance with continuing treatment.

Within the general areas of teaching mentioned above will be included the reasons for procedures, as well as instruction and supervised practice.

In marked contrast to Skeet's (1970) finding that the most frequent advice given to patients on leaving hospital was 'Don't do too much' and 'Take care of yourself', is Raphael's (1978) finding that patients expressed the wish to know precisely which activities they can perform and which they cannot.

The importance of such information is evident when it is seen that loss of strength due to inactivity is liable to affect all patients to some extent (Wilson-Barnett and Fordham, 1982). If inactivity has been prolonged the problem of muscular weakness may be aggravated by stiffening of joints due to shortening of soft tissue or the laying down of connective tissue within joints. Thus the importance of activity must be taught alongside information about which activities to avoid and when they may be resumed. Methods of lifting to cause least strain should also be taught. Increasing development of strength due to their own efforts is rewarding to patients, giving them a sense of achievement and control.

Another important area of information required by the patient being discharged can be deduced and extrapolated from the literature relating to hospital and surgery, i.e. the patient requires sensory information about how he or she will feel during convalescence and recovery. We know that most patients suffer feelings of tiredness, spells of boredom, mood changes, and spells of weepiness. Many suffer sleeplessness. They need to be told this so that they are prepared for it and not worried that something has gone wrong if it occurs. Any persisting symptoms should also be prepared for by explanation. For example, Wilson-Barnett (1981) found that patients experienced pain in the sternotomy site for up to a year following coronary artery bypass operation. We need research of this kind for other conditions so that we can pass such information on to other patients. However ex-patients may be able to help others directly through self-help groups. Thus, giving patients information about the existence of such groups and how to contact them is very useful.

Patient teaching during the period in hospital prepares the patient for coping on leaving hospital. It thus helps to strengthen coping, reducing the likelihood of stress occurring during recovery and thus delaying recovery.

The degree of re-adjustment required

Unfortunately not all patients are restored to their former level of health as a result of treatment in hospital. A period in hospital may be just one of many such admissions during the course of a chronic illness. Seemingly dramatic, one-off operations such as lower limb amputation are more likely in practice to be the latest in a series of such operations which started with toe amputation (Crowther, 1982).

The illness itself or the treatment may have resulted in the loss of some part of the body structure or an organ, e.g. mastectomy. As a result the demands made on the patient in the recovery period include coping with such loss. A grieving process has been described (Parkes, 1972) and going through this process is a form of coping, which may lead to re-adjustment to the new circumstances of life.

For some patients, loss or change in physiological or behavioural functioning means that normal activities of daily living, far from being routine, now pose major problems and effort must be expended in re-learning skills which contribute to functional independence, although for some they may never actually be achieved. Examples are patients who have had a stroke and who may have to re-learn how to move around within the home, or how to balance, whilst carrying out activities such as dressing, cooking and washing up. For patients who have developed diabetes mellitus, normal activities may be hampered initially by the need to calculate dietary components, test urine, monitor activity levels etc.

The problems of coping with a new life style may leave patients vulnerable to stress from demands they would once have coped with easily. Social support and practical help may make the crucial difference between the ability to cope at home and the need for re-admission to hospital.

Arrangements for continuity of care

In a study of stress amongst the families of children with chronic illness, Harrisson (1977) found that the need for long-term treatment, lack of communication, problems of finance and occupation and the absence of supportive services were identified as stress-provoking factors. She claims that these stress factors, not only apply in any illness but at any age.

The importance of social support can best be illustrated by a quote from a patient taken from the book by Gay and Pitkeathley (1979).

> A few years ago I came out of hospital after major surgery in Portsmouth. It took a long time to recover even though that operation wasn't as big as the one I've just had. Having people interested in you acts like a tonic. That time no one outside the family cared a damn whether I lived or died. It makes a difference to the way you recover, and how quickly, if you feel outsiders care. Somehow you make an effort. I know it sounds funny, but you make an effort so when they come in to ask how you are for the sixth or seventh time you say 'Yes, I'm getting on famously' even if you don't feel up to much. And saying that makes you feel just a tiny bit better somehow.

The study by Wilson-Barnett and Carrigy (1978) showed that at discharge some patients worried that they would be unable to cope at home without help. That their worry is justified is confirmed in the study by Skeet (1970) in which 533 patients who had been recently discharged from hospital were surveyed. She found that double the number of community services had been called upon within 2 weeks of discharge compared with the number arranged by the hospital staff at the time of discharge. She also found that 45% of the newly discharged patients were not receiving the nursing they needed. Nearly one-third of the sample had required help with personal care on first returning home and 6% still needed it some 8 weeks later. Almost all patients relied on families and friends for care. Therefore it can be seen what problems may be created for discharged patients who live alone with no relatives at hand. Gay and Pitkeathley (1979) suggest that voluntary services can fulfil some of these needs.

Roberts (1975) found that some of the patients in her sample of 164 who had recently left hospital were unable to carry out some activities without help, although they were judged by the researcher to be physically capable of doing so. This inability was attributed to the individual's perceptions influenced by their experience of dependence in the past, personality etc. Activities which gave this sample the most problems were cleaning, preparing meals and laundry, suggesting that volunteers could be of considerable help to patients in coping after discharge.

Whenever an individual is to any extent handicapped in his capacity to look after his own daily needs he becomes dependent upon other people to supply help. When there is no caring and competent relative or friend at hand, and no acceptable substitute, the adverse consequences of dependence may be only trivial personal discomfort. At the other extreme, they can entail high risk of physical deterioration or damage. For instance, without suitable nourishment or adequate warmth a person must eventually suffer progressive impairment of bodily functions whilst attempting, if he can to fend for himself in spite of, or in ignorance of, any risk to his health or safety. Obtaining the right help in such circumstances is a practical problem for anyone sufficiently disabled to be dependent upon others and often, also for members of his household or circle of friends whose resources of strength, skill, time and goodwill do not meet the evident demands of the situation. Adequate solution of the problem requires practical planning and the recruit-ment of appropriate human or mechanical assistance, It cannot always be achieved without the intervention of some health service, local authority or voluntary agency (Roberts, 1975).

7.3 SUMMARY

In this chapter the experiences of patients during admission to hospital have been discussed. The relationship between stress and negatively toned emotions has been explored. In general measures of emotional states have been used in research studies as operational indicators of stress experienced by patients and as outcome measures of interaction designed to prevent or alleviate stress. The difference between trait and state anxiety is crucial in such research. Evidence suggests that an individualized approach to admitting a patient to hospital can modify anxiety on admission. Patients' experiences occurring in hospital and which arouse negative emotions have been explored in some research studies which have been quoted. In particular the experience of undergoing a special test is a crucial one for patients. The importance of giving patients information in helping them to cope with demand has been explored. In particular the importance of giving sensory information is supported by research showing improved outcomes following such information.

Finally the importance of teaching and planning for discharge, and of continuity of care has been discussed in relation to patient recovery.

REFERENCES

Ahmadi, K. S. (1985) The experience of being hospitalised: stress, social support and satisfaction, *Int. J. Nurs. Stud.*, **22**(2), 137–48.

Anderson, B. J., Mertz, H. and Leonard, R. C. (1965) Two experimental tests of a patient centred admission process, *Nursing Research*, **14**(2), 151–7.

Armitage, S. K. (1981) Negotiating the discharge of medical patients, *J. Advanced Nursing*, **6**, 385–9.

Baderman, H., Corless, C., Fairey, J. M., Modell, M. and Ramsden, Y. (1973) *Admission of Patients to Hospital*, King Edward's Hospital Fund for London.

Buchanan, A. (1979) *A Study of the Liaison Nursing Service: Elderly Patients Discharged Home From Hospital in One Area Health Board 1976–78*, Greater Glasgow Health Board, Glasgow.

Cartwright, A. and Anderson, R. (1981) *General Practice Revisited: A Second Study of Patients and Their Doctors*, Tavistock Publications, London.

Clarke, M. (1984) Stress and coping: Constructs for nursing, *J. Advanced Nursing*, **9**(1), 3–13.

Cohen, F. and Lazarus, R. S. (1983) Coping and adaptation in health and illness, in *Handbook of Health, Health Care and the Health Professions* (ed. D. Mechanic), Free Press, New York, N.Y.

Coser, R. L. (1962) *Life in the Ward*, Michigan State University Press, MI.

Crowther, H. (1982) New perspectives on nursing lower limb amputees, *J. Advanced Nursing*, **7**(5), 453–60.

Elms, R. R. and Leonard, R. C. (1966) Effects of nursing approaches during admission. *Nursing Research*, **15**(1), 39–48.

Engström, B. (1984) The patient's need for information during hospital stay, *Int. J. Nurs. Stud.*, **21**(2), 113–31.

Eysenck, S. B. and Eysenck, H. J. (1972) The questionnaire measurement of psychoticism, *Psychol. Med.*, **2**, 50–5.

Ferguson, T. (1961) Aftercare of the hospitalised patient, *Brit. Med. J.*, **1**, 1242–4.

Franklin, B. L. (1974) *Patient Anxiety on Admission to Hospital*, RCN, London.

Gay, P. and Pitkeathley, J. (1979) *When I Went Home . . .*, King Edward's Hospital Fund for London.

Harrisson, S. (1977) *Families in Stress*, RCN, London.

Hockey, L. (1966) *Feeling the Pulse: A Study of District Nursing in Six Areas*, QIDN, London.

Horsley, J. A., Crane, J., Reynolds, M. A. and Haller, K. B. (1981) *Distress Reduction Through Sensory Preparation*, CURN Project, Grune and Stratton, New York, N.Y.

Johnson, J. E. (1973) Effects of accurate expectations about sensations on the sensory and distress components of pain, *J. Pers. Soc. Psych.*, **29**, 710–18.

Johnson, J. E. (1983) Preparing patients to cope with stress, in *Patient Teaching*, (ed. J. Wilson-Barnett), Churchill-Livingstone, Edinburgh, pp. 19–33.

Karsh, E. B. (1970) Fixation produced by conflict, *Science*, **168**, 873–5.

Kornfield, D. S. (1979) The Hospital environment and its impact upon the patient, in *Stress and Survival* (ed. Charles A. Garfield), pp. 154–61, Mosby, St Louis, MO.

Lazarus, R. S. and Launier, R. (1978) Stress-related transactions between person and environment, in *Perspectives of Interactional Psychology* (eds L. A. Pervis and M. Lewis), Plenum Press, New York, N.Y., pp. 287–327.

Ley, P. and Spelman, M. (1967) *Communicating with the Patient*, Staples Press, St Albans.

Locker, D. and Dunt, D. (1978) Theoretical and methodological issues in sociological studies of consumer satisfaction with medical care, *Soc. Science Medicine*, **12**(4), 283–92.

McCaffery, M. (1979) *Nursing Management of the Patient with Pain*, (2nd edn), Lippincott, PA.

Mathews, A. and Ridgeway, V. (1984) Psychological preparation for surgery, in *Health Care and Human Behaviour* (eds A. Steptoe and A. Mathews), Academic Press, London, pp. 231–62.

Mayou, R., Costa, A. and Williamson B. (1978) Psycho-social adjustment in patients one year after myocardial infarction, in *J. Psychometric Res.*, **22**, 447–53.

Mishel, M. H. (1984) Perceived uncertainty and stress in illness, *Research in Nursing and Health*, **7**, 163–71.

Naismith, L. D., Robinson, J. F., Shaw, G. B. and MacIntyre, M. M. (1979) Psychological rehabilitation after myocardial infarction, *Brit. Med. J.*, **1**, 439–41.

Newman, S. (1984) Anxiety, hospitalization and surgery, in *The Experience of Illness* (eds J. Fitzpatrick, S. Hinton, G. Newman, J. Scambler, J. Thompson), Tavistock Publications, London.

Nuckalls, L. B., Cassel, J. and Kaplan, B. H. (1972) Psychosocial assets, life crises and the prognosis of progress, *Amer. J. Epidemiology*, **95**, 431–44.

Pallidla, G. V., Grant, M. M., Rains, B. C., Hanson, B. C., Bergtrom, N., Wong, H. L., Hanson, R. and Kubo W. (1981) Distress reduction and the effect of preparatory teaching films and patient control, *Research in Nursing and Health*, **4**, 375–87.

Parkes, C. M. (1972) Components of the reaction to loss of a limb, spouse or home, *J. Psychosomatic Research*, **16**, 343–9.

Raphael, B. (1978) Psychiatric aspects of hysterectomy, in *Modern Perspectives in the Psychiatric Aspects of Surgery* (ed. J. G. Howells), Macmillan, London.

Reynolds, M. (1978) No news is bad news: patients' views about communication in hospital, *Brit. Med. J.*, **1**, 1673–6.

Roberts, I. (1975) *Discharged from Hospital*, RCN, London.

Rosillo, R. H. and Fogel, M. L. (1970) Correlation of psychologic variables and progress in physical rehabilitation. 1. Degree of disability and denial of illness, *Archives of Physical Medicine and Rehabilitation*, **51**, 227–32.

Rutter, B. M. (1978) *Psychological Aspects of Chronic Bronchitis*, PhD Thesis, University of London.

Skeet, M. (1970) *Home From Hospital*, Dan Mason Nursing Research Committee; reprinted by Macmillan Journals Ltd., London.

Spielberger, C. (1979) *Understanding Stress and Anxiety*, Harper and Row, London, pp. 76–7.

Viney, L. L. and Westbrook, M. T. (1982) Psychological reactions to chronic illness-related disability as a function of its severity and type, *J. Psychosomatic Med.*, **35**, 513–23.

Viney, L. L., Clarke, A. M., Bunn, T. A. and Bonjamin, Y. (1985) An evaluation of three crisis intervention programmes for general hospital patients, *Brit. J. Med. Psych.*, 75–86.

Volicer, J. V. and Bohannon, M. M. (1975) A hospital stress rating scale, *Nursing Research*, **24**, 352–9.

Wilson-Barnett, J. (1976) Patients' emotional reactions to hospitalization: an exploratory study, *J. Advanced Nursing*, **1**, 351–8.

Wilson-Barnett, J. (1978) Patients' emotional responses to barium X-rays, *J. Advanced Nursing*, **3**(1), 37–46.

Wilson-Barnett, J. (1979) *Stress in Hospital*, Churchill-Livingstone, Edinburgh.

Wilson-Barnett, J. (1981) Assessment of recovery: with special reference to a study with post-operative cardiac patients, *J. Advanced Nursing*, **6**, 435–44.

Wilson-Barnett, J. and Carrigy, A. (1978) Factors affecting patients' responses to hospitalisation, *J. Advanced Nursing*, **3**, 221–8.

Wilson-Barnett, J. and Fordham, M. (1982) 'Recovery of fitness', in *Recovery from Illness*, Ch. 2, J. Wiley, Chichester.

Wong, J. (1979) An exploration of a patient-centred nursing approach in the admission of selected surgical patients: a replicated study, *J. Advanced Nursing*, **4**(6), 611–19.

Yerkes, R. M. and Dodson, J. D. (1908) The relation of strength of stimulus to rapidity of habit-formation, *J. Comparative Neurology and Psychology*, **18**, 459–82.

CHAPTER EIGHT

Patients undergoing surgery

Physical illness involves a deviation from homeostasis, the response to which in itself can be characterized as physiological stress (Clarke, 1984). In Chapter 7 we discussed the issues related to the patient's psychological response to hospital admission. In this chapter we wish to examine the relationship of stress and coping to surgery and recovery. For the majority of people undergoing surgery, there is likely to be pre-existing disturbance of homeostasis and the problem which has caused that is the very reason for undergoing surgery. Leaving that aside, it is important to note that a surgical operation *is* trauma of a physical kind, albeit trauma inflicted under ideal and controlled conditions, and therefore in itself is a stressor. In man, stress is 'an unavoidable consequence of surgery' (Selye, 1976). 'Surgery threatens homeostasis and elicits a stress response or the General Adaptation Syndrome' (Marcinek, 1977). Schlaus and Pritchard (1949) cited by Janis (1958) classified stress situations as mild, moderate or severe. Surgical operations were classified within the severe category alongside the death of a loved one.

The physiological risks of undergoing surgery are by no means uniform and surgeons are anxious to identify and minimize these risks. Surgical risk has been defined as 'the probability of morbidity or mortality resulting from pre-operative preparation, anaesthesia, operation and post-operative convalescence' (Feigal and Blaisden, 1979). They go on to detail the factors which influence surgical risk. These include: type of anaesthesia and operation; urgency; the experience of the surgical team and the hospital resources including equipment for specialized monitoring of homeostatic indicators and critical nursing care.

Selye (1976) has argued on the basis of research literature that the physiological manifestations of stress resulting from surgery are usually complicated by pre-operative medication, analgesia and loss of blood.

Aiken and Henrichs (1971) list surgical stress risk factors in open heart surgery as: anaesthesia time; cardiopulmonary by-pass time; total units of blood needed; degree of hypothermia; duration of hypothermia; and multivalve replacement.

From this and similar evidence physiological stress in uncomplicated surgery can be related to length of time of anaesthesia, type of anaesthetic, amount of blood loss, degree and amount of trauma to tissue, and total time of operation.

Following surgery, many indicators of the patient's physiological status reflect dimensions of the general adaptation syndrome. For example there is increased secretion of adrenaline and noradrenaline associated with tachycardia, increased blood pressure, cool, pale skin, bronchial dilatation and raised blood sugar due to hepatic glycogenolysis. Adrenocorticotrophic Hormone (ACTH) secretion is increased leading in turn to higher levels of circulating glucocorticoids and mineralocorticoids. Glucocorticoids bring about a catabolic response in relation to body proteins, releasing amino acids which can then be available for tissue repair, and intracellular K^+ (potassium), which may be excreted. In addition the immunological response is depressed. Platelet production is increased. Secretion of ACTH, together with enhanced secretion of renin from the juxtaglomerular tissue leads to increased secretion of aldosterone followed by increased secretion of antidiuretic hormone, conserving body fluid but also possibly causing oliguria (Marcinek, 1977).

Whilst (some of) these actions are functional in maintaining or restoring homeostasis (in particular, the maintenance of blood volume to the brain), if prolonged, this response has deleterious effects. For example, the depressed immunological response predisposes to infection; the increased platelet count is a risk factor in relation to deep vein thrombosis and the catabolic response, if extreme, and exacerbated by pre- and post-operative starvation can lead to protein calorie malnutrition. Protein calorie malnutrition in turn delays healing, leads to muscular weakness and delayed return to full motor power.

It can be seen how surgical risk can be affected by the pre- and post-operative period. Pre-operative preparation is vitally important to physiological coping with surgery and recovery from operation.

So far all that has been said about stress and surgery would apply if a human being was a mere physiological system with no intelligence, imagination or coping skills. However, in real life, undergoing an operation is as much a psychological process as a physiological one. It has been described as

> a potential threat to a person's integrity and thus may produce both physiologic and psychologic stress reactions. The physiologic stress reaction is directly related to the extent of the surgery, that is, the more extensive the surgery the greater the physiologic response. The psychologic response, however, is not directly related. (Long and Phipps, 1985)

8.1 PSYCHOLOGICAL THREAT

In considering surgery in humans we have to take account not only of the degree of disturbance to the maintenance of homeostasis but also the degree of psychological threat posed by the operation to the individual (Janis, 1958, p. 10).

> From a psychological standpoint, a major surgical operation constitutes a stress situation which resembles many other types of catastrophes and disasters in that the 'victim' faces a combination of three major forms of imminent danger: the possibility of suffering acute pain, of undergoing serious body damage and of dying.

Appraisal of threat or loss in the face of the impending surgery is frequently manifested as anxiety and fear. Wolfer and Davis (1970) in a study of 76 female patients undergoing gynaecological surgery and 70 male patients undergoing major abdominal surgery found that at least 15% of males and 30% of female patients reported a high degree of fear and anxiety the night before surgery. Asking 47 patients in medical, surgical or cancer wards to rank stressors, Volicer (1974) found that amongst the highest ranking stressors were several which are associated with surgery. Rank 1 was possibility of loss of an organ. Rank 6 was the possibility of disfigurement and rank 8 was admission for surgery.

Carnevali (1966) found that pre-operative patients most fear pain, the unknown, death, destruction of body image, loss of control and separation from their normal environment.

Graham and Conley (1971) found that patients facing major surgery manifest many of the behaviours and signs commonly believed to represent anxiety, as portrayed in the psychiatric or psychological literature on anxiety and fear. Whilst they recorded both physiological and behavioural indicators of anxiety and fear they found that the most useful and frequently occurring indications of pre-operative fear were the subjective expressions of this by the patients.

Theoretically it might be argued that anticipatory fear could mobilize physiological components of stress so that the body was prepared for surgery.

Janis (1958) investigated the effects of anticipatory pre-operative fear on the post-operative emotional state of patients in a retrospective study, using a questionnaire to elicit information about a previous surgical experience. He classified the patients into three groups: a denial or low fear group who showed little or no fear before surgery; a vigilance or high fear group who showed extreme fear reactions prior to surgery; and a moderate fear group. Post-operatively it was the moderate fear group who coped best during the recovery period. Janis suggested that this group used their fear constructively to engage in what he called the 'work of worrying'. This involves cognitive preparation for what happens in the post-operative period. The denial group showed anger and disappointment post-operatively and they resisted efforts to promote their recovery. The vigilant or high fear group also showed a poor level of coping in the recovery period. This research suggested an inverted U relationship between the degree of anticipatory fear and recovery and fits well into a model suggesting that it is extremes of stress which impair psychological and physical recovery from surgery. Unfortunately the relationship described by Janis has not been supported by later research where it has more frequently been the case that an inverse linear relationship has been found between pre-operative fear and post-operative recovery (Newman, 1984), i.e. low fear is associated with good post-operative recovery and increased fear is associated with poor post-operative recovery.

An example of a study showing this was one by Cohen and Lazarus (1973) who studied 71 surgical patients. These were classified into three groups according to their predominant method of coping: a denial group, a vigilant group and a neutral group. The crucial difference between these groups was the amount of information which they sought about the peri-operative period. The denial group showed reluctance to seek information and denied that they felt disturbed in any way, whilst the vigilant group actively sought information. However, the authors suggested that the way in which they sought information was unrealistic and neurotic.

In addition to identifying the patients' psychological reactions post-operatively some more objective indicators of recovery were used in this study. These were number of days in hospital after the operation and frequency of minor complications. Findings were that the denial group recovered best and the vigilant group had the worst recovery rates. Similar findings have occurred in studies by Wolfer and Davies (1970), Sime (1976), and Johnston and Carpenter (1980).

However, some support for Janis' work comes from a study by Chapman and Cox (1977) who compared pain, anxiety and depression on a sample of kidney donors, kidney recipients and general surgical patients. The kidney donors were found to have the lowest anxiety prior to surgery but developed a more volatile anxiety reaction following surgery than the other groups.

This study can be seen to support the cognitive–phenomenological–transactional (CPT) model of stress and coping. It can be argued that kidney donors have volunteered for the operation and are highly motivated. Therefore they viewed the operation positively and were found to be least anxious pre-operatively. However, physiological disturbance and pain post-operatively may occur in the same way as for the less motivated patients and it may also have been the physiological effects of circulating hormones which affected anxiety levels.

Nonetheless, in spite of later conflicting findings, Janis' work has been both influential and valuable, pointing as it does to the relationship between the pre-operative emotional state of the patient and post-operative recovery.

This has led to many studies in which the effect of pre-operative intervention to prepare the patient psychologically has been evaluated for its effectiveness post-operatively.

Some of the early studies of this type will be included here, since, as it has become increasingly accepted that psychological preparation for surgery is an important variable affecting recovery, so forms of psychological preparation have been increasingly incorporated into the routine pre-operative care of patients. This makes the effectiveness of additional psychological preparation more difficult to demonstrate.

It is often difficult to compare studies of this type since the research designs may differ; the form of intervention may be inadequately described and it may have included more than one mode of psychological preparation for operation. Studies also vary in the extent to which they have controlled for any experimental manipulation. In many studies the 'control' group has received only the routine and somewhat random psychological preparation normally received by pre-operative patients. The psychological preparation received by the experimental group of patients may then be confounded by the additional attention they have received from a researcher or a special member of staff. The more careful studies have controlled for this by ensuring that the control patients have received an equal amount of attention.

It is made equally difficult to compare results of studies because different indicators of recovery (i.e. different dependent variables) have been studied. The type of measure which has been used includes days in hospital, numbers of injections of narcotics, number of post-operative days before getting out of bed, demandingness, co-operativeness and number of post-operative complications (Dziurbejko and Larkin, 1978), in-patient ambulatory activity immediately post-operational, activities of daily living on first post-operative day, activities of daily living on the third post-operative day, time elapsed before returning to work or usual level of activity, post-operative analgesic consumption, comfort, satisfaction, length of hospital stay after operation and re-admission before 33 days' post-operatively (Fortin and Kirouac, 1976). Other researchers have used some of the measures mentioned above but others in addition, such as post-operative pain ratings, anxiety levels (Hayward, 1975), body temperature, urinary 17-hydroxycorticosteroids and feelings of wellness (Boore, 1978).

Studies which use more than one indication of the post-operative progress are to be commended since a measure such as day of discharge from hospital can reflect the hospital and ward or surgeon's policy as much as the patient's well being. Also there may not always be a good association between subjective and objective measures and psychological measures and physiological measures. Recently Johnston cited by Newman (1984) has identified the degree of association between 16 measures of post-operative outcome. The results showed the measures grouped into higher level factors. One of these was 'well-being' and included self-rating of sleep and energy, positive mood and independent washing. Another factor was the patients' attitude to the hospital and a distress factor. Interestingly pain was not associated with other measures.

It should be noted, however, that many of the indicators of recovery used in these studies are indicators of stress levels and thus of adaptation and coping effectiveness. Theoretically this follows, since excessively high levels of stress can be expected to impede recovery. Not all the studies in this area of work have related the experimental manipulation of the findings to stress.

One study which did this was that of Boore (1978) which has already been mentioned above. Boore used the Neuman Health-Care Systems Models of nursing as the theoretical framework for her study. This is one of several nursing models based on concepts of stress. In Neuman's case it is Selye's concept of stress which is used.

The study sample was two matched groups of 40 patients undergoing herniorrhaphy, cholecystectomy, cholecystectomy with exploration of the common bile duct or appendicectomy.

Pre-operatively the following measures were taken: 3-hour urine sample for 17-hydroxycorticosteroid estimation, and body temperature. Experimental group patients were given information about pre-operative starvation and the premedication, transfer to theatre, induction of anaesthesia and the recovery room. The post-operative presence of drains and IVI were explained. The problem of pain and the availability of analgesia was discussed and the importance of early ambulation was stressed. Patients were taught by demonstration and practice how to inspire and expire fully, how to cough and how to splint the wound whilst coughing. They were also taught relaxation of abdominal muscles. Patients were encouraged to express their own anxieties and where possible reassurance was given by offering specific information. This study was well controlled as the control group were visited for an equivalent period of time during which the researcher talked about topics unrelated to the hospital.

Post-operative measures were collected from days 1–14 of the post-operative period. For each of the first 4 days post-operatively, a 3-hourly urine sample was tested for 17-hydroxycorticosteroids and $[Na^+]/[K^+]$ was estimated. The body temperature was recorded and patients were assessed as to their own subjective condition. Information about any analgesics given and post-operative complications was collected from medical/nursing records.

Doctors' and nurses' assessments of the patients were completed at the time of the patients' discharge from hospital.

The patients' subjective assessment of their own condition included the following items which were assessed on a six-point scale from very poor to excellent: sleep, strength and energy, presence or absence of gastric symptoms, state of bowels, appetite, urination, ability to help themselves and ease in movements, interest in surroundings and general mood. Patients were also asked to indicate how much pain they had by using the pain thermometer (Hayward, 1975).

The most interesting of these measures from the point of view of stress and coping are the measures of urinary 17-hydroxycorticosteroids and $[Na^+]/[K^+]$ ratios. (The latter are affected by the mineralocorticoid effects of glucocorticosteroids and directly by the mineralocorticosteroids. It will be recalled that increased secretion of gluco- and mineralo-corticosteroids occur as part of the general adaptation syndrome (Selye, 1956).)

Results showed that post-operatively the patients in the experimental group had lower mean 17-hydroxycorticosteroid excretion levels than the control group. This difference was statistically significant on days 2 and 3 post-operatively.

Significantly more patients in the control group than in the experimental group developed wound infection and among those patients undergoing cholecystectomy more control patients developed complications (wound, respiratory or urinary infection or urinary retention). There was no difference in complication rate between the experimental or control patients who underwent herniorrhaphy or appendicectomy – $[Na^+]/[K^+]$ ratios and other dependent variables failed to distinguish between experimental/control patients.

Since Boore specifically used a stress formulation as a basis for her study, some of her discussion of results is interesting. She suggests that her results indicate that the magnitude of the rise of glucocorticoid secretion which is a usual response to operation can be modified. This appeared to be the case for the herniorrhaphy and appendicectomy patients where the amounts of excreted hormone were down to the pre-operative level by day 2 post-operatively in the experimental group. The difference in excreted cortico-steroid levels between the experimental group of cholecystectomy patients and the control group was smaller and here Boore suggests that the predominant factor governing these results is the physiological stress which is severe in a moderately serious operation, reducing the difference between the control and experimental groups. Thus Boore is attributing the difference in excreted corticosteroid levels between the experimental and control groups to psychological factors which had been affected by the pre-operative intervention levels. In the patients undergoing the less severe operation the stress measure reflected the psychological stress component to a greater extent, thus revealing differences between the experimental and control groups.

Boore was particularly interested in one patient amongst those in the control group undergoing cholecystectomy. This particular patient had lower urinary corticosteroid levels after operation than before (unlike the other patients). Of all the patients this one made very poor progress and had to remain in hospital for many weeks. Boore remarks that this patient supports the literature which states that an increase in corticosteroid secretion in physical threat is essential for successful adaptation.

We have mentioned above the research in which specific psychological preparation for operation has been evaluated and a particular example (Boore, 1978) has been quoted in some detail.

8.2 PREPARATION FOR SURGERY: A BASIS FOR COPING

We now wish to examine some of this literature in relation to coping. Psychological preparation for operation can be viewed in terms of improving patients' coping skills with the threat posed by operation.

Giving pre-operative information can be seen as helping coping strategies to be developed and identified. This is consistent with the secondary appraisal stage of the CPT model. One of the first studies of this type was one by Egbert *et al.* (1964) whose subjects were patients due to have elective abdominal surgery. The anaesthetist visited all patients included in the study and informed them of the method of preparation for anaesthesia, time and duration of surgery, and about waking up in the recovery room. The control group received no further information but the experimental group were told about the location, severity and duration of pain they should expect and that some pain after operation was normal. Mechanisms of pain production were explained, together with how muscular relaxation can help. They were shown how to move in order to place the least strain on abdominal muscles.

In the post-operative period the patients receiving the special preparation required a significantly smaller amount of narcotic drugs and were rated as being more comfortable, in a better emotional and physical condition and were discharged from hospital sooner than those in the control group.

It is important to note that in this early study patients were given two different types of information: **procedural**, i.e. about the events involved in operation; and **sensory**, i.e. how they would feel. In addition they were also given instruction in how they could help themselves.

Later research studies have attempted to evaluate the effect of these different components of psychological preparation for operation.

Giving procedural information

There are few studies in which procedural information alone has been evaluated and those that have been carried out have been poorly controlled, since they have compared patients who have received additional procedural information with patients who have been prepared for operation in the usual hospital way: Andrew (1970); Vernon and Bigelow (1974); Reading (1982);

and Anderson and Masur (1983). However, results have shown that patients receiving the additional information either gained no benefit or only a little compared with those prepared in the normal way.

This result is unsurprising within the framework of a CPT view of stress and coping. To be told when, where and what will happen to you is better than being told nothing, since it normalizes events, aids appraisal of events and prevents them from appearing threatening. However, this type of information is information given from the point of view of the staff and is not specially selected and designed to help patients to cope with coming events. For patients to rehearse their coping strategies, they need information from their point of view, i.e. what it will feel like, and what they need to do to help (Altschul, 1975).

Procedural information fails to allow the individual to develop coping strategies and treats the patient as a passive receiver of care rather than the perceiving, appraising, anxious, and potentially coping person that he can be.

Giving sensory information

Instead of (or as well as) giving procedural information, it is possible to give a patient information which describes the physical sensations he will experience. That is, telling the patient what is to be felt, seen, heard, tasted and or smelled during the procedure (Horsley, 1981). Such information 'describes an event from the patient's point of view' (Johnson et al., 1975).

A programme of research to investigate the effects of sensory information upon distress experienced by patients undergoing various procedures has been (and is still being) carried out by Johnson and colleagues in laboratory studies. They have demonstrated effectiveness in relation to ischaemic pain induced by the inflation of a blood pressure cuff applied to the non-dominant arm to a pressure of 250 mm Hg (Johnson 1972, 1973, 1975; Johnson and Rice, 1974).

Clinical tests of sensory information-giving were carried out in relation to endoscopic examination (Johnson et al., 1973) in a controlled experimental study which included a test of procedural information alone as well as sensory information alone. Both information groups required significantly less tranquillizer to achieve sedation than the control group but the sensory information proved superior in reducing the behavioural signs of distress.

Similar findings were obtained in a study of children aged 6–11 years undergoing removal of a plaster cast (Johnson et al., 1975). However, these studies were concerned with single procedures, whereas we are concerned with patients undergoing surgical operation which involves many different procedures.

In a fairly complex experimental design Johnson et al. (1978b) investigated the effects of sensory information upon the recovery of patients undergoing cholecystectomy.

The experiment was designed as a two-level factorial study. Any patient in the study could receive either (a) procedural information in addition to the information routinely given by staff, or (b) sensory information and procedural information in addition to the routine information, or (c) routine information alone. In addition patients could have either (1) instruction in the exercises they were to perform post-operatively, or (2) no such instruction.

The effects of each of these six treatments were evaluated by a Mood Adjective Check List (MACL), amount of ambulation, doses of analgesic received, length of hospitalization following operation, and length of time between discharge and going out from the house.

Results showed that only those patients whose pre-operative scores on the MACL were above the median showed a post-operative effect on this measure due to the experimental manipulations and each of the experimental manipulations produced an effect, reducing anger in particular.

Instruction about exercises had the strongest effect on emotional response and this group of patients also tended to use less analgesic and to ambulate more than those who did not receive the instruction. Those patients who received the additional sensory information had a shorter hospitalization and a reduced time interval before venturing out of the house. The patients who received both sensory information and instruction in exercise had the shortest hospitalization.

There have been other studies which have shown the effect of sensory information on post-operative recovery measures, although the evidence is not consistently convincing (Newman, 1984).

The reason for detailing the study by Johnson *et al.* (1978a), is that it brings out the complexity and difficulties involved in assessing the efficacy of any one component of pre-operation preparation, and it is a useful study to discuss in the light of theories of stress and coping.

Some significant issues

First it should be noted that no patient in the study received additional sensory information alone since in a topic as complex as the peri-operative period more than one procedure is involved and so each must be mentioned to make sense of the sensory information. Therefore some procedural information was given as well.

From the theoretical point of view, Johnson (1975) has stated that the sensory information acts upon cognitive processes involving expectations about sensations to be experienced and that the expectation of atypical sensations tends to increase a patient's distress, whilst expectations that sensations are typical decreases distress (i.e. it acts by reducing the mismatch between expected sensations and actual sensations).

However, Johnson's experiments with surgical patients were designed to test a theoretical assumption based upon Lazarus (1966), Lazarus and Launier (1978), and Leventhal (1970). From this Johnson divided coping into emotion regulation and instrumental transactions (indirect and direct coping in our terms). She argued that emotion regulation coping does not ensure that instrumental transactions will be achieved and that instrumental transactions do not ensure regulation of emotion.

However, Johnson also suggested that a high level of emotional reaction could disrupt instrumental function. Thus she is suggesting relative independence of emotional and instrumental coping (indirect and direct) except in a negative sense where lack of coping with high emotional reactions may interfere with instrumental coping.

From this Johnson hypothesized that instruction in direct or instrumental coping activities would facilitate instrumental coping whilst sensory information would facilitate emotion regulation or coping.

The experiment detailed above does not fully support this, and Johnson (1983) discussed this. First, results support the role of cognitive appraisal processes in coping with stress related to surgery. Secondly, there is support for suggesting that coping can serve two functions: regulation of emotional response and regulation of instrumental transaction with the environment and that these functions are relatively independent. This is supported by evidence that intervention which reduces emotional response does not always affect instrumental behaviour and that therefore reduction of emotional response alone is not always sufficient to ensure direct coping. Thirdly, the research showed that each of the pre-operative interventions helped patients to maintain or achieve personal control, but that the processes of achieving control varied with each type of intervention. Fourthly, the research suggests something in line with the bulk of research in this general area that the emotional response can be affected by a wide variety of different psychological interventions.

These findings and the inferences which Johnson made from them support the CPT model of stress and coping outlined in Chapter 2.

Behavioural instruction

To an extent this topic has already been discussed since both Boore (1978) and Johnson et al. (1978a) included instructions on post-operative exercise in their pre-operative psychological preparation of the patient and this has been the case in other studies, e.g. Egbert et al. (1964), Fortin and Kirouac (1976) and Healey (1968). One study was carried out by Lindeman and Van Aernam (1971) to evaluate the effect of pre-operative teaching of deep breathing, coughing and exercise.

The study was poorly controlled however since the comparison group received only the routine instruction given to all pre-operative patients: 135 patients receiving routine preparation were compared with 126 patients who received additional structured teaching pre-operatively. Results showed that their ability to deep breathe as measured by vital capacity and to cough was significantly increased amongst the patients given additional teaching compared with the control group. The mean length of hospital stay from the day of operation was also significantly reduced in the group which received additional teaching. Analgesics needed post-operatively by the two groups showed no significant difference. Conclusions reached by Mathews and Ridgeway (1984) in a review of studies on psychological preparation for surgery was that the evidence in favour of the effectiveness of behavioural instruction upon recovery is more impressive than that for information.

Further areas of behavioural instruction which can be included pre-operatively are instruction in obtaining post-operative analgesia (included in most evaluative studies of pre-operative preparation), leg exercises, how to move in bed and how to splint the wound whilst coughing. Relaxation techniques may be included as well, but these will be discussed separately as they have an additional importance for stress and coping.

The types of instruction listed above can all be expected to have a positive effect upon physiological recovery and so the reader may wonder why they are included as methods of psychological preparation for operation. This is for three reasons: firstly such techniques give the patient a feeling of personal control which can be exercised over recovery and this of course has a direct psychological effect. It also gives the patient a method of direct coping. Teaching the technique pre-operatively rather than post-operatively allows cognitive preparation and ensures that the patient is taught at a time when he is more likely to be able to learn than he would be when drowsy, in pain or otherwise distressed in the post-operative period. Finally, it suggests that there are important psycho–physiological interrelationships affecting recovery.

General psychological preparation for operation

We have examined studies in which different elements of pre-operative preparation have been evaluated separately, these being procedural information, sensory information and behavioural instruction. Whilst at least some studies have shown the efficacy of each of these interventions, the evidence has not been entirely unequivocal and in any case the intervention used has often been 'contaminated' or poorly controlled.

In real life the distinctions between these different types of preparation may be artificial although if research could prove that one method of preparation alone was effective this would obviously have great practical importance.

We now wish to discuss a study in which the different methods of preparation used in combination were evaluated. This is a study by Fortin and Kirouac (1976) which has already been referred to very briefly.

In this study male and female patients between 20 and 59 years of age who were to be admitted for herniorrhaphy, cholecystectomy or pelvic surgery under general anaesthetic were matched and randomly assigned to an experimental or a control group; 58 patients were studied overall. Pre-operative teaching for the experimental group included the following elements:

1. Orientation to surgery in general and to the study hospital in particular.
2. Elementary biological facts.
3. The effects of smoking on respiratory function during and after anaesthetics.
4. The importance of early ambulation after surgery.
5. The purposes and techniques of respiratory and muscular exercise including routines to follow pre-operatively both at home and in hospital, and those appropriate to the immediate post-operative period.
6. The technique of changing position in the immediate post-operative period.
7. How to anticipate and cope with post-operative nausea, vomiting, pain, dizziness and weakness.
8. Practical suggestions on self-care.

Teaching was started before admission in groups of seven and patients were offered a tour of the hospital before admission.

The study was not well controlled since the controls received only routine preparation. The outcome measures used have already been detailed. Results showed that there were statistically significant differences between the groups on measures of physical functioning, comfort measures, satisfaction, and the amount of post-operative analgesia by injection. There were no statistically significant differences in length of post-operative hospital stay, oral analgesic consumption or days lost from work or school to day 33 post-operatively.

Nonetheless the study does show that from the patients' point of view and indeed from the point of view of the hospital staff, the pre-operative intervention was well worthwhile.

From the nursing point of view we can conclude that the provision of procedural and sensory information and pre-operative instruction in relevant post-operative behaviour has sufficient research support to justify its routine use, not just for humanitarian reasons but to ensure greater cost-effectiveness of patient care in surgery.

8.3 SUPPORT OF FAMILY

In the study by Fortin and Kirouac we have examined above, the patient's family was not mentioned, but since patients were involved in pre-operative preparation before admission to hospital it is likely that their families' commitment and support were forthcoming. On theoretical grounds the support of the family is important since any apprehension or anxiety on the part of relatives or friends may increase the patient's emotional response. Conversely they can potentially do much to help the patient to cope by reinforcing the information or instruction given by staff.

A small experiment to evaluate the benefit of including the patient's family in pre-operative teaching was conducted by Dziubejko and Larkin (1978): 21 female patients aged between 25 and 55 years were randomly assigned to one of three groups. In one group, both family and patient were given pre-operative teaching; in another group only the patient was taught and the third group of patients acted as a control receiving no additional teaching.

The pre-operative teaching which was given included sensory and procedural information and instruction on coughing, splinting the wound, deep breathing, leg exercises and the mechanics of turning without causing strain on abdominal muscles. Where the family was included in the teaching they were also informed of the importance of encouraging the patient to move.

Results showed that where significant effects of the intervention occurred they were greater for the group of patients whose family had been included in the teaching. Teaching of the patient alone showed superiority over the outcome for the control group.

The following post-operative dependent measures showed statistical significance:

(a) Days in hospital from the time of operation to discharge
(b) Days from the operation to the day of getting out of bed
(c) 'Demandingness'
(d) Family apprehension.

Some pre-operative measures also showed the effectiveness of the intervention and this is important since teaching which occurs some time before operation could be expected to have a pre-operative as well as a post-operative effect. Significant differences in pre-operative measures were found for:

• Co-operation during procedures
• Anxiety
• Ability to relax

- The number of questions asked
- Family anxiety

8.4 EMOTIONAL SUPPORT

From a nursing point of view giving emotional support to patients who are anxious, by listening to them and answering their questions, could be expected to be important as a means of psychological preparation for operation. However, in the main, research to evaluate the effectiveness of such intervention has failed to convince of its efficacy. Dumas and Leonard (1963) found some small beneficial effects but a later study by Dumas and Johnson (1972) failed to demonstrate these. One other study, where effects were shown, included behavioural instruction. Mathews and Ridgeway (1984) conclude that the evidence for the effectiveness of 'emotional support and non-directive discussion of patients' worries is extremely weak'.

So far we have discussed the effectiveness of pre-operative psychological preparation of the patient which is well within the competence of nurses and which would be accepted as a nursing responsibility even if it is not always carried out systematically.

From our stress and coping perspective there are more specialized interventions which in theory would be expected to influence recovery. Some of these have been investigated and the research will now be discussed.

Relaxation

Whilst instruction about relaxation has been included in some of the studies discussed above (e.g. Egbert *et al.*, 1964), studies in which the benefit of systematic relaxation has been evaluated are rather more recent. Theoretically such relaxation training comes from the work on desensitization by Wolpe and Lazarus (1966) and has been discussed in Chapter 3 on coping strategies for nurses. An early study of this kind was one by Aiken and Henrichs (1971). Patients were undergoing open-heart surgery and they were encouraged to practise systematic relaxation daily during a session in which they were also encouraged to ask questions which were readily answered.

Unfortunately, whilst the outcome measures did show significant differences between the experimental and control groups, it was not possible to claim that these were due to the intervention, since the control patients showed more severe physiological surgical stress factors than the experimental patients. However, Flaherty and Fitzpatrick (1978) did demonstrate that a simple form of relaxation can produce useful effects. Wilson (1981) compared the effects of relaxation training with the effects of providing sensory information. The relaxation training group scored rather better on an index of general recovery and also required less analgesia for pain.

Cognitive restructuring

Since we have accepted a view of stress and coping which emphasizes the importance of an individual's own beliefs and knowledge (cognitions) about events, it is particularly interesting to identify the effectiveness of cognitive pre-operative interventions designed to help patients to view surgery more positively than they might do otherwise.

Two general techniques have been used in research studies. One attempts to direct the patient's attention away from the threatening aspects of surgery and the other encourages re-evaluation (or re-appraisal) of any threatening cognitions about surgery (Newman, 1984).

A study of the first type was carried out by Pickett and Clum (1982). In this study there were two intervention groups and a control group. One intervention group was taught relaxation and the second group was first taught to focus attention upon their worries about surgery and then to redirect their attention to imagined pleasant situations. This latter group were found to have lower anxiety levels post-operatively than either the relaxation or control groups.

Langer *et al.* (1975) carried out a study of the second type mentioned above. In this, a group of patients was asked to replace their worries about surgery with thoughts about the positive aspects of the hospital experience and to rehearse these positive thoughts. This group of patients was rated by nurses to have lower levels of anxiety and stress than patients given procedural and sensory information, or than the control group. They also required lower levels of post-operative analgesia.

A rather complex experiment by Mathews and Ridgeway (1984) involved female patients admitted for hysterectomy. They were interviewed on admission, following which they were assigned into one of three groups: (a) an information group; (b) a group which received attention from the investigator, together with information about the ward layout; (c) a group which was given instructions about a strategy to imagine the positive aspects of surgery and to re-appraise negative aspects in a positive manner. A fourth group, smaller than the other groups, comprised patients who said they did not wish for pre-operative information.

The pre-operative intervention comprised the distribution of a booklet with equal amounts of written material giving the information relevant to the group to which all but the fourth group of patients was randomly assigned. In addition to the booklet patients were asked if they had read and understood the contents and further elucidation was given if necessary.

Results showed clearly that the cognitive coping strategy produced the best outcome, in terms of pain, analgesia consumption, and total post-operative symptoms.

Interestingly, the patients receiving the procedural and sensory information were the ones who rated the booklets the most highly. The group which did worst post-operatively whilst in hospital were those who had refused information. They were confident that they were well informed but a test of knowledge showed them to be badly informed and they suffered greater pain and worse wind than the other groups, as well as developing a higher post-operative pyrexia than the other patients in the study.

Individual differences

Using the CPT model of stress and coping, individual differences in appraisal of threat and coping would be expected to make a difference to a person's experience of surgery. However, in the research studies which have been reviewed so far, individual differences have been obscured by the assignment of patients to groups in a random fashion. There are, however, some research studies in which individual differences amongst patients have been examined. Indeed Janis' (1958) study can be considered to be within that category.

When psychologists talk about individual differences they are considering differences between people in terms of behaviour, intelligence, mood, emotional reactivity, perceptual style, attitudes and values (see Chapter 2). The totality of these differences is termed personality, and people are often described by the score they obtain on a personality test which compares individuals along one or more dimensions (or traits).

One of the most well-established of such tests is the Eysenck Personality Inventory (EPI) and this has been used to identify those people who are the most likely to suffer from anxiety when undergoing surgery. The EPI measures two personality traits which are said to be independent of each other: extraversion–introversion (E scale) and stability–neuroticism (N scale). It is this latter N scale which has been found to be an indicator of how individuals may respond to surgery. In general a high neuroticism score has been found to show considerable promise in identifying those patients more likely to have a delayed or complicated recovery from surgery (Mathews and Ridgeway, 1981).

Two measures of anxiety are commonly used in research with patients. One of these measures state anxiety which is said to identify how an individual feels at the time of measurement and thus reflects any anxiety in response to threat which has been appraised as operating at the time of the test. The other measure of trait anxiety reflects a more permanent disposition to respond readily with anxiety and is said to be a personality trait. Trait anxiety measures have been found to correlate well with the neuroticism scores of the EPI (e.g. Hayward, 1975). However, studies which used measures of trait anxiety have by no means shown consistent results in predicting response to surgery.

A measure of a personality dimension of particular interest in relation to stress and coping is that of coping style. This has already been mentioned earlier. The dimension classifies people according to whether they use vigilant or denial modes of coping. As with most such scales the majority of individuals would be expected to use a mode of coping lying between those two extremes. Vigilant individuals are likely to scan the environment for threat and to perceive ambiguous stimuli as threatening. Individuals using a denial style of coping are less likely to seek out threat or to perceive ambiguous stimuli as threatening. Indeed they are likely to deny as threatening circumstances which the average majority see as threatening.

Studies in which the individual's coping style has been linked to the outcome of surgery have shown, on balance, that the subjects using a denial strategy have tended to recover more rapidly. However the evidence here is far from unequivocal and it could well be that the studies which demonstrate this relationship were merely reflecting the fact that 'deniers' are less likely to experience anxiety (Mathews and Ridgeway, 1981).

Another personality dimension of particular interest to the present authors is that of locus of control (Rotter, 1966). This dimension describes at the extreme ends people who believe strongly in their own personal control over what happens, as opposed to those who believe that their own actions have little or no effect on events, which these people believe are controlled externally. Again, however, according to Mathews and Ridgeway (1984), there is no clear-cut evidence of the impact of this personality variable on recovery from surgery.

8.5 THE RELATIONSHIP BETWEEN PERSONALITY AND THE EFFECTIVENESS OF PSYCHOLOGICAL PREPARATION FOR OPERATION

The early research by Janis (1958) showed that the patients who responded best to surgery were the moderate fear group, whilst both the low fear group and the high fear group did less well. As mentioned earlier this result has not been substantiated in subsequent work which for the most part has shown a linear relationship between increased fear and poorer recovery. How do people who differ in relation to pre-operative fear respond to psychological preparation for operation?

A study by Johnson et al. (1978a) grouped patients into a high fear or a low fear group. Behavioural instructions and sensory information given pre-operatively gave an improved score on a mood measure for the high fear group but gave a worse score post-operatively for the low fear group, suggesting that emotional arousal had been increased post-operatively for this group.

Such a relationship is also suggested by a study by Delong (1970). Patients in this study who used a vigilant coping style appeared to benefit more from pre-operative psychological preparation than those patients who used a denial coping style.

Confirmation comes from a study by Sime and Libera (1985) in relation to 113 patients undergoing gingivectomy. Patients were assigned to one of four groups and these received interventions before the operation as follows: a technique for self-instruction; sensory information; sensory information and a technique of self-instruction; control – no intervention. Levels of trait and state anxiety were assessed. The three types of intervention helped those patients who scored high on state anxiety but produced negative effects with those patients who scored low on state anxiety.

Locus of control

All psychological methods of preparation for surgery have one effect in common: that is they give the individual a method of exerting personal control. (A possible exception here is procedural information.) Thus one would expect pre-operative intervention methods to affect those who demonstrate internal locus of control beliefs in a different way from those who demonstrate external locus of control beliefs.

The expectation gains confirmation in the study by Pickett and Clum (1982) which has been mentioned above. In this study the interaction effects between locus of control and pre-operative intervention were analysed. Patients who demonstrated internal locus of control benefited from learning a cognitive restructuring strategy whilst patients who demonstrated external locus of control beliefs benefited from relaxation training. Clearly this is another area where further research is needed.

8.6 CONCLUSION AND SUMMARY

From the evidence so far the case for giving patients sensory information and instruction in behavioural manoeuvres, exercise, coughing, breathing, etc. pre-operatively is very strong indeed.

This appears to have a beneficial effect upon post-operative recovery. The suggestion is that it reduces the components of stress due to the appraisal of threat. Whilst this effect may be shown more strongly in comparison to patients not given pre-operative teaching when the operation is relatively minor, it is most important when the operation is serious. In this latter case the physiological stress will be great and additional stress through negative appraisal may delay recovery severely.

An area in which insufficient research has been carried out so far is that of the optimum timing of pre-operative psychological care. Most studies have delivered patient teaching within the hospital and on the immediate pre-operative day. The study by Fortin and Kirouac (1976) showed quite powerfully the benefit of patient teaching prior to entry to hospital.

Another area in which there is insufficient evidence is the extent to which pre-operative measures of anxiety (often used as a baseline in the studies quoted) are themselves already showing increased state anxiety due to admission to hospital and appraisal of surgery. Studies in which repeated measures of anxiety have been taken over a period of hospitalization suggest that anxiety is increased pre-operatively.

The techniques of distraction, cognitive restructuring, self-instruction, and systematic relaxation show promise as methods of pre-operative intervention but more careful studies to identify those patients most likely to benefit are required.

An explanation of some of the contradictory research findings in this area has been put forward by Johnson (1983, p. 31). She suggests that

> the characteristics of situations that patients encounter during hospitali-zation and the nature of demands made on them have received inadequate attention. Some situations provide little opportunity for patients to exert active control. In these situations the patient maximizes benefits by being passive and co-operative, while in other situations the patient benefits by taking an active role. Each situation should be examined with respect to the demands on patients and the role they can play to maximize their benefits.

Perhaps those patients who use denial as a method of coping prefer to put themselves completely in the hands of professionals and let the professionals do the worrying! Similarly, in hospitals, most circumstances are ones in which internal locus of control beliefs undermine the role of doctors and nurses who exert control over the environment for care, and during the peri-operative period over the person's body!

Clearly a note of caution in the general enthusiasm for pre-operative psychological care is that the small number of patients who continue to use denial as a method of coping will probably not benefit.

In this chapter, then, we have examined the physiological stress associated with surgery. For patients who are undergoing an operation, an additional source of stress is the appraisal of the threat which surgery poses. Pre-operative psychological preparation has been shown to affect the post-operative levels of excreted 17-hydroxycorticosteroids, post-operative pain levels, indicators of post-operative recovery, and the post-operative emotional state of patients.

Investigations to identify the types of psychological preparation which are effective suggest that sensory information alone, or behavioural instruction alone are useful interventions. By behavioural instruction is meant: breathing exercises; leg exercises; coughing; splinting the wound; movement in a manner causing the least tension on the wound; and the importance of activity and early ambulation.

The most effective pre-operative intervention appears to be patient teaching which includes procedural and sensory information and behavioural instruction. Teaching systematic relaxation techniques, cognitive distraction, or cognitive restructuring as forms of coping, appear to be effective ways of helping patients who are undergoing surgery. However, the use of these methods and the pre-operative teaching mentioned above appears to be most effective with those who are anxious pre-operatively and least effective with people who consistently use denial as a coping strategy.

REFERENCES

Aiken, L. H. and Henrichs, T. F. (1971) Systematic relaxation as a nursing intervention technique with open heart surgery patients, *Nursing Research*, **20**, 212–17.

Altschul, A. (1975) *Psychology for Nurses* (4th edn), Baillière Tindall, London, p. 108.

Anderson, K. A. and Masur, F. T. (1983) Psychological preparation for invasive medical and dental procedures, *J. Behav. Medicine*, **6**, 1–40.

Andrew, J. M. (1970) Recovery from surgery, with and without preparatory instruction, for three coping styles, *J. Pers. Soc. Psychol.*, **15**, 223–6.

Boore, J. (1978) *Prescription for Recovery*, Royal College of Nursing, London.

Carnevali, D. F. (1966) Pre-operative anxiety, *Amer. J. Nursing*, **66**, 1536–8.

Chapman, C. R. and Cox, G. B. (1977) Determination of Anxiety in Elective Surgery Patients, in *Stress and Anxiety* (eds. C. G. Spielberger and I. G. Sarason), Vol. 4, Hemisphere, Washington.

Clarke, M. (1984) The constructs 'stress' and 'coping' as a rationale for nursing activities, *J. Advanced Nursing*, **9**, 267–75.

Cohen, F. and Lazarus, R. S. (1973) Active coping processes, coping dispositions and recovery from surgery, *Psychomatic Medicine*, **35**, 375–89.

DeLong, R. D. (1970) *Individual Differences in Patterns of Anxiety Arousal, Stress-relevant Information and Recovery from Surgery*, Doctoral Dissertation, University of California, Los Angeles.

Dumas, R. G. and Leonard, R. C. (1963) The effect of nursing on the incidence of post-operative vomiting, *Nursing Research*, **12**, 12–15.

Dumas, R. G. and Johnson, B. A. (1972) Research in nursing practice: a review of five clinical experiments, *Int. J. Nursing Studies*, **9**, 137–49.

Dziurbejko, M. M. and Larkin, J. C. (1978) Including the family in pre-operative teaching, *Amer. J. Nursing*, (November), 1892–4.

Egbert, L. D., Battit, G. C., Welsh, C. E. and Bartlett, M. K. (1964) Reduction of post-operative pain by encouragement and instruction of patients: a study of doctor–patient rapport, *New England J. Med.* **270**, 823–7.

Feigal, D. W. and Blaisden, F. W. (1979) The estimation of surgical risks, *Medical Clinics of North America*, **63**, 1131–43.

Flaherty, C. G. and Fitzpatrick, J. C. (1978) Relaxation technique to increase comfort level of post-operative patients, *Nursing Research*, **27**, 352–5.

Fortin, F. and Kirouac, S. (1976) A randomised controlled trial of pre-operative patient education, *Int. J. Nursing Studies*, **13**, 11–24.

Graham, L. E. and Conley, E. M. (1971) Evaluation of anxiety and fear in adult surgical patients, *Nursing Research*, **20**, 113–22.

Hayward, J. (1975) *Information – A Prescription Against Pain*, Royal College of Nursing, London.

Healey, K. M. (1968) 'Does pre-operative instruction make a difference?' *Amer. J. Nursing*, **68**, 62–7.

Horsley, J. A. (1981) *Distress Reduction Through Sensory Preparation*, CURN Project, Michigan Nurses' Association, Grune and Stratton, New York, N.Y.

Janis, I. L. (1958) *Psychological Stress*, J. Wiley, New York.

Johnson, J. E. (1972) Effects of structuring patients' expectations on their reactions to threatening events, *Nursing Research*, **21**, 499–504.

Johnson, J. E. (1973) Effects of accurate expectations about sensations on the sensory and distress components of pain, *J. Pers. Soc. Psychol.*, **27**, 261–75.

Johnson, J. E. (1975) Stress reduction through sensory information, in *Stress and Anxiety* (eds I. G. Saranson and C. D. Spielberger), Vol. 2, Hemisphere, Washington.

Johnson, J. E. (1983) Preparing patients to cope with stress, in *Patient Teaching* (ed. J. Wilson-Barnett), Churchill-Livingstone, Edinburgh, pp. 19–33.

Johnson, J. E., Morrissey, J. F. and Leventhal, H. (1973) Psychological preparation for an endoscopic examination, *Gastrointestinal Endoscopy*, **19**, 180–2.

Johnson, J. E. and Rice, V. H. (1974) Sensory and distress components of pain: implications for the study of clinical pain, *Nursing Research*, **23**, 203–9.

Johnson, J. E., Kirchoff, K. T. and Endress, M. P. (1975) Altering children's distress behaviour during orthopaedic cast removal, *Nursing Research*, **24**, 404–10.

Johnson, J. E., Rice, V. H., Fuller, S. S. and Endress, M. P. (1978a) Sensory information, instruction in coping strategy and recovery from surgery, *Research in Nursing and Health*, **1**, 4–17.

Johnson, J. E., Fuller, S. S., Endress, M. P. and Rice, V. H. (1978b) Altering patients' responses to surgery: an extension and replication, *Research in Nursing and Health*, **1**, 111–21.

Johnston, M. Dimensions of recovery from surgery, *J. Appl. Psych.*, cited by Newman (1984).

Johnston, M. and Carpenter, L. (1980) Relationship between pre-operative anxiety and post-operative state, *Psychological Medicine*, **10**, 361–7.

Langer, E. J., Janis, I. L. and Wolfor, J. A. (1975) Reduction of psychological stress in surgical patients, *J. Exp. Soc. Psychol.*, **11**, 155–65.

Lazarus, R. S. (1966) *Psychological Stress and the Coping Process*, McGraw-Hill, New York, N. Y.

Lazarus, R. S. and Launier, R. (1978) Stress-related transactions between person and environment, in *Perspectives of Interactional Psychology* (eds. L. A. Pervin and M. Lewis), Plenum Press, New York, pp. 287–327.

Leventhal, H. (1970) Findings and theory in the study of fear communications, in *Advances in Experimental Social Psychology* (ed. L. Berkowitz), Vol. 5, Academic Press, New York, N.Y., pp. 119–86.

Lindeman, C. A. and Kanaernam, B. (1971) Nursing intervention with the pre-surgical patient. The effects of structured and unstructured pre-operative teaching, *Nursing Research*, **20**, 319–32.

Long, B. C. and Phipps, W. J. (1985) *Essentials of Medical Surgical Nursing*, Mosby, St Louis, MO, p. 292.

Marcinek, M. (1977) Stress in the Surgical Patient, *Amer. J. Nursing*, **77**, 1809–12.

Mathews, A. and Ridgeway, V. (1981) Personality and surgical recovery: a review. *British J. Clinical Psychology*, **20**, 243–66.

Mathews, A. and Ridgeway, V. (1984) Psychological preparation for surgery, in *Health Care and Human Behaviour* (eds A. Steptoe and A. Mathews), Academic Press, London.

Mayou, R., Foster A. and Williamson, B. (1978) Psychosocial adjustment in patients one year after myocardial infarction. *J. Psychosomatic Research*. **22**, 447–53.

Newman, S. C. (1984) Anxiety, hospitalisation and surgery, in *The Experience of Illness* (eds R. Fitzpatrick, J. Hinlon, S. Newman and S. Scambler), Tavistock, London, pp. 132–53.

Pickett, C. and Clum, G. A. (1982) Comparative treatment strategies and their interaction with locus of control in the reduction of post-surgical pain and anxiety, *J. Consult. Clin. Psychology*, **50**, 439–44.

Reading, A. E. (1982) The effects of psychological preparation on pain and recovery after minor gynaecological surgery: a preliminary report, *J. Clin. Psych.*, **38**, 504–12.

Ridgeway, V. and Mathews, A. (1982) Psychological preparation for surgery: a comparison of methods, *Brit. J. Clin. Psychol.*, **21**, 243–60.

Rotter, J. B. (1966) Generalized expectancies for internal versus external control of reinforcement', *Psych Monographs*, **80**, 1.

Schlaus, R. and Pritchard, J. (1949) Situational stresses and extrapyramidal disease in different personalities. Life stress and bodily disease', *Assoc. Research in Nervous Mental Disease*, pp. 48–60 (as cited in I. L. Janis, *Psychological Stress*, 1958).

Selye, H. (1956) *The Stress of Life*, McGraw-Hill, New York, N.Y.

Selye, H. (1976) *Stress in Health and Disease*, Butterworths, Reading, MA.

Sime, M. (1976) Relationship of pre-operative fear, types of coping and information received about surgery to recovery from surgery, *J. Personal Soc. Psychol.*, **34**, 716–24.

Sime, A. M. and Libera, M. B. (1985) Sensation information, self-instruction and responses to dental surgery, *Research in Nursing and Health*, **8**, 41–7.

Vernon, D. T. and Bigelow, D. A. (1974) Effect of information about a potentially stressful situation on responses to stress impact, *J. Personal Soc. Psychol.*, **29**, 50–9.

Volicer, B. J. (1974) Patients' perceptions of stressful events associated with hospitalization, *Nursing Research*, **23**, 235–8.

Wilson, J. F. (1981) Behavioral preparation for surgery: benefit or harm?, *J. Behav. Medicine*, **4**, 79–102.

Wolfer, J. and Davis, C. (1970) Assessment of surgical patient: pre-operative emotional condition and post-operative welfare, *Nursing Research*, **19**, 402–14.

Wolpe, J. and Lazarus, A. A. (1966) *Behaviour Therapy Techniques*, Pergamon Press, New York, N.Y.

CHAPTER NINE

Patients with coronary heart disease

Out of the many clinical conditions which can affect people, we have chosen to discuss coronary heart disease (CHD) and its relationship with stress at some length. Indeed we have devoted a whole chapter to this condition. We believe this to be merited for several reasons.

Coronary heart disease assumes a high place in the league table of causes of death within the developed world, especially amongst males within the age group 45–64 years (Lee and Franks, 1980). Within the UK 41% of male deaths from the ages of 45–54 years can be attributed to CHD and overall 32% of all male deaths and 24% of all female deaths are certified as caused by CHD (Donaldson and Donaldson, 1983).

More important perhaps is the morbidity caused by the disease. Black and Pole (1975) developed an index of disease burden in which CHD was ranked as the third most serious (after mental illness and handicap and respiratory disease). Donaldson and Donaldson (1983) claim that in the year 1978 in England and Wales nearly 90 000 people became hospital inpatients due to CHD and were responsible for occupying more than 3500 hospital beds each day. In the same year the annual incidence rate in the London Borough of Tower Hamlets was 3.2 per 1000 of the male population and 1.0 per 1000 of the female population.

CHD is a condition affecting people at an age which results in great impact upon their entire family and indeed upon the nation as a whole in terms of reduced productive employment.

Patients with acute coronary heart disease consume a significant share of scarce NHS resources. It follows that if the incidence of CHD could be reduced through preventive measures this would be beneficial not only to potential sufferers and their families but also to the nation.

Apart from considerations of the importance of CHD in mortality and morbidity statistics it is a particularly appropriate condition to discuss in a book devoted to stress and coping, since stress is believed to play an important role in its aetiology. Although there is evidence for such a statement the link between stress and CHD is far from being the clear-cut type of cause–effect relationship that one finds, for example, between the measles virus and measles. Discussion of evidence relating stress to the aetiology of CHD provides a useful example of the kind of work which is needed in establishing links between stress and disease.

Concepts of stress and coping are extremely important for an understanding of the patient's experience of CHD and form a framework within which rehabilitation and the nurse's role can be considered.

9.1 PATHOPHYSIOLOGY OF CHD

First the pathophysiology of CHD will be described before we turn to an identification of the way in which patterns of behaviour may link with disorders of physiology.

The underlying pathological condition in coronary heart disease is athero-sclerosis. Atherosclerosis affects large and medium-sized arteries, the most commonly affected being the aorta, the iliac, femoral, coronary and cerebral arteries. Atherosclerosis exists without any overt signs or symptoms until a mass of artherosclerotic plaque reduces the blood flow through the involved artery to such a level that it compromises the function of the tissue lying distal to the blood vessel (Wolinsky, 1982). By the time the plaque is large enough to cause a problem it comprises: (a) a mixture of cells which are mainly smooth muscle in origin; (b) connective tissue such as elastin, collagen and glycos-aminoglycans; (c) lipid deposits, both intra- and extra-cellular complexes of cholesteryl ester, cholesterol, triglycerides and phospholipids. Cell necrosis is prominent, calcification is often present and haemorrhage from small ingrowing vessels may have occurred. Finally, there has usually been a transient or progressive deposition of platelet clumps or actual thrombus on the irregular luminal surface provided by the plaque. The plaque may have ruptured, releasing its components into the lumen of the vessel. Alternatively there may have been haemorrhage into the plaque or into the vessel wall.

Within the coronary arteries the reduction in blood flow associated with such a lesion can lead to angina pectoris (angina), myocardial infarction (MI) or both (Willerson, 1982). It is these conditions which are referred to by the term coronary heart disease (CHD). In angina, the severe narrowing of the lumen of the coronary vessels results in a decreased ability to deliver the levels of oxygen (0_2) needed by the myocardium to cope with increased cardiac output demanded under conditions of exercise, emotional stress, exposure to cold, or after a heavy meal. Angina is diagnosed from the symptom of pain which occurs when the cardiac muscle demand for oxygen is greater than that received.

Myocardial infarction is the term used to describe the irreversible cellular damage and necrosis which is the consequence of prolonged ischaemia. Ischaemia in its turn is due to an absolute inadequacy of the blood supply to the area. The consequence to the sufferer may vary from pain to sudden death depending upon the amount of myocardial tissue which becomes ischaemic.

Risk factors and coronary heart disease

From what has been described of the pathophysiology of this condition it will be obvious that we need to consider on the one hand the long-term factors which are associated with the development of atherosclerosis and on the other hand the precipitating factors which alter the calibre of the coronary vessels, the composition of the blood within the coronary vessels, or the demand made on the myocardium.

Since atherosclerosis may have been present for a considerable period of time before problems present themselves, evidence identifying the cause or causes may be difficult to obtain. Evidence does show however that there is no one single factor which reliably 'causes' CHD. Instead multiple risk factors have been identified through the use of both retrospective and prospective studies (Donaldson and Donaldson, 1983). These risk factors are as follows:

1. Cigarette smoking

Post-mortem studies have shown that cigarette smoking increases the extent of atheroma in coronary arteries. It is a behaviour which is associated with myocardial infarction and angina in both sexes and the greater the number of cigarettes smoked in unit time, the greater the risk of CHD. When comparing the incidence of myocardial infarction between groups of smokers and non-smokers the greatest difference is in the younger age groups. This is thought to be because other risk factors begin to assume a role in the condition amongst the older age group. In all probability smoking acts synergistically with hypertension and raised blood cholesterol levels. Sudden death from myocardial infarction in particular is strongly related to cigarette smoking.

2. Hypertension

Rises in both systolic and diastolic blood pressure have been shown as important in increasing the risk of CHD.

3. Serum cholesterol levels and dietary fat

There is a fairly clear-cut relationship between higher serum cholesterol levels and risk of death from myocardial infarction. The relationship between serum cholesterol levels and the intake of saturated fats in the diet is disputed however.

4. Other dietary factors

There is some evidence that a high fibre diet reduces the risk of CHD.

5. Lack of exercise

Regular exercise appears to protect the individual from CHD.

6. Obesity

Whilst obesity is certainly associated with risk of CHD, the relationship may be a complex one since obesity is frequently associated with hypertension.

7. Diabetes mellitus

There is an increased risk of CHD amongst diabetics.

8. Other factors

Other factors associated with increased risk of CHD include Type A personality (see below), stress, living in a soft-water area, and increased consumption of coffee.

It is interesting to note that individual behaviour is a factor underlying almost all of the risk factors mentioned above. However the link between the risk factors and the pathophysiology of atheroma has not been explained. In practice this link is not fully understood and exactly which physiological processes trigger the development of atheroma or precipitate coronary heart disease is still unknown. It can be claimed, however, that most of the risk factors already enumerated affect blood vessels or blood composition.

As an example, nicotine, self-administered by inhalation in cigarette smokers has a complex effect upon the size of blood vessels. Hypertension increases the work of the myocardium in delivering an adequate blood supply to tissues. This in turn increases the amount of blood required from the coronary vessels. Increases in serum cholesterol and the disease diabetes mellitus alter the normal blood composition.

On the other hand, there is some evidence that a high fibre diet reduces the absorption of fat from the diet. Regular exercise increases the demand of the myocardium for blood over short periods of time (unlike hypertension which acts similarly for long periods of time). It may act by 'training' cardiovascular control mechanisms to respond more readily to demand for coronary artery vasodilatation. Regular exercise also tends to increase the efficiency of the cardiovascular system so that it can cope with the body's needs at rest at a lower level of heart rate and blood pressure.

Clearly these factors are complex and the underlying mechanism through which behaviour affects physiology is still speculative.

Stress and CHD

It will be apparent by now that the role of stress in the aetiology of CHD is far from simple. Stress was listed amongst the 'other' factors involved in the risk of the disease and this may appear to assign it a fairly insignificant role. However, it is not possible to dismiss stress so lightly since:

(a) stress plays a role in the development of hypertension;
(b) it has been implicated in the development of mature onset diabetes mellitus;
(c) many people claim that they smoke cigarettes to relieve stress;
(d) finally the personality type cited as affecting risk of CHD appears to describe the individual's way of handling stress.

Physiological components of stress and CHD

Before going on to discuss personality and CHD it is worth reminding the reader of the physiological components of stress which were detailed in Chapter 1.

Those aspects which are relevant to our present discussion are as follows:

(a) Arousal is mediated through the reticular activating system (RAS)
(b) Sympathetic nervous system activity occurs and is reinforced by the secretion of the catecholamines, adrenaline and nor-adrenaline from the adrenal medulla
(c) Increased levels of secretion from the adrenal cortex also occur, especially the glucocorticoids but the mineralo-corticoids are also affected

The physiological actions consequent upon these processes which are of relevance here include:

1. increased blood pressure;
2. increased heart rate;
3. release of free fatty acids into the bloodstream;
4. a shift of the equilibrium of the blood toward clotting

There is some evidence that such mechanisms are of clinical relevance. Firstly this evidence comes from animal studies where it has been shown that animals which have been actively coping with environmental stressors have myofibrillatory degeneration of the heart, atherosclerosis, arterial hypertension and increased levels of serum cholesterol. In animals subjected to stressors, but deprived of an effective means of coping, observed pathophysiology comprised ventricular arrest, bradycardia, hypotension, renal defects and gastrointestinal ulceration (Herd, 1978; Schneiderman, 1978).

It is interesting to note that gastrointestinal ulceration is associated in animals and humans with high levels of circulating glucocorticoids.

In humans, environmental stressors have been shown to increase serum cholesterol, blood pressure and heart rate. Carruthers (1969) suggested that the free fatty acids mobilized by sympathetic activity in stress are converted to triglycerides. Where there is an absence of metabolic need (for example in the absence of intense skeletal muscular activity serving 'fight' or 'flight') they are incorporated into atheromatous plaque. Lewis *et al.* (1974) correlated hypertriglyceridaemia with the tendency to develop overt coronary artery disease. Also in a study of motor racing drivers Taggart and Carruthers (1971) found that raised plasma free fatty acids and raised plasma catecholamines occurred together. Later there were rises in plasma triglycerides and reduced free fatty acid levels.

Raab (1971) suggested that in coronary artery insufficiency sympathetic activity increases demand and this leads to myocardial hypoxia. He proposed that any subsequent adrenocortical activity affected myocardial electrolytes by encouraging K^+ and Mg^{2+} excretion and Na^+ retention. Any resulting low K^+ levels within myocardial cells leads to severely reduced cardiac contractility.

Type A personality and CHD

In a retrospective study 100 young patients with coronary heart disease were compared with 100 matched healthy controls by Russek and Zohman (1958). Results showed that prolonged stress in their job had been experienced by 91% of the patients prior to the study but by only 20% of the controls; 25% of the CHD group had been coping with two jobs and 46% had been working for 60 hours or more a week for some time; 20% of this group said they felt insecure, frustrated, restless or inadequate at work. Russek and Zohman also found that the CHD patients were aggressive, ambitious and living beyond their 'normal' capacity.

Russek (1962) also compared doctors in more or less stressful specialities and found the incidence of CHD greater in the more stressful specialities. Hours of work were shown to be important in relation to mortality under the age of 45.

However, whilst these studies suggest a tentative relationship between personality, work and CHD their retrospective nature makes them difficult to interpret. It could well be that people who have suffered a heart attack perceive the period of work leading up to it as more stressful than it really was because they themselves are looking for an explanation, or because they are depressed and/or anxious and this colours all their perceptions.

A research programme which was prospective rather than retrospective was carried out by Rosenman *et al.* (1964, 1975, 1976). This provided better evidence for a link between personality, stress and CHD. However, before discussing this study it is appropriate to define Type A and Type B personality. These are described in terms of behaviour.

Type A (or coronary prone) behaviour

This includes hard driving behaviour, excessive job involvement, time urgency, competitiveness, aggression and hostility (Rosenman and Friedman, 1974). Type A people feel the need to work to achieve self-selected but poorly defined goals which include a desire for recognition and advancement. They appear to have a need to involve themselves in multiple and diverse functions which are constantly subject to time restrictions. They show extraordinary mental and physical alertness and a tendency to accelerate the speed of many physical and mental functions.

Type B individuals

These do not show the characteristics outlined above and display a much more relaxed approach to life and work.

Rosenman *et al.*'s study mentioned above is also known as the Western Collaborative Group Study (WCGS) and was carried out in the USA. In it 3154 males aged 39–59 years and free of clinical CHD were followed up for 8½ years. Approximately 50% were classified as Type A personality on entering the study. Results showed that the Type A subjects were twice as likely to develop CHD than the Type B subjects. Analysis of the results controlling for age, serum cholesterol level, blood pressure level and smoking still showed this two-to-one risk amongst Type A subjects.

The study allowed the identification of the key characteristics of the Type A behaviour which typified those who developed CHD and distinguished them from those who did not develop CHD. These were: potential for hostility, irritability, impatience, competitiveness and vigorous voice stylistics. Rather than relying upon the individual's own account of behaviour, personality classification by these defining behaviours is best carried out through observation in circumstances where there is challenge or provocation to which the subject responds.

Friedman and Rosenman have classified extreme Type A people as Type A_1 and have contrasted them with Type B behaviours as follows.

Type A$_1$ individuals

These individuals

- showed increased urinary and serum levels of noradrenaline during the working day in response to challenge and competition
- had raised serum cholesterol levels
- showed elevated serum triglyceride levels both before and after the ingestion of a fatty test meal. They also showed 'sludging' of erythrocytes after a meal
- exhibited higher serum levels of ACTH and low secretion of 17-hydroxycorticosteroids when injected with ACTH
- showed diminished levels of growth hormone both before and after arginine administration
- displayed a hyperinsulinaemic response when given glucose although there was no abnormal glucose tolerance
- showed more rapid blood clotting

This study is interesting as it shows physiological differences between groups of people who were classified into those groups on the basis of behavioural characteristics and this strengthens the concept of links between behaviour and physiology.

Other studies also suggest the link between Type A behaviour, prevalence and incidence of CHD, recurrent myocardial infarction, and severity of atherosclerosis. For example Glass (1977) associated the occurrence of severe non-controllable stressors with CHD prevalence in Type A people (an example of such a stressor is job loss). This suggests that such stressors have a greater effect on Type A than Type B people. Hames (1975) carried out a long-term prevalence study of CHD in Evans County, Georgia. He found that those individuals who developed CHD were involved in roles which were in the process of changing. They were also less active physically and smoked more than those individuals who did not develop CHD. Significantly, in the light of the discussion above, he found the people who developed CHD to have an exaggerated physiological response to stress, producing twice as much adrenaline in 24 hours as the non-CHD prone group.

CHD and evidence as to 'causes'

It will be obvious that there are many pitfalls in obtaining evidence of the factors leading to the development of CHD. Whilst atheroma and areas of infarcted myocardium can be seen post-mortem, the processes which lead to these pathological states cannot be so easily identified. One of the problems is the time scale over which the condition develops. Any attempt to identify factors which might have been present in a patient's past are not only subject to selective memory but also to the possibility of those memories being re-interpreted through the effects of emotions felt at the time of illness. They may even be affected by the patient or control subject attempting to please the investigator by telling him/her what it is believed they wish to hear. For such reasons scientists are usually extremely cautious about relying on such studies.

Prospective studies are regarded far more favourably but they are not without their problems. Firstly they are expensive since very large samples of subjects must be included to make sure that some will eventually become 'patients' with the diagnosis in which the researchers are interested and also to allow for refusals and drop-outs. Using a large sample not only makes a study expensive but it usually means that several centres and investigators must collaborate. Problems of the reliability and comparability of data must be solved as a consequence. A further problem is that one cannot control the environment and lives of subjects who have agreed to take part in the study as one could laboratory animals. Therefore there may be many variables (events, behaviour) which occur during the course of the study affecting the sample. Some of these variables may be relevant but unknown to the investigator. Others may be relevant and known to the investigator but of such complexity and perhaps low frequency as to make statistical comparisons difficult.

In both retrospective and prospective studies, researchers infer that all significant differences between the CHD group and the controls are relevant to the development of the condition. This is not necessarily the case (Cromwell and Levenkron 1984).

Prevention of CHD

From what is known about risk factors in the development of CHD it follows logically that individuals could reduce the risk of developing CHD themselves quite considerably by altering specific behaviour patterns or the total life style. Unfortunately it seems difficult to convince people of this. For example, Friedman (1979) has argued that Type A behaviour can only be successfully changed in patients who have suffered myocardial infarction rather than individuals who are clearly at risk but who have not suffered symptoms. This is supported by studies carried out by Roskies *et al.* (1978, 1979), Jenni and Wollersheim (1979) and Suinn and Bloom (1978) in which there was an attempt to modify the life style of Type A people who had no overt coronary symptoms. Such people appear to deny that their behaviour leads to a risk of CHD. However, in the research cited one strategy using a teaching programme which was more successful, was that of an attempt to modify components of the individual's behaviour.

The teaching programmes designed for post-infarction patients are often aimed at instruction about specific behaviours, and these also seem to be more effective than those programmes aimed at counselling or changing value systems underlying Type A behaviour. Examples of effective programmes include instruction in exercise, relaxation techniques, the recognition of signs of tension and guided imagery.

The implications of this appear to be that individuals may respond more positively to teaching about ways in which they can themselves do something to prevent disease (e.g. exercise, stopping smoking, stress management, taking a high fibre diet, reduction in alcohol consumption) than more general methods aimed at getting them to be less competitive, less aggressive, and generally to take it more 'easily'. It could be argued that learning about specific behaviours gives individuals a method of active control.

In this country today the media is promoting the idea of healthy living to a much greater extent than in the past. Articles, books, radio and TV programmes deal with aspects such as diet, methods of losing weight, the importance of exercise and stress and its management. Sponsored runs and jogging are organized. Social pressure is gradually making smokers aware that cigarette smoking is an antisocial activity, apart from its effects upon health. There are increasing numbers of non-smoking areas in restaurants and public transport. Hospitals are introducing 'no-smoking' policies. Advertisements emphasize the benefits of polyunsaturated fats and fibre-rich food.

It will be interesting to see if these changes in the values promoted through the media and public opinion generally result in any effect upon the incidence of CHD. However, without properly controlled study cause and effect relationships cannot be elucidated.

However, this does show the ways in which professionals within the NHS could help in the prevention of CHD. This might be first of all through their own good example in being non-smokers, eating healthily and taking regular exercise. Secondly, whenever there is an opportunity for health education at an individual or a group level, it should be taken. In this context it is particularly disappointing that health visitors concentrate so much of their time on the under-five's that they have little time left for others who could benefit from their advice. Thirdly, nurses could possibly teach patients stress management techniques such as relaxation as for coping with pain, sleep-lessness or anxiety during the course of their treatment. Techniques taught in a specific context could then be used later by the individual to cope in other situations where relaxation techniques would be beneficial.

9.2 THE CHD PATIENT DURING ADMISSION TO HOSPITAL

In Chapter 7 we have seen that many patients develop increased anxiety on admission to hospital. A patient who suffers myocardial infarction is likely to be anxious long before reaching hospital. He or she will probably have experienced a crushing pain in the chest and may have collapsed. Such events lead to certainty that something serious has happened. Anxiety may also be experienced as a consequence of the physiological effects of low blood pressure and increased levels of circulating catecholamines. If breathlessness is present it may have resulted in the administration of oxygen by means of a mask. This frequently leads to feelings of panic in patients who are unused to polymasks.

Patients with a diagnosis of myocardial infarction are usually admitted to a coronary care unit (CCU) where the electrical events in the heart are monitored and an intravenous infusion (IVI) is set up. The implications of being admitted to a CCU may in themselves frighten patients (and relatives) apart from the fear which may be evoked by high-tech equipment and procedures (Hay and Oken, 1972). From this we can predict that many patients with myocardial infarction will undergo an increase of anxiety on admission over and above an already high level of anxiety.

It should be remembered, however, that not all patients experience anxiety on admission to hospital. To some it is comforting. Certainly, many patients with myocardial infarction will be relieved to get the expert care and treatment which is available within the CCU. The administration of an opiate to relieve pain will also reduce anxiety. Nonetheless anxiety levels are likely to rise as the realization of what has happened makes its impact.

It seems fairly obvious that under such conditions the phychological aspects of care become all important. Yet, there appear to be few research studies into the early period of hospitalization after myocardial infarction. One programme of research into the psychological care within the CCU was known as the Vanderbilt/Holy Cross Project as it was a collaborative project between Vanderbilt University and Holy Cross Hospital, Silver Spring, Maryland.

The Vanderbilt/Holy Cross Project

A total of 229 patients admitted to the CCU were judged suitable and comprised the initial study population. However, some 20% of these were discharged before the study was completed, leaving 183 patients who participated throughout the research period. Independent and retrospective diagnosis of these patients resulted in 51% being allocated alternative diagnosis such as congestive cardiac failure, pancreatitis or duodenal ulcer. This provided an excellent control group for the other 49% admitted to the CCU whose diagnosis of myocardial infarction (MI) received independent validation.

A further control group, however, comprised 80 patients who were admitted to other wards in the hospital and had no disorder of the cardio-vascular system.

A complex research protocol was designed to investigate the effects of different psychological treatments in a 2 × 2 × 2 factorial design. Each patient entering the study was assigned to receive high or low levels of psychological care on each of three dimensions. These dimensions of psychological care were:

1. receiving high or low amounts of information about the nature and severity of the condition;
2. being allowed high or low diversional activity and stimulation;
3. being permitted to carry out high or low levels of self care.

It is important to note that low levels of psychological care on any dimension meant receiving the normal ward care. Staff in the CCU were instructed as to their role in the low information condition. Interestingly this meant that nurses were asked not to answer factual questions but to refer such questions to the physicians. It is worth noting that Volicer and Bohannon (1975) found that 'not having your questions answered' was ranked quite high as a stressor. In contrast, the high information condition included the provision of a tape recording with extensive information about heart attacks, their course and treatment. A shorter tape focused upon support, reassurance and a description of the CCU. Both tapes were available for further listening as requested. Extensive literature was also made available explaining heart attacks, how the heart works and the treatment. A house physician was assigned to explain this same information and all medical and nursing staff were encouraged to be as informative as possible.

For the 'high diversion' condition, the patient was assigned a bed area near a large window, given a TV set and positioned near to the entrance to the ward so that the comings and goings offered stimulation. An art 'mobile' was hung outside the window. Magazines, books, and newspapers were readily available and extended visiting was allowed unless the patient himself wished to curtail this. Nursing and other staff of the CCU were asked to engage patients in this condition in friendly conversation and the relevant clergy were encouraged to visit for unlimited time.

Each patient assigned to the 'high participation' condition was instructed to activate the ECG tape of the cardiac monitor whenever a symptom was felt. They were asked to carry out a daily regime of mild isometric exercise to prevent embolism, and a fast pedalling exercise was to be done whilst being monitored for heart rate, blood pressure and ECG. In general the attitude that the patient was a full participant in his/her own recovery was fostered. One criticism of this regime is that it could well be that the actuation of the ECG monitor when symptoms occurred actually reinforced more frequent occurrence of symptoms.

As well as being assigned to one of the eight treatment groups patients were identified at a point on each of three personality scales. These scales were: Repression – Sensitization (see Chapter 2), Environmental Scanning, which refers to the rate at which an individual processes information within the environment, and Locus of Control (see Chapter 8).

Dependent or outcome measures of psychological interventions included many indices of recovery, comfort and compliance with treatment and advice.

Such a complex research design was used because it was believed that personality variables and psychological intervention would interact together. It was also hypothesized that the different types of psychological intervention would also interact together. For example, high participation might be effective with an individual who was high on internal locus of control but not with an individual who was high on external locus of control. Another example might be that high diversion and high participation were ineffective together but that either was effective with low levels of other psychological interventions.

It was hoped that this research design would produce results which gave more precise guidance about which patients should be given information, a self-care role, or diversion, and whether such interventions might actually prove harmful to some.

Since all these psychological interventions were designed to be included as part of the nursing role, the study has important implications for nursing.

Results of the study

Firstly, the study was able to demonstrate that the effectiveness of a high level of one type of psychological intervention depended very much upon the level of the other two psychological interventions which were included in the study. For example, if high information was given to a patient who was also assigned either high self-care or high diversion but not both, then the outcome was favourable, both in terms of the length of stay in the CCU and in terms of the length of stay in the hospital itself. On the other hand, high information levels with low diversion and low self-care participation was associated with a longer stay both in the CCU and the hospital. The authors of the study interpreted this to mean that high levels of diversion and self-care gave the patient the means of coping with the information they had received about their condition. This interpretation was supported by other data. For example, patients who were given much information and assigned to the high participation condition exhibited few cardiac monitor alarms for abnormal heart rate. If, however, information was low and participation high or information high and participation low then the number of alarms was greater. Effects of the psychological interventions were not apparent after the patient left hospital but this was most probably because of the relative insensitivity of the measures used in this period (deaths and re-admission rates).

Turning to the exploration of any interaction between personality and psychological intervention, four findings supported the hypothesis that these would prove important. One outcome however, which was striking, could not be submitted for statistical evaluation. Each of the patients who died or developed a further infarction during the 12-week follow-up were either internal locus of control with low participation in self-care or external locus of control with high participation in self-care, both combinations could be predicted to be incongruent and therefore psychologically uncomfortable. The authors speculate as to whether this prevented patients from seeking early help if the symptoms of further infarction occurred as they wished to avoid further hospitalization.

Interestingly the authors of this study also argue that there was evidence from the study that the repression–sensitization scale measured anxiety levels and not repression–sensitization. Those which were labelled as sensitizers by this scale were those with the high levels of anxiety.

Further findings from the study were that sensitizers (or those with high anxiety) who received low information and repressors (those with low anxiety) who received high information levels, displayed a greater number of monitor alarms per day than the opposite combinations. It should be noted that these findings are congruent with those quoted in Chapter 8 from studies by Johnson *et al.* (1978), Delong (1970) and Sime and Libera (1985) in relation to surgical patients.

As for the scanning dimension of personality, the number of monitor alarms was greater in those low on scanning given low diversion and those high on scanning given high diversion. It was also the case that more of the patients who died in the follow-up period, regardless of their score on the personality scales, had been subject to the high diversion condition. The researchers suggest that this might be because the high diversion provided had led some of the patients not to take their cardiac illness seriously and they might therefore not have complied with the advice they received about management after discharge from hospital.

Prediction or prospective study

In addition to the analysis referred to above, the authors also used the information which they collected during the course of the study to identify its usefulness in the prediction of outcome during the 12-week period after discharge. This therefore became a prospective study for the development of complications, further infarction or death.

It was found that death during the follow up period was predicted by (a) a low score for social affection on the Nowlis Mood Adjective check list at the end of the CCU stay, and (b) the level of plasma non-esterised fatty acids. The low social affection score was interpreted by the researchers as a sign of 'giving up'.

Re-admission to hospital with a further infarction was predicted by four psychological variables and three biological ones. The relevant psychological variables were: extensive scanning; the number of cards guessed during a solvable guessing game; level of depression at the beginning of the stay in CCU; and high anxiety. Biological predictive variables were: sedimentation rate; 17-hydroxycorticosteroid level at 3.30 pm following an unsolvable card guessing game which had taken place between 10.45 and 11 am; the highest recorded systolic blood pressure during the stay in CCU. (The lower this was, the more likely the patient was to have been re-admitted to hospital.) Interestingly, in this study, the psychological variables mentioned here were more powerful predictors than were the biological variables.

MI PATIENTS VERSUS CONTROLS

Reference was made above to card guessing games. These were used with both the MI patients and the controls to identify responses during stress. The games were simple and designed to produce slightly less of an autonomic response than an exciting TV programme. They were used at the same time in the morning on two consecutive days. On the first occasion the game was solvable and the patients experienced success, whilst on the second occasion the game was unsolvable and the patient experienced failure. The most interesting of the differences in response between the MI patients and the controls was in the 17-hydroxycorticosteroid levels. On both days the non-MI controls showed an immediate but slight increase in plasma levels which had returned to normal within 70 minutes of the game. By way of contrast the MI patients showed only a minimal increase in 17-hydroxycorticosteroid levels immediately after the game but a marked elevation some 70 minutes later on both days. This pattern is similar to that seen in hospitalized depressed patients.

Further analysis of data included identification of the differences on a complex of variables between the MI patients and the non-MI patients in the CCU. Many of these differences proved not to be predictive of outcome for the MI patients and so the authors advise caution in the interpretation of studies in which two groups of people are studied, one group of which has the diagnosis in which the researchers are interested. The pattern in such studies is to identify the differences on many variables between the two groups and then to assume that the differences which are found are relevant to the diagnosis of interest. There is an error of logic in such reasoning but the Vanderbilt/Holy Cross study has produced evidence of the dangers of that type of study.

Findings in the Vanderbilt/Holy Cross study of relevant differences between the MI patients and the controls were that the MI patients were more likely:

- to have been male

- to have a history of heart disease themselves and for their family to have such a history
- to bottle up tension
- to score for external locus of control
- to get little exercise
- to have greater self-control

This particular study of psychological intervention within the CCU has been explained at length here for several reasons. Firstly it was concerned with the effectiveness of nursing care of a psychological nature. Secondly it is one of the few studies to investigate psychological care in the CCU systematically. This may well indicate that psychological care is of less importance to staff than physiological care during the acute stage of myocardial infarction. Yet the patient is likely to suffer the greatest degree of psychological discomfort during this stage.

In contrast, many studies have been carried out into the psychological care of patients with myocardial infarction before their discharge from hospital. Indeed routine programmes of psychological care and education for discharge which occur once the patient has left the CCU are fairly commonplace. It is to a discussion of re-education and rehabilitation that we now turn.

Re-education and rehabilitation after myocardial infarction

As was demonstrated by the Vanderbilt/Holy Cross study, recovery from myocardial infarction does not protect the sufferer from further attacks. On the contrary, the risk of further attacks is high. This is why it is common to teach the patient before discharge from hospital about actions which he or she can take to reduce the risk of further myocardial infarction.

Obviously no teaching or advice is of use unless the individual complies with it and continues to comply over a long period of time. Indeed the issue which has already been discussed, that of Type A people failing to take advice before myocardial infarction, is largely a problem of compliance. There is a vast literature on compliance (see for example Dimatteo and Dinicola, 1982), but one of the basic principles is that the individual must believe

(i) that he/she has a health problem;
(ii) that following advice, taking the prescribed drug or changing one's life style will help to alleviate the problem (Rosenstock, 1966; Becker and Maiman, 1975).

As mentioned above, most hospitals attempt a teaching programme for patients with myocardial infarction before their discharge from hospital. This often takes the form of an information leaflet. Such leaflets or booklets are extremely useful to back-up face-to-face teaching but are no substitute for such informative communication.

In general, the teaching programme should be planned so that it can include the patient's family. Information should be given gradually, i.e. over several days, with plenty of time for consolidation and questions. The purpose or aim of the teaching is two-fold:

(i) to give information about behavioural changes which will help to prevent further myocardial infarction;
(ii) to prevent invalidism and morbidity.

One such programme has been fully reported in the nursing literature (Howard and Erlanger, 1983). Important aspects of such a teaching programme are:

1. Assessment of the patient's educational needs, educational level and readiness to learn.
2. Keeping careful records of the assessment and of each teaching session.
3. Careful planning of each session.
4. Reinforcement of the previous teaching before giving new information.
5. Ensuring uninterrupted time with the patient during which the teaching can be carried out.
6. Careful planning to suit the information to the patient's needs.

The information which is usually included comprises:

- an account of the anatomy and physiology of the heart
- the nature of myocardial infarction, the development of atheroma and sudden occlusion
- healing, the formation of scar tissue within the myocardium and the development of a collateral circulation
- risk factors and how to cope with these for the future (specialists such as a dietician may be brought in to give advice)
- how long each phase of hospital care will take
- instructions for care after leaving hospital, in terms of precise guidelines on activity and mobility, driving, sexual activity and returning to work
- information about medication and what to do if there is any pain

Throughout the teaching programme both the patient and the family should be given every opportunity to ask advice. The entire programme should be evaluated in terms of the knowledge gained and the compliance with advice.

Other psychological care

We have discussed above the provision of systematic education for the patient who has had a myocardial infarction. This will usually be carried out by nursing staff although sometimes medical staff may wish to do it themselves. Clearly such information is an important component of psychological care since it includes much information about the condition as well as specific advice on coping in the future. However the part of the individual teaching which the patient most welcomes may be the opportunity to ask questions and also to express their anxieties to a member of staff who shows a willingness to listen. Since only those patients who wish to do so will open up in this way there is nothing here which contradicts those research studies which suggest that different types of psychological care should be provided to suit the different coping styles of patients. It is important to allow those patients who wish to express their feelings to do so. This means that staff must be prepared to encourage this by the use of open questions not closed ones, and by their non-verbal communication through which they indicate that they have time for the patient.

9.3 SUMMARY

In this chapter we have discussed coronary heart disease (CHD) and its relationship with stress. Statistics on mortality and morbidity show CHD to be an important condition within the developed world in general and within the UK in particular. In terms of the number of deaths attributed to CHD, the age group in which it assumes prominence, and the morbidity associated with it, the disease is one which causes great concern both to the health services and in relation to the economy.

The pathophysiology of CHD has been described and an account of the risk factors implicated in its causation given. Some of the evidence which points to an association between stress and CHD led us to a discussion of Type A or coronary prone personality.

We next turned to a consideration of the type of research evidence available to identify the causes of the disease and an account of factors which might help in the prevention of the condition.

In the latter part of the chapter consideration was given to the psychological care (or stress-reduction methods) given to patients admitted to hospital with acute myocardial infarction. This centred mainly upon a detailed account of one programme of research, the Vanderbilt/Holy Cross study. Some of the findings of this study, in identifying the interaction between personality type and response to psychological intervention, reinforce similar findings in studies of patients undergoing surgery which were discussed in Chapter 8.

Finally, education for discharge from hospital following acute myocardial infarction can be seen as acting by giving patients a range of coping strategies for the future.

REFERENCES

Becker, M. H. and Maiman, L. A. (1975) Sociobehavioural determinants of compliance with health and medical care recommendations. *Medical Care*, **13**, 10–24.

Black, D. A. K. and Pole, J. D. (1975) Priorities in biomedical research: indices of burden. *Brit. J. Prev. Soc. Med.*, **29**, 222–7.

Carruthers, M. A. (1969) Aggression and atheroma. *Lancet*, **ii**, 1170.

Cromwell, R. L. and Levenkron, J. C. (1984) Psychological care of acute coronary patients, in *Health Care and Human Behaviour* (eds A. Steptoe and A. Mathews), Academic Press, London.

DeLong, R. D. (1970) *Individual Differences in Patterns of Anxiety, Arousal, Stress – Relevant Information and Recovery from Surgery*, Doctoral Dissertation, University of California, Los Angeles.

Dimatteo, M. R. and Dinicola, D. D. (1982) *Achieving Patient Compliance*, Pergamon Press, New York, N.Y.

Donaldson, R. J. and Donaldson, L. J. (1983) *Essential Community Medicine*. MTP, Lancaster.

Friedman, M. (1979) The modification of Type A behavior in post-infarction patients. *Am. Heart J.*, **97** 551–66.

Glass, D. C. (1977) *Behavior Patterns, Stress and Coronary Disease*, Lawrence Erlbaum, Hillsdale, N.J.

Hames, C. (1975) Most likely to succeed as a candidate for a coronary attack, in *New Horizons in Cardiovascular Practice* (ed. H.I. Russek), University Park Press, New York, N.Y.

Hay, D. and Oken, D. (1972). The psychological stresses of ICU nursing. *J. Psychosomatic Medicine*, **34**, 109–18.

Herd, J. A. (1978) Physiological correlates of coronary prone behavior, in *Coronary-Prone Behavior* (eds T. M. Dembroski, S. M. Weiss, J. L. Shields *et al.*), Springer-Verlag, New York, N.Y.

Howard, J. A. and Erlanger, H. (1983) Teaching methods for coronary patients, in *Patient Teaching* (ed. J. Wilson Barnett), Churchill-Livingstone, Edinburgh.

Jenni, M. A. and Wollersheim, J. P. (1979) Cognitive therapy, stress management training and the type A behavior pattern. *Cog. Ther. Res.*, **3**, 61–73.

Johnson, J. E., Rice, V. H., Fuller, S. S. and Endress, M. P. (1978) Sensory information, instruction and coping strategy and recovery from surgery. *Research in Nursing and Health*, **1**, 4–17.

Lee, P. R. and Franks, P. E. (1980) Health and disease in the community, in *Primary Care* (ed. J. Fry), Heinemann, London.

Lewis, B., Chait, A, Oakley, C. M. O. *et al.*, (1974) Serum lipoprotein abnormalities in patients with ischaemic heart disease; comparisons with control population. *Br. Med. J.*, **3**, 489.

Raab, W. (1971) Cardiotoxic biochemical effects of emotional–environmental stressor-fundamentals of psychocardiology, in *Society, Stress and Disease*, Vol. 1 (ed. L. Levi), Oxford University Press, Oxford.

Rosenman, R. H. and Friedman, M. (1974) Neurogenic factors in pathogenesis of coronary heart disease. *Med. Clinics North Amer.*, **58**, 269–79.

Rosenman, R. H., Friedman, M., Strauss, R. *et al.* (1964) A predictive study of coronary heart disease: the Western Collaborative Group Study. *J. Amer. Med. Assoc.*, **189**, 15–22.

Rosenman, R. H., Brand, R. J. Jenkins, C. D. *et al.* (1975) Coronary heart disease in the Western Collaborative Group Study: final follow-up experience of 8½ years. *J. Amer. Med. Assoc.*, **223**, 872–7.

Rosenman, R. H. Brand, R. J., Scholtz, R. I. and Friedman, M. (1976) Multi-variate prediction of coronary heart disease during 8.5 year follow up in the Western Collaborative Group Study. *Am. J. Cardiology*, **37**, 903–10.

Rosenstock, I. M. (1966) Why people use health services. *Milbank Memorial Fund Quarterly*, **44**, 94–127.

Roskies, E., Spevack, M., Surkis, A. *et al.* (1978) Changing the coronary-prone (Type A) behavior pattern in a non-clinical population. *J. Behav. Med.*, **1**, 201–16.

Roskies, E., Kearney, H., Spevack, M. *et al.* (1979) Generalizability and durability of the treatment effects in an intervention program for coronary-prone (Type A) managers. *J. Behav. Med.*, **2**, 195–207.

Russek, H. I. (1962) Emotional stress and coronary heart disease in American physicians, dentists and lawyers, *Am. J. Med. Sci.*, **243**, 716.

Russek, H. I. and Zohman, B. L. (1958) Relative significance of hereditary, diet and occupational stress in CHD of young adults. *Am. J. Med. Sci.*, **235**, 266.

Schneiderman, N. (1978) Animal models relating behavioral stress and cardiovascular pathology, in *Coronary-Prone Behavior* (eds. T. M. Dembroski, S. M. Weiss, J. L. Shield *et al.*), Springer-Verlag, New York, N.Y.

Sime, A. M. and Libera, M. B. (1985) Sensation information, self-instruction and responses to dental surgery. *Research in Nursing and Health*, **8**, 41–7.

Suinn, R. M. and Bloom, L. J. (1978) Anxiety management training for Type A patients. *J. Behav. Med.*, **1**, 25–35.

Taggart, P. and Carruthers, M. (1971) Endogenous hyperlipidaemia induced by emotional stress of racing driving. *Lancet*, **i**, 363.

Volicer, J. V. and Bohannon, M. M. (1975) A hospital stress rating scale. *Nursing Research*, **24**, 352–9.

Willerson, J. T. (1982) Angina pectoris and acute myocardial infarction, in

Cecil Textbook of Medicine (16th edn) (eds J. B. Wyngaarden and L. H. Smith), W. B. Saunders, PA.

Wolinsky, H. (1982) Atherosclerosis, in *Cecil Textbook of Medicine* (16th edn) (eds J. B. Wyngaarden and L. H. Smith), W. B. Saunders, PA.

CHAPTER TEN

Patients with chronic/disabling conditions

Medical technology and nursing care have advanced to the position where people survive injuries and diseases which would once have been fatal. However, once the person has progressed to the point where his or her life is no longer in danger they and their families are faced with an enormous task of adaptation to an entirely new mode of living. Such adjustment is necessary if the life which has been saved is to possess any quality at all. This process of adjustment can be defined as a process employed toward the goal of achieving harmony between the person and the new circumstances (Trieschmann, 1980a). In the terms used in this book it can be seen as a process of coping.

Since the late 1930s medical science has achieved enormous progress in the eradication of acute disease due to infection within developed countries. This has changed the pattern of mortality and morbidity with far-reaching consequences. In the highly industrialized countries what people suffer from mostly are chronic conditions (Strauss et al., 1984). The 10 leading causes of limitation of activity in the USA in 1977 (Strauss et al., 1984) were, in order of magnitude of the number affected:

1. Heart disease
2. Arthritis and rheumatism
3. Impairments of the back or spine
4. Impairments of the lower extremities or hips
5. Other musculoskeletal disorders
6. Hypertensive disease
7. Asthma
8. Diabetes
9. Senility
10. Emphysema

In Britain in 1976 the main causes of severe and very severe handicap in adults of working age (Donaldson and Donaldson, 1983) were, again in order of magnitude of numbers affected:

1. Arthritis
2. Rheumatoid arthritis
3. Stroke and Parkinsonism
4. Cardiorespiratory disorders
5. Trauma and amputations
6. Disorders of infancy and youth (e.g. cerebral palsy)
7. Multiple sclerosis
8. Other rheumatic disorders
9. Other systems
10. Miscellaneous including paraplegia/hemiplegia, neoplasms, and sensory disorders

It is obvious that from the medical or nursing point of view we are classifying together very disparate types of condition. What they all have in common is the effect upon the sufferer's life of limiting their range of activity in some way. This imposes a need for coping and that is our concern in this chapter.

From the point of view of the sufferer there are many problems and demands consequent upon chronic illness. These have been listed by Strauss *et al.* (1984) as:

- the long-term nature of the conditions
- the uncertainty associated with prognosis and with some conditions and their episodic nature
- the requirement for great effort in palliation of the condition
- consequences tend to be multiple
- the conditions are extremely intrusive on the lives of the patients and families, causing changes in lifestyle and household routine
- they create social isolation
- they require a wide variety of ancillary services
- they are expensive
- multiple problems of daily living occur
- medical crises must be prevented or managed if they occur
- symptoms must be controlled
- prescribed regimens must be carried out and these may in turn create attendant problems
- adjustment to changes in the course of the disease is needed if it gets worse or if there are remissions

Coping which is required to maintain the quality of life under such circumstances includes:

- efforts to normalize interaction with others and life style
- finding the necessary money to pay for treatment or survive complete or partial loss of employment
- confronting psychological, marital and familial problems

Some of the issues concerned with those disease states which become gradually or rapidly severe will be discussed in other chapters. In this chapter we wish to consider the adjustment and coping required when an individual must learn to live with relatively suddenly imposed physical limitations, but where there is not normally any implication of gradual deterioration thereafter. The prime examples of such circumstances are major accidental injury, or stroke, but in the past, poliomyelitis causing severe paralysis also illustrated the same type of changed lifestyle.

One accidental injury about which there has been a fair amount of research is that of spinal cord injury resulting in paraplegia or quadriplegia. Consequently, discussion in this chapter will focus mainly around this condition, with some illustrations from work on other traumatic physical conditions where it is available and appropriate.

10.1 SPINAL CORD INJURY

It is interesting to speculate on the reasons for the amount of research on spinal cord injury. It is a considerable problem in financial terms, especially in the USA where much of the research has been carried out. In 1984 in the USA there were between 120 000 and 150 000 persons with spinal cord injury and it is estimated that about 10 000 new cases occur each year (Brackett *et al.*, 1984). It is a problem which affects males predominantly (80% are male) and which occurs mainly within the younger age group (80% are under 40 years). Thus it affects a group who would normally be economically active. Approximately 50% of the spinal injured population are paraplegic and 50% quadriplegic (Brackett *et al.*, 1984). Causes are motor traffic accidents, dives into shallow water, gunshots or other criminal woundings. War veterans are included among the spinal injured population.

In Britain the problem is less prominent. This can partly be attributed to legislation on the wearing of seat belts and drink-driving and the lower incidence of crime involving firearms.

As suggested above, spinal cord injuries do pose a problem in war time and it was the medical and nursing care developed during the Second World War under the leadership of Guttman in the UK which has ensured that, under normal circumstances, those who survive the immediate post-trauma period live to within 10% of their pre-injury life expectation.

The process of adjustment of people who suddenly sustain severe spinal cord injury can be classified into three phases which parallel phases of contact with health services. The initial phase occurs during the immediate period after injury, i.e. during intensive care. Rehabilitation follows this and the third phase is adjustment back to life in the community, albeit a very different life from that enjoyed before injury.

Phase 1: The acute, intensive care phase

If we imagine what it must be like to be in the intensive care unit having suffered a spinal cord injury our reactions are probably as extreme as those displayed in the professional literature. 'Few non-fatal injuries have as devastating a physical and psychological aftermath as those created by trauma to the spinal column and its contents' (Franco, 1986). 'The impact embodies two of mankind's greatest fears; physical helplessness and sexual impotence' (Friedman-Campbell and Hart, 1984). However it is unlikely that the full impact of the condition in this devastating form is felt by the patient immediately.

The intensive care/accident and emergency environment itself, however, may be extremely threatening, as may the medical intervention necessary to save life on admission. It takes little imagination to identify the impact of the following (Brackett *et al.*, 1984):

> Once the emergency breathing and circulation support is established, appropriate roentgenograms are taken (X-rays). If it is necessary for the patient to be moved, a special mobilizer with an electrically driven top is used, which can scoop up and place a patient without any risk of spinal motion. Cervical fractures will be stabilized in the emergency room with halo or tong traction and the patient placed directly on a kinetic treatment table on which he is then wheeled to the intensive care unit. The kinetic treatment table is a bed that oscillates slowly and continuously from side to side with the patient being secured between foam packs. . . Once the nursing team has established the intravenous and all other lines and has the patient stabilized, the protocol then calls for notification of respiratory and physical therapy, the psychologist and such ancillary specialists and personnel as may be necessary.

There is little in the literature about how the patient feels at this time but much speculation about the impact not only of the life-saving techniques and environment but the gradually dawning realization of the extent of the injury which involves paralysis.

Theoretically it is believed that the individual in such circumstances will grieve for the loss of self (Friedman-Campbell and Hart, 1984). A model for grieving by Worden (1982) has been adapted to apply to the spinal cord injured person by Friedman-Campbell and Hart (1984). This is a stage model.

In the first stage there is acceptance that the loss of part of the body function is final. The individual moves through shock and denial to the second stage in which there is the experience of the pain of grief. This has been termed 'grief work'. Experience of the present loss may reactivate experience of past losses as well and these all contribute to the grieving process. During the third stage the individual begins to develop strategies which help in adapting to altered relationships, the environment and decreased physical and financial independence. Goals are re-defined. The fourth stage occurs when the injured person withdraws his or her emotional energy from the loss and reinvests it in other relationships and activities. This stage is called 'restitution' and it may occur one to two years or even as many as four years after injury.

Friedman-Campbell and Hart (1984) believe that crisis intervention is a useful model to use for the provision of support to the patient and family. Crisis intervention is a therapeutic approach which is used to analyse and to aid psychological functioning during situations in which emotional stability is at great risk. The goal of intervention is the resolution of the immediate crisis through a focus upon the present. The individual is helped in exploring the meaning of the crisis and their personal responses to it. Coping behaviour and support networks which have been helpful in past threats are identified and an individual plan is formulated to handle the current crisis. Thus both internal and external coping support systems are mobilized. The technique aids grieving since it allows for discussion of the traumatic event and its meaning. It also has the value that it familiarizes the family with the mourning process and legitimizes their own grief.

Obviously the stage model of grief outlined above extends considerably beyond the immediate period after the injury. There are many other stage models of the patient's emotional adjustments described in the literature. However, the validity of such models has been called into question (Trieschmann, 1980b). Many models suggest that a period of denial of the extent of damage occurs in the early weeks after injury, but Trieschmann argues that there are no data to substantiate this. Indeed she argues compellingly that there is likely to be clouding of consciousness at this time from anaesthesia, analgesia, sensory deprivation and sleep deprivation and this prevents full realization of the extent of functional loss. Certainly this suggestion is supported by Braakman et al. (1976) who showed that patients actively wish for information about their prognosis within two weeks of injury.

The problem with stage models of emotional responses is the implications which people draw from them that the individual will fail to recover if each stage is not experienced or worked through. In particular it is believed that initial denial must be followed by profound depression. However research has suggested that those who are least depressed in the early stages are most likely to function better during rehabilitation and after discharge, whilst Hohmann (1966) suggests that the spinal injury itself may disrupt the autonomic nervous system, reducing the experience of emotion. A study by Bodenhamer et al. (1983) is interesting in this context. In this study, in two rehabilitation units in Dallas (Texas), both staff and patients completed the same questionnaire about emotional responses after spinal cord injury. The staff were asked to complete the questionnaire in the way they thought the average patient would. Results showed that staff overestimated the amount of depression and social discomfort experienced by patients but underestimated the degree of anxiety patients experienced. They also underestimated the patients' positive outlook. Interestingly the staff who most accurately reflected patients' reactions were the least experienced, all but one having had less than one year's experience in rehabilitation.

Thus it can be argued that staff should be very careful about attributing emotions to patients but should be sensitive to and assess carefully the emotions actually experienced. This is particularly important since anxiety can probably be helped more easily than depression.

Regardless of the accuracy of stage theories of emotion there is no doubt that the patient's period in intensive care will be a stressful one. Staff quite rightly see their first priority as establishing physiological stability and so psychological care may be pushed to one side. Psychological care which accompanies physical items of care can be of enormous benefit in helping the patient to cope during this time and can also serve to reduce the degree of stress experienced. Brackett *et al.* (1984) have described psychological care in a spinal cord injury treatment centre in Florida.

First of all, three principles underly all care in this centre. These are:

1. The person with spinal cord injury has dignity, value and importance.
2. Detailed explanation of what is being done and why is important, as is the constant presence and reassurance of staff. Explanation to the family is also important and they are given insight into the anatomy and physiology of spinal cord injury. Staff concern for the patient's physical and psychological well-being is expressed frequently.
3. It is helpful to talk about interests, hobbies and habits which concerned the patient before injury with the patient and family. Knowledge of these can be used in conversation and interaction with the patient to give reassurance about concern for him/her as an individual.

Staff actions can also be used to enhance psychological care. For example, staff are encouraged to sit when feeding the patient and when talking and also to maintain eye contact. (It should be pointed out that the position in which the patient is being nursed makes this more difficult than it may appear.) During kinetic therapy there is no way that the patient can wipe his/her own tears and these may track into the ears. Nursing staff are briefed to wipe tears frequently and also to hold the patient's hand and assure him/her that tears are acceptable and that staff are with him to help. Active listening is employed to allow the patient to express fears. Staff are expected to announce their presence before entering the patient's room. Reassurance of patients is achieved by:

- making sure that each patient feels that staff are with him/her physically and psychologically
- ensuring that patients know that help is available if there is any breathing difficulty

- encouraging staff to touch the patient on the forehead or cheek
- staff asking direct questions about what fears the patient has and being accepting of these fears
- explaining the knowledge and expertise of the staff

In this paper (Brackett *et al.*, 1984) the authors discuss problem behaviour which might be displayed by patients, but point out that such behaviour in terms of its goal may well be serving an important psychological need for the patient, for example, gaining a sense of mastery or control. By attempting to identify the function such behaviour is performing for the patient, empathy can be aroused and other less disruptive ways of achieving the same goal may be found. For example, finding opportunities where the patient can legitimately exert control, e.g. in choice of food at mealtimes, participation in care planning, negotiation of times for therapy. Staff in the Florida unit are encouraged to deal honestly and openly with their own feelings, even to the extent of expressing them to patients.

Trieschmann (1980b) has documented the problems which patients experience initially after severe spinal cord injury; these are mainly related to physiological experiences and knowing what these are leads to an understanding of strategies which may help.

Trieschmann argues that immediately the paralysis is realized there may be a feeling that the limbs have been cut off. Allowing the individual to see and touch the affected limbs removes this feeling and it may rekindle hope. Disturbances in sensation may occur, and pain may be a problem. There are changes in body image. Sensory deprivation is a potential problem, partly at least because the sensory input from a part of the body is no longer reaching the brain. The actual restriction of movement causes distress, body discomfort and thinking difficulties, but additional sensory deprivation increases the distress significantly. Physical exercise helps to counteract sensory deprivation and is associated with significantly lower levels of impairment on intellectual, perceptual and motor tasks. There are also fewer EEG changes when exercise is carried out.

Therefore it appears that there are many ways in which patients can be helped during the initial phase after injury. Such help however needs to be based on accurate assessment of the individual patient and family and insightful sensitivity to his emotional state. Attention to psychological needs when attending to physical needs is probably a most helpful strategy to use.

In an interesting study Bracken *et al.* (1981) attempted to identify psychological reactions to spinal cord injury at the time of discharge from acute care: 190 patients were involved in the study and information about motor and sensory function on admission, at discharge and at one year following injury was obtained from case notes. Patients were young with one-third of the sample being under the age of 21 years. The average age was 33.1

years and 158 were males. Discharge was an average 46 days after admission but with a range of 8–242 days.

Psychological variables which were investigated were levels of denial, anger, anxiety and depression, although the measures used appear rather simplistic. Other aspects on which information was obtained include dependency on the sick role, degree of adaptation to injury, acceptance of therapy, positive attitude about the future, and adaptation to life in general (e.g. resilience and locus of control). Results showed considerable denial, anger, anxiety and depression but average dependency on sick role. Ego resilience and internal locus of control were around the theoretical or population means. Intercorrelations between measures showed that those with high levels of denial showed low levels of depression but in turn those with high levels of denial were less well adapted to the injury. Patients who were more adapted to life in general were also more positive about their future and more likely to be accepting of their therapy. Interestingly, greater dependence on the sick role was also associated with acceptance of therapy. The most depressed of the patients were less likely to accept therapy. Those who scored highly on anger, anxiety and depression were significantly more uncertain about the future and less well adapted to life in general. Patients who scored high on ego resilience and internal locus of control were significantly low on anger, more likely to accept therapy and better adapted to life in general.

Denial of injury was unrelated to the severity of motor and sensory function, although strong emotional responses were associated with a greater loss of motor function. Those who had a severe loss of neurological function at discharge scored low on adaptation to the injury.

Whilst this study should be regarded with caution because of the lack of independent validity of the measures and the correlational nature of the relationship between variables, it does support Trieschmann's view that severe depression is related to poor adjustment. The study was carried out at a crucial point in the patient's career, at the transition from acute care to rehabilitation.

Phase 2: Rehabilitation

Rehabilitation is an important phase in the transition of the spinal cord injured person back into the community. Trieschmann (1980a and b) defines rehabilitation as 'the process of learning to live with one's disability in one's own environment. This learning is a dynamic process starting at the moment of injury and continuing for the rest of life', whilst Crowther (1985) in a study of people who have undergone lower limb amputation, defined rehabilitation as 'the restoration of the man to a proper condition . . . which was seen in terms of the usual interests and activities of all people in society'. Trieschmann argues that the newly spinal cord injured person requires at least 18–20 months before the new methods of coping with activities of daily living and mobility become routine. She also believes that the traditional medical model of rehabilitation with its concentration on mobility and activities of daily living alone is inadequate and that social, recreational and emotional adjustment is also important. She argues that the traditional medical model tends to dispense rehabilitation in units of treatment; that the term 'motivation' used about patients in rehabilitation is synonymous with 'co-operation' and that a patient is labelled as unmotivated if too active or too passive. This is certainly borne out in Crowther's (1985) study of the walking training class for lower limb amputees. A double message is conveyed in such settings: 'Learn to take care of your body'; 'all decisions will be taken for you' (Trieschmann, 1980a). Indeed, Trieschmann (1980b) argues that the treatment environment accounts for more variability in patient behaviour than individual patient characteristics do. She argues that a large part of a patient's day is typically spent alone or in a non-therapeutic activity. Whilst aides and orderlies spent the most time in contact with patients they have the least training. This results in patients being rewarded for dependent non-assertive behaviour and ignored or punished for trying to be independent.

This was certainly what Crowther (1985) found in her study within walking training classes for lower limb amputees. Indeed she showed quite clearly that rehabilitation was not taking place. Encouragement of rehabilitation was observed as only 0.16% of the total activity going on in the class and the more limited physical therapy accounted for only 10% of activity in each session. Even the patients who successfully accomplished the therapists' goals were incapacitated at home and the training was having no useful bearing upon the requirements of their daily lives. She observed one patient who despite satisfactory artificial limb replacement and good walking progress still found it easier to undertake home chores before putting on the limb.

She also found that amputee patients were handled by numerous members and grades of staff whose duties were frequently ill co-ordinated and incompatible. Crowther argued that one reason for the problems she identified in these classes was that the therapists had a primary responsibility for patient safety as well as therapy and so their duties were both custodial and restorative. In line with safety requirements staff restricted patients' movements, lifted them (in a walking training class!) and reached for items which patients had inadvertently dropped. Thus staff goals were conflicting and were incompatible with patient goals but staff did not realize this. As a result patient motivation to be restored to active life was not harnessed and mobility training which began in a safe and private environment ended also in the same private and safe environment, leaving patients still unprepared for the rigours of daily living. Perhaps this is understandable in the light of the stated aim of therapy in one instance: to enable the patients to potter about a bit at home.

Interestingly, in view of the discussion above about staff inaccuracy in identifying patients' emotional responses to spinal cord injury, Crowther observed instances of staff exaggerating the irremedial nature of the loss of a limb and so failing to give urgency to the task of uniting patient and the replacement limb. This resulted in therapists storing limbs before allowing their use, and removing limbs to get patients to take part in limbless activities. They failed to make positive comments which would have placed value on the artificial limbs.

In the light of the problems posed by a medical model in rehabilitation, both Trieschmann and Crowther believe that an educational model is far more appropriate in such settings.

A study in which a programme of education was used for both spinal cord injured patients and their families during rehabilitation in Poland was reported by Pachalski and Pachalska (1984). The educational programme focused upon tasks, recreation, the direct goal of movement, creative motor expression and problems. An individual plan was devised for each patient in three areas: medical, kinesitherapeutic and psychosocial. Each person involved in the programme was assigned a specific role.

The therapist's role was:

- to give necessary information
- to solve and interpret problems
- to set the patient tasks
- to teach patients to cope

The role of the family was:

- to teach everyday activities
- to overcome psychophysical and social barriers
- to create motivation for rehabilitation
- the organization of leisure time

The role of the patient was:

- to co-operate with the therapist and the family
- to form proper attitudes and motivation to gain independence
- to undertake a job
- participate in sport, recreation
- to help others.

A total of 38 patients were involved in this educational programme (18 males and 20 females), whilst a control group of 37 patients (19 males and 18 females) was given the same semi-structured interview before and after therapy. As well as the semi-structured interview several scales were administered to each group before and after therapy. These were:

1. Self-evaluation of adaptation to environment
2. Evaluation of psychological integration

3. Social independence
4. Frustration–aggression test

Results showed the effectiveness of the educational programme. The group of patients who had participated in this programme showed improvement in terms of adaptation to the environment; more saw a future, and had found a goal and evaluated positively their own work. Feelings of guilt, threat and fear had diminished. There was a clear decrease in aggression and frustration, whilst dependence had decreased. The differences in the measures taken before and after the educational programme for this group were statistically significant whilst there were no statistical differences in the before and after measures for the control group. There were significant differences between the two groups on the measures used after the treatment.

The number of patients who were not working decreased among the group who had received the educational programme, the number using a bus, tram or train had increased and they had been helped in organizing their own activities and free time.

The areas of physical coping which are relevant to spinal cord injured patients during rehabilitation are:

- managing fluid intake and bladder emptying (which may involve intermittent catheterization)
- managing diet and bowel emptying
- strengthening of upper limbs through exercise and push-ups
- prevention of pressure sores
- developing mobility skills

In addition to this patients must begin coping in terms of social, sexual, recreational, work and family relationships. Clearly, a great deal of learning is required and this underlines the appropriateness of an educational model rather than a medical model during rehabilitation.

The final test of rehabilitation is how well the patient copes with life back in the community after being discharged from rehabilitation. Interestingly most studies of coping or adjustment after discharge seem concerned with progress not as an aid to evaluation of the rehabilitation programme but as a means of identifying the characteristics of patients who respond well to rehabilitation. This seems to be another example of the process which both Crowther (1985) and Trieschmann (1980a) have identified; namely that of blaming the individual's lack of motivation for poor progress rather than identifying the processes in rehabilitation which block progress.

A study by Malec and Neimeyer (1983) attempted to correlate results on several psychometric tests with the subject's progress at an average of 7 months after discharge from rehabilitation. Subjects were 28 spinal cord injured people who were tested on admission to rehabilitation. Tests used were a symptom check list paying special attention to the patient's current psychological state, the MMPI (Minnesota Multiphasic Personality Inventory) and the Beck Depression Inventory. Outcome measures were the length of in-patient stay, ratings by staff in terms of patients' self-care performance (in particular the bladder and skin care programme) and similar ratings at follow up.

Findings showed that there was a high correlation between distress and depression ratings suggesting that the difference between distress and depression was not a qualitative one but one of degree. The more distressed patients required a much longer period of care in the rehabilitation unit and they showed lower levels of self-care competence at discharge. By the follow-up at approximately 7 months after discharge, only previously demonstrated self-care ability and dwelling on somatic concerns in the absence of general distress was predictive of their present performance at self-care. One can argue from this that most patients had caught up with the 'best' patients, in self-care skills, at follow up about 7 months after discharge from rehabilitation. The authors of this study, whilst accepting the limitations of a small sample, suggest that it is worth attempting to ameliorate feelings of distress and depression during rehabilitation since this may help to reduce length of stay and improve self-care ability on discharge.

Coping at home

From what is known about the tendency to focus upon physical tasks in both acute care and rehabilitation it follows that social, recreational, sexual, and emotional adjustment is to a large extent dependent upon the patient's own resilience and coping skills together with support from family and friends.

One type of injury in which the impact for the family may be even greater than that of spinal cord injury is brain injury where personality has been affected. Indeed family members have rated the consequent personality and behavioural changes as being more distressing than cognitive, intellectual and motor changes (Mauss-Clum and Ryan, 1981). Personality change is a relatively frequent problem after head injury (Rogers and Kreutzer, 1984). Lezak (1978) has identified some attitudinal principles underlying counselling help for families with a brain-damaged member. These can equally be applied in helping the families of other severely injured patients.

The six principles are:

1. Anger, frustration and sorrow are natural emotions for close relatives of severely injured patients.
2. Care-taking persons must take care of themselves first if they are going to be able to continue giving the patient good care.
3. The care-taker must ultimately rely on his own conscience and judgement in conflicts with the patient or other family members.
4. Role changes that inevitably take place when an adult becomes dependent or irresponsible can be emotionally distressing for all concerned.

5. A family member can probably do little to change the brain-damaged patient and thus need not feel guilty or wanting when care does not result in improvement.
6. When it appears that the welfare of dependent children may be at stake, family members must explore the issue of divided loyalties and weigh their responsibilities.

Group therapy for the families of brain-damaged patients, and indeed the patients themselves, is advocated by Kimball (1981). Again this is useful for patients following other types of severe injury. It gives patients an opportunity to help others which may lead to improved self-esteem and independence. A protected environment is provided in which feelings can be expressed freely and new relationships explored. An understanding that their own problems are not unique is gained, together with support and help from other patients. Definition and discussion of inappropriate behaviour can take place in a non-threatening environment.

The initiation of a support system for the family of brain damaged patients has been described by Rogers and Kreutzer (1984). They argue that support is necessary in the light of several studies which have indicated that the ability of the family to help is crucial to the level of recovery achieved by a brain-damaged person. The family of such a person faces enormous demands such as financial difficulties, changed roles within the family and a future which is uncertain. In addition, prolonged dependency of a family member with significant personality change, inappropriate social behaviour, and physical disability, is unrewarding and frequently exhausting to those upon whom he/she is dependent.

The specific family support system which Rogers and Kreutzer (1984) describe is called networking and is a technique adapted from work with schizophrenic patients. A frequent problem faced by a family caring for a disabled dependent member is that of isolation. Networking helps to overcome this as well as providing support.

The process of initiating the network intervention usually begins during acute hospital care when the first of three sessions is arranged. Family members are asked to list potential participants from amongst relatives and friends and are helped in setting up the first meeting. During this initial meeting, the primary focus is on the structure of the network through building on pre-existing relationships. Family and friends receive education about the effects of injury and the likely long-term outcome. During a brain-storming session members participate in identifying potential problems and generating possible solutions. A series of goals is formulated and each participant identifies his/her own responsibilities. Two further sessions are held at which professional staff are present and progress toward goals is assessed and new goals and responsibilities are identified and assigned. If the network has been successfully created it then maintains itself although crises may give rise to the need for more professional involvement beyond the first three meetings.

Difficulties associated with setting up such networks are (1) the logistics of arranging the meetings and (2) families may not see the need at an early stage because of denial and/or lack of knowledge of the stress levels which will be generated within the family in caring for the brain injured person.

Evaluation of the benefits of such a social network shows that conflict is reduced, crises are averted, mutual growth within the family is possible and emotional stress is reduced.

Whilst few situations of caring for the dependent person create such distress as that involving the loved one whose personality change has turned him/her into a stranger, it is well worth considering the support needed by the family of anyone who has become severely disabled. Formal networking may not be possible but the resources available for support could well be identified for the family.

Phase 3: Adjustment to disability in the long term

Following rehabilitation severely injured people must begin to live again within the context of the constraints and problems posed by the consequences of the injury.

It is against a background in which normal activities of daily living may create enormous demands that day to day life must go forward. Disabled people are not exempt from the stress which all of us experience within our lifetimes. Indeed a study by Caplan *et al.* (1984) suggests that stressful life events occur with a greater frequency than average for the disabled and indeed did occur more frequently after than before injury in the lives of the same people.

The subjects in this study had all been discharged from a rehabilitation unit between 6 months and 13 months previously: 158 subjects were invited to participate in the study but only 71 did so and of these only 50 returned usable questionnaires. Among the 71 respondents, 30 had suffered spinal cord injury, 11 a stroke, 4 head injury and 2 patients had a tumour resection. Of the remaining subjects one had undergone lower limb amputation, one had multiple trauma and one suffered from Guillain–Barré syndrome. Each person who participated was asked to complete a Recent Life Change Questionnaire (based on the social readjustment rating scale developed by Holmes and Rahe (1967)) with respect to (a) the 6-month period before the onset of illness/injury and (b) the 6-month period following discharge from rehabilitation.

Results showed that the life change units experienced in the 6-month period before hospitalization were in the range 0–417 with an average of 75.4 whilst in the 6-month period after discharge the range was 17–555 with an average of 259.1 (where a level of 150 or more is considered risky). This difference was highly significant. On comparing spinal cord injured patients with brain injured patients it was found that the spinal cord injured had the higher scores in both periods.

The number of stressful life events was also greater in the period after hospitalization than before. Life changes units identified after discharge included changes in recreation, personal habits, social activities, financial status, sleeping or eating habits and major decisions regarding the future. Average scores for the spinal cord injured group barely fell short of the major crisis level.

There are problems in this study however. One of these is the large number of non-respondents. Would these have changed the results in any way? Another is the retrospective nature of the study given that individual perception was the main focus of the study. Were patients inclined to forget events or interpret them more favourably in relation to the period before injury? In particular this may have been the case for the brain-injured patients.

Nonetheless the result of the study underlines the enormous task of adjustment faced by the newly disabled person. Nonetheless, of course, people do adjust to the most adverse circumstances and several studies have investigated long-term adjustment among spinal cord injured people.

A comparatively large study by Woodrich and Patterson (1983) was carried out to identify the degree of acceptance of disability among spinal cord injured people. This was quite an important study in that data were collected from women, since a good deal of the data following spinal cord injury have been obtained predominantly from men. A total of 432 spinal cord injured people in vocational rehabilitation in Florida were contacted and asked to participate in the study. Injury had been sustained at least 6 months previously. There was quite a low response rate, with only 251 usable and 15 unusable responses obtained. Instruments which were used were (a) Linkowski's Acceptance of Disability Scale which measured the individual's perception of their adjustment to injury (a high score on this means a high acceptance of disability) and (b) a specially designed questionnaire to collect demographic information.

The respondents comprised 176 males and 75 females with an age range of 17–52 years and a mean age of 29.4 years; 192 respondents, however, were 35 years or less; 165 respondents were single, 61 married and 25 were divorced or separated at the time of injury, whilst at the time of data collection, 135 were married. The duration of disability ranged from 6 months to 21 years with an average of 4.7 years. All respondents required a wheelchair as the primary means of mobility. Many needed an attendant. Among the sample were 114 quadriplegic and 137 paraplegic persons; 210 were Caucasian, 33 were Black and 8 were of other ethnic groups.

On looking at the results for adjustment it was found that there was a significantly greater level of acceptance of disability among the women than among the men, whilst amongst the group as a whole there was significantly less acceptance of disability among the older subjects compared with the younger ones. Not surprisingly it was found that the longer the time elapsed since the individual had suffered injury, the greater the acceptance. Finally those with the greatest educational attainment were more accepting of disability than those with low educational attainment.

The reasons for these significantly different levels of acceptance among different subgroups of the study population could not be ascertained from the study data itself, so any suggestions are purely the results of speculation. However, regardless of the fact that women are no longer mainly carrying out a role within the home, it is nonetheless true that the range of activities both in terms of work and recreation which women engage in outside the home is smaller than that of men, whilst the range of activities available to women inside the home may be greater than that for men. This could make it easier to adjust to a restricting disability. The finding that both the younger and the more educated are more accepting of disability is probably a function of resilience and learning ability, although it is also the case that education provides a greater range of potential sedentary, intellectual sources of satisfaction.

Acceptance of disability contributes toward acceptance of a changed body image which in turn is crucial to the self concept. A study carried out by Green *et al.* (1984) explored the self concept amongst a group of spinal cord injured people who had sustained their injury at least four years previously. They argued that for adjustment to have taken place completely, a new self concept must have been reached. A total of 71 persons took part in the study, of whom 34 were quadriplegic and 37 were paraplegic. The average number of years since injury was 11 and 73% of the sample had been injured before the age of 30 years. There were 53 men and 18 women respondents. Only 13 were in full-time employment; 1 was employed part-time, whilst the remainder were supported from government funds, insurances or trusts; 47 lived with a spouse, 10 lived alone, 5 with relatives and the remainder in a variety of other settings. The sample was asked to complete the Tennessee Self Concept Scale which comprises Lickert type items on six subscales: physical self; moral–ethical self; personal self; family self; social self; and self criticism. The total score was a measure of self esteem. In addition, a specially-designed questionnaire was used to collect other information.

Results showed that as a group the respondents in this study had very positive self esteem. They seem to have accepted the injury and had re-defined themselves in positive terms. Interestingly on personal self, social self and moral–ethical self the sample average score was significantly higher than the average of the norm population for the instrument. Conversely, and not surprisingly, the sample average was significantly lower than the norm average for physical self. Scores were higher but not significantly so for self criticism and family self.

Relationships between results on this scale and the additional information collected showed that the greater the perceived independence, the higher the scores for physical self, personal self, social self and self-esteem, whilst those respondents requiring more assistance with activities of daily living had significantly higher moral–ethical self scores than those requiring little help. Although this is a difficult relationship to account for the authors suggest it results from a process of self analysis and searching for the meaning of life said to relate to adaptation to injury.

A finding compatible with the results of the study previously discussed (Woodrich and Patterson, 1983) was that the older the individual, and especially the older the individual was at injury the lower the physical self score. This reflected perceptions of physical appearance, physical skill, health and sexuality. Another compatible finding was that those with the highest levels of educational achievement also scored highly on self concept scales including self esteem. Overall this study shows that adjustment does indeed take place after spinal cord injury and suggests that quality of life can be satisfactory.

Most of the studies which have been mentioned here have used specially designed or standard questionnaires on a population of spinal cord injured people, followed by intercorrelating and comparing the results. The meaning of such results can only be a subject for speculation. A British study used a different method in which a small group of spinal cord injured people were interviewed and the themes abstracted from these interviews were then used to formulate a questionnaire to produce some quantitative data. This method allows greater insight into the meaning of the process of adjustment for the individuals concerned.

The purpose of this study (Ray and West, 1984a, b) was to identify the long-term implications and the coping strategies employed among a sample of 22 paraplegics. An attempt was made to obtain information from women paraplegics in particular and to this end these were chosen first and a sample of men was then chosen to match. Subjects had to be aged 20–40 years and to reside in or near London. For the female sample ($n = 11$) the mean number of years since onset of disability was 9.5 years and for the males ($n = 11$) it was 12.2. Subjects were interviewed in their own homes and interviews were unstructured except for being centred upon their experience of paraplegia with regard to social, sexual and personal adjustment. Interviews were recorded and transcribed. Questionnaires based on these transcriptions were then posted to the same sample but only 18 responded, 2 of the non-respondents being in hospital by then.

Results showed that in terms of meeting others and developing friendships, 4 found it easier, 9 more difficult, and 4 the same as before the accident. Difficulties in meeting people related to physical problems of negotiating stairs, doors, and toilets etc., but also of being 'captive' in a gathering, it being more difficult to interact with those selected by the subject as potentially interesting. Only a few respondents mentioned lack of confidence, or the rudeness or ignorance of others as a barrier. Since the accident, 9 had lost some or many friends, and 6 had fewer friends now. Many found that whilst friends had initially found difficulty in coping they had learned to do so with the passage of time. Only 2 of the sample had no disabled friends and half the sample attended groups or events specially organized for the disabled.

In terms of sexual intercourse, 2 found it a great problem, and for 13 it was a 'bit of a problem'; 16 felt a need for sex and most had had some sexual experienced since injury, 8 with more than one partner. Only 4 had experienced difficulty with position and 4 with spasms during intercourse. The problem of achieving and then maintaining an erection was mentioned by 8 out of the 11 males. However, sexual feelings, one's partner's pleasure, and feelings of closeness were cited as sources of sexual pleasure. None felt sex to be impossible but it was complicated by the disability, requiring practice, imaginative technique and perseverance. It was seen by most as having a status similar to, or less than, the other difficulties experienced.

As for personal adjustment, 11 had experienced depression from time to time. One had attempted suicide, whilst several alleviated depression by imbibing alcohol. Frustration at their slowness in carrying out ordinary tasks was a problem as was other people's lack of understanding about this. They felt that their self image was affected by a feeling of being set apart but only 3 felt that their feelings toward self had changed for the worse, with half being more positive toward themselves. They reported that they now feel more confident, more patient and stronger, having been forced to face an enormous challenge and come through.

With respect to coping with social relationships, the major problem seems to be the attitudes of others who impose inappropriate stereotypes upon the disabled. The physically disabled are often treated as if they are also mute, deaf or mentally handicapped. Many treat the disabled with pity and this causes pain. Such people often interfere to give unsolicited help. This encourages dependence. Coping strategies employed by these subjects included being self assertive, educating others, putting others at their ease and giving cues so that others know how to behave. In this context Caywood (1974) cited by Trieschmann (1980a) believes that the injured person's ability to put others at ease is critical in the ultimate adjustment to disability. Many of Ray and West's (1984a, b) subjects had become very sensitive to other's reactions and were extraverted since the accident.

Ray and West (1984b) discuss coping mechanisms used by their subjects in making their personal adjustment in the face of helplessness, anxiety, frustration and regret. They argue that each person has a personal style of coping but included among these are:

Suppression

This is described as cultivating consciously, an appearance of not caring and of being able to cope. Such a style of coping is encouraged in hospital. It involves a 'bottling up' of feelings. It is used as a defence against showing true feelings.

Denial and repression

This is similar to suppression, but is a less conscious process. Here the individual refuses to acknowledge the fact of disability and its implications. There is a focusing upon the present and the future rather than the past. Individuals do not allow themselves to think about their feelings and they may be reluctant to associate with other disabled people.

Resignation and acceptance

This involves coming to terms with the limitations imposed by the injury, i.e. the changed lifestyle, the limited horizons. It means learning patience and not wishing to do more than one can.

Positive thinking

This is an extension of acceptance, since here the individual makes the most of his/her circumstances. The importance of the effort made in coping is emphasized. There is a counting of blessings and a developing confidence in one's ability to cope.

Independence and assertiveness

This appears to be a strategy developed against the pressures exerted by individuals and society in general for the disabled to become dependent and to rely on others. Individuals in the study argued that whilst not rejecting help where it is needed, coping on one's own enhances self respect and confidence. To some extent people using this coping method are rebelling against the situation, but in a constructive way.

The authors of this study believe that counselling could help patients to explore the different ways of coping with disability and suggest that such counselling could be done by specialist nurses, psychologists or volunteers.

One final study showing that good levels of long-term adjustment to physical disability can be attained will be cited here. This was a study by Schulz and

Decker (1985) who interviewed 100 middle-aged and elderly people with spinal cord injury on average 20 years after the injury. Respondents were all Caucasian and male, aged 40–73 years. No respondent was living in an institution. They were asked about various aspects of adjustment and satisfaction.

Respondents reported on their health status which was poor in the case of only 7%, moderate for 34%, fair for 18%, good for 30%, and excellent for 11%.

Subjects reported degrees of well-being only slightly lower than that of non-disabled adults. Those subjects with high levels of social support were very satisfied with social contacts and those with high levels of social contact in turn reported high levels of well-being. These factors were highly associated with adjustment.

More important perhaps was some of the qualitative data from this study showing strategies used by the respondents in maintaining their feelings of well-being.

Firstly, they made favourable social comparisons not with less fortunate others, but between themselves and the non-disabled. This they did by selectively focusing on attributes in which they were favoured or could excel, e.g. 'brain is more important than brawn', and 'relationships and sensitivity to others is important'.

Secondly, they did not create hypothetical worse worlds with which they could compare themselves. They did, however, attach meaning to the accident and many felt they had even benefited as a result of it.

Trieschmann (1980a) proposed that there are three areas of functioning which are crucial to a successful life whether or not one is disabled. These are:

1. The prevention of medical complications and the utilization of activity of daily living skills, and mobility skills.
2. The maintenance of a stable living environment.
3. Productivity defined in terms of vocational endeavours, education, volunteer activities and non-vocational pursuits.

The literature reviewed in this chapter suggests that the coping skills required to achieve this level of functioning following severe injury can be attained. However, severely injured individuals must make enormous personal efforts in the process. They could be helped more by the caring professions in facilitating this process than they are at present.

10.2 SUMMARY

In this chapter the focus has mainly been on the literature relating to adjustment of those with spinal cord injury to life with their disablement.

The process of adjustment which involves many individual coping skills has been classified into three main phases. The first of these was the initial impact of the injury and the stressful environment of the accident and emergency and intensive care departments. Major adjustments during this phase are to the highly technical care environment, the physiological interventions and to the impact of the prognosis. Whilst staff tend to concentrate on obtaining physiological stability during this time, ways in which psychological interventions may be employed to help have been identified.

Rehabilitation is the second phase of adjustment. The appropriateness of an educational rather than a medical model of therapy has been discussed along with some of the problems associated with staff adopting a medical model and an orientation toward tasks. Research identifying patient characteristics which are associated with a successful outcome from rehabilitation has also been discussed. However it is believed that it may be more appropriate to identify successful and unsuccessful strategies of therapy in relation to patient characteristics rather than to label patients as more or less likely to respond well to therapy.

Finally, adjustment to everyday life has been discussed. The family have an important role here and ways in which the family may be helped were mentioned. In particular the families of those who have suffered head injuries, and in whom there is a consequential personality change need a great deal of help.

One study has been cited which suggests that the disabled may be subject to a greater number of stressful life events during the first 6 months after discharge from rehabilitation than an average population. This underlines the need for adjustment skills. Areas in which adjustment are important spread into all aspects of life. Coping in terms of social, familial, physical, recreational, sexual and personal areas of life has been explored in relation to several research studies.

In general, the evidence suggests that the spinal cord injured population do attain a good quality of life and the majority eventually develop a positive self-image.

REFERENCES

Bodenhamer, E., Achterberg-Lawlis, J., Kevorkian, G., *et al.* (1983) Staff and patient perceptions of the psychosocial concerns of spinal cord injured persons. *Amer. J. Physical Medicine,* **62**(4), 182–93.

Braakman, R., Orbaan, J. and Dishoeck, M. (1976) Information in the early stages after spinal cord injury. *Int. J. Paraplegia,* **14**, 95–100.

Bracken, M. B., Shepard, M. J. and Webb, S. B. (1981) Psychological response to acute spinal cord injury: an epidemiological study. *Paraplegia,* **19**(5), 271–83.

Brackett, T.O., Condon, N., Kindelan, K. and Bassett, J. (1984) The emotional care of a person with a spinal cord injury. *Journal of the American Medical Association*, **252**(6), 793–5.

Caplan, B., Gibson, C. J. and Weiss, R. (1984) Stressful sequelae of disabling illness. *Int. Rehabilit. Med.*, **6**, 58–62.

Caywood, T. (1974) A quadriplegic young man looks at treatment. *J. Rehab.*, **22**, 5.

Crowther, H. (1985) *An Investigation of Rehabilitation with Special Reference to Lower Limb Amputation*, PhD Thesis, University of Hull.

Donaldson, R. J. and Donaldson, L. J. (1983) *Essential Community Medicine*, MTP, Lancaster.

Franco, L. (1986) Spinal cord injury, in *Trauma Nursing* (ed. V. D. Cardona), Wright, Bristol, pp. 61–8.

Friedman-Campbell, M: and Hart, C. A. (1984) Theoretical strategies and nursing interventions to promote psychological adaptation to spinal cord injuries and disability. *J. Neurosurg. Nursing*, **16**(6), 335–42.

Green, B. C., Pratt, C. C. and Grigsby, T. E. (1984) Self-concept among persons with long-term spinal cord injury. *Arch. Phys. Med. Rehab.*, **65**, 751–4.

Hohmann, G. C. (1966) Psychological aspects of treatment and rehabilitation of the spinal injured person. *Clinical Orthopaedics*, **112**, 81–8.

Holmes, T. H. and Rahe, R. H. (1967) The social readjustment rating scale. *J. Psychosom. Res.*, **11**, 213–18.

Kimball, C. P. (1981) *The Biopsychosocial Approach to the Patient*, Williams and Wilkins, Baltimore, MD.

Lezak, M. D. (1978) Living with the characterologically altered brain injured patient. *J. Clinical Psychiatry*, **39**, 592–8.

Malec, J. and Neimeyer, R. (1983) Psychologic prediction of duration of inpatient spinal cord injury, rehabilitation and performance of self care. *Arch. Phys. Med. Rehab.*, **64**(8), 359–63.

Mauss-Clum, N. and Ryan, M. (1981) Brain injury and the family. *J. Neurosurg. Nursing*, **13**(4), 165–9.

Pachalski, A. and Pachalska, M. M. (1984) Programme of active education in the psycho-social integration of paraplegics. *Paraplegia*, **22**(4), 238–43.

Ray, C. and West, J. (1984a) 1. Social, sexual and personal implications of paraplegia. *Paraplegia*, **22**(2), 75–86.

Ray, C. and West, J. (1984b) 2. Coping with spinal paraplegia. *Paraplegia*, **22**(4), 249–59.

Rogers, P. M. and Kreutzer, J. S. (1984) Family crises following head injury. A network intervention strategy. *J. Neurosurg. Nursing*, **16**(6), 343–6.

Schulz, R. and Decker, S. (1985) Long-term adjustment to physical disability: the role of social support, perceived control and self blame. *J. Personal Social Psych.*, **48**(5), 1162–72.

Strauss, A. L., Corbin, J., Fagerhaugh, S. *et al.* (1984) *Chronic Illness and the Quality of Life* (2nd edn), Mosby, St Louis, MO.

Trieschmann, R. B. (1980a) *Spinal Cord Injuries: Psychological, Social and Vocational Adjustment*, Pergamon, New York, N.Y.

Trieschmann, R. B. (1980b) The psychological social and vocational adjustment to spinal cord injury, *Annual Rev. Rehabilit.*, **1**, 304–18.

Woodrich, F. and Patterson, J. B. (1983) Variables related to acceptance of disability in persons with spinal cord injuries, *J. Rehab.*, **49**(3), 26–30.

Worden, J. W. (1982) *Grief Counselling and Grief Therapy*, Springer-Verlag, New York, N.Y.

CHAPTER ELEVEN

Cancer, stress and coping

The word 'cancer' has been shown to have negative connotations, arousing negative emotions such as anxiety and fear (Brooks, 1979; Charlton, 1981). To be told that one has cancer is a major life event demanding major coping resources. Several authors have commented on this, for example:

> The news of a cancer diagnosis often sets off a crisis in the patient. (Feigenberg, 1970)

> Psychological reactions in patients affected by cancer are understandable. The reactions are characterised by the patient's psychological helplessness and what cancer and its location really mean – consciously and unconsciously to the victim. The reactions with which we are concerned here are of the same type as others released by a traumatic experience such as natural catastrophes, fire, war-time experiences and the like . . . (Caplan and Grunebaum, 1967)

> however, the patient's emotional response to cancer may best be described by what has been termed death images. Cancer, perhaps, more than any other disease, presents images of primordial suffering and terror that make it a uniquely devastating entity, both psychologically and physically. It is not as though no other disease kills, but this disease. . . has long been associated with man's most unspoken and primitive fears, those of boundless suffering. (Wellisch, 1981)

This suggests that the diagnosis of cancer in itself creates such distress that it commands major coping forces in its own right without the added demands of undergoing treatment techniques, some of which may be termed 'heroic', which are used in the fight against cancer.

Thus, the characteristics of the psychological response of people to this disease are such as to warrant serious discussion in a book devoted to stress and coping. However, the prevalence of the disease, or more accurately, groups of diseases, is another reason for devoting a whole chapter to the subject. Its prevalence means that it affects a large number of people at any one time.

In the developed countries of Europe, in the USA and Canada, in Austra-
lia and New Zealand and in Japan, the major causes of death are cardiovascular diseases, malignant neoplasms and accidents. In most
industrialised countries cardiovascular diseases and neoplasms account
for two thirds of the total mortality in both sexes . . . The three leading
causes of death by age, with infancy excluded are accidents from age 1
to 44, and malignant neoplasms and cardiovascular disease in middle
age and old age. (Lee and Franks, 1980)

One hundred and eighty thousand new cases of cancer and 125 000
deaths from cancer occur each year in England and Wales. Around one
in three people in Great Britain could expect to develop cancer at some
time during their lives and one in five will die from it. (Donaldson and
Donaldson, 1983)

However, it is important to emphasize that 'rather than a single entity,
cancer actually represents a large heterogeneous group of diseases characterized by the uncontrollable proliferation of cells' (Irwin and Anisman,
1984)

The cancer group of diseases varies in terms of site, degree of malignancy
and cell of origin. However, statistics compiled from cancer registrations and
death certificates classify the cancers according to site. This gives a good idea
of the common sites of cancer (see Table 11.1). There is a different distribution of site frequencies for men and women.

Table 11.1   Common sites of cancer in Britain based on registrations in 1974

Women	Frequency	Men	Frequency
Breast	24%	Lung	30%
Large intestine and rectum	13%	Large intestine and rectum	11%
Skin	10%	Skin	11%
Lung	8%	Stomach	8%
Stomach	6%	Prostate	8%
Ovary	5%	Bladder	6%
Cervix	5%	Leukaemias and lymphoma	6%
Leukaemias and lymphoma	5%		

Based on Donaldson and Donaldson, 1983.

Later in this chapter, the impact of the diagnosis upon the individual suffering from cancer will be discussed, as will coping with cancer and the treatment. Before this, however, there is another issue which should be discussed
in relation to stress and cancer, since there has long been a suggestion that
the onset of cancer may be associated in some way with stress.

11.1 STRESS AND THE DEVELOPMENT OF CANCER

There is a considerable amount of literature about the possibility that the onset of cancer may be triggered by stress (for example Crisp, 1970; Fox, 1978; Cox and McKay, 1982). The idea appears in Galen's writings as well as re-appearing in work published from 1701 onwards (Rosch, 1984). Modern research on this hypothesis is subject to more pitfalls of methodology and logic than is the work linking the concept of the Type A personality with chronic heart disease (Temoshok and Heller, 1984).

Temoshok and Heller (1984) have identified some of the methodological issues which create such problems in identifying the link, if there is one, between stress and the development of cancer. There are potentially two ways in which stress might be related to cancer: (1) it could be implicated in the causation of cancer; and/or (2) it could aid the progression of the disease.

The issues of research methodology identified by Temoshok and Heller (1984) will now be discussed briefly.

1. Independent variables

It was pointed out above that cancer is not a single diagnosis but a large group of diseases which vary not only as to site but also in terms of tissue of origin and degree of malignancy. Yet, much of the research into the relationship between psychosocial variables and cancer has treated cancer as if it were a single entity and has disregarded these complexities.

Frequently the case is that in such research the role of physical factors, age and heredity has been ignored. If, however, the onset of cancer could be explained by toxic substances in the environment, heredity or age, there would be very little of a role for psychosocial factors to play in the aetiology. In practice, biological risk of cancer is associated with contact with carcinogens, heredity and age, and these should be taken into account in research studies.

2. Dependent variables

Initiation versus progression

A research report should clearly state whether it was concerned with elucidating factors leading to the onset of cancer or to its progression/spread. Clearly the identification of evidence of a link between stress and the spread of cancer gives no proof of a link between stress and the onset of cancer.

Severity of disease

When the focus of the study is the link between stress and progression of the disease, accurate measurement of the severity and spread of the disease is crucial to using it as a dependent variable. However, professionals working in the field of oncology realize only too well the difficulty of making such measurements. Even if they can be made, it is rare for psychology researchers to be given access to them.

Methodological design

Many of the relevant points discussed by Temoshok and Heller (1984) have been discussed in Chapter 9. Suffice it to remind the reader here that prospective studies are extremely expensive and difficult to mount. In the case of the cancers, their heterogeneous nature means that the probability of any sizeable group of people developing a similar cancer is remote. Consequently researchers tend to treat all cancers as if they were the same.

RETROPROSPECTIVE STUDIES

These are ones which are frequently made use of in types of research such as cancer. In this research design the investigator uses personality measures collected years before for other purposes to attempt to identify relationships between personality style and the onset of cancer. Many problems arise from this. For example, since the test was intended for a different purpose, it may be one of little relevance to those dimensions of personality style believed to link with the onset of cancer. The MMPI (Minnesota Multiphasic Personality Inventory) for example, serves little relevant purpose. Indeed the concept of links between personality and cancer are nebulous and few people who develop cancer in this country at least, will have had personality tests in the past, the results of which would be available.

QUASI-PROSPECTIVE STUDIES

This is a term coined by Temoshok and Heller (1984) to describe a type of study which has been used quite frequently in research into stress and cancer. The example of breast cancer can illustrate the principle. Women who have lumps in their breasts are assessed in terms of psychosocial variables before biopsy. Once the results of the biopsies are known, a comparison on psychosocial variables can be made between those with benign lumps and those with malignant growths.

Such studies are useful, since the time period involved between collecting data and drawing conclusions from it is quite brief. However, it is important to note that these are not true studies of onset since data is collected at a time when the malignancy had developed sufficiently to cause palpable lumps.

More importantly, though, all women in the sample will have been worried at the time of testing that they had cancer. Thus their memories and mood may have been affected, giving results reflecting their current state rather than more permanent traits.

RETROSPECTIVE STUDIES

Studies of psychosocial factors and cancer are subject to the usual problems attendant upon retrospective studies. The nature of any control group is absolutely crucial and the pitfall of assuming that all differences between the cancer group and the control group are relevant to the diagnosis should be avoided.

CONTROL OR COMPARISON GROUPS

Comparison groups used in different studies may vary enormously, making comparison between studies extremely difficult. In some studies the 'comparison' group may merely be the group of subjects on whom the norms for a personality test were established. This is quite clearly inappropriate.

THEORIES AND CONSTRUCTS

The theoretical assumptions made by different researchers in relation to psychosocial variables may make comparisons between studies quite impossible. An example is where the theoretical assumptions lead to the use of the social readjustment scale in a study, whilst another researcher's theory base leads to the use of MMPI. Obviously comparison is impossible. Reviews of the literature frequently fail to record such differences.

Types of measure

The same psychosocial variable may be measured in different ways, for example an in-depth interview by a clinical psychologist as contrasted with a self-administered questionnaire. Is it valid to compare the results even where the same construct is being explored?

From such an analysis and a more detailed critique of individual studies Temoshok and Heller (1984) have identified seven main themes which are crucial to an evaluation of issues in this area of study. These are:

1. In spite of an enormous number of studies and a large number of variables studied, there is a paucity of positive findings. There is, however, one consistent theme, and that is that people who develop cancer have a history of difficulty in expressing emotions or even of feeling them.
2. There is a constellation of factors which appears to predispose some individuals to develop cancer, or to proceed through the stages of cancer development more rapidly.

3. Recent controlled studies support earlier hypotheses derived from clinical impressions.

4. In general, the evidence suggests that the individual's knowledge of having cancer does not result in physiological or psychological reactions which compromise the validity of retrospective studies.

5. Apart from the difficulty in expressing emotion already mentioned, other personality traits associated with the onset of cancer, or its rapid development, include 'niceness', industriousness, perfectionism, sociability, conventionality and more rigid mental defences.

6. Those people in whom cancer takes an unfavourable course show a tendency to respond with helplessness or hopelessness or giving up. In contrast, those whose cancer takes a more favourable course show a tendency to fight it and to be aggressive.

7. The mere number of past or recent life events appears to be less important to the development of cancer than the style in which those events which occurred were dealt with cognitively, emotionally or behaviourally.

The conclusion reached by Temoshok and Heller (1984) from a rigorous examination of the relevant research is that there is a core of evidence favouring a link between psychosocial events and cancer.

Two large-scale prospective surveys which appear to support these conclusions were reported by Grossarth-Maticek et al. (1984). One of these was carried out in a Yugoslavian town with a population of 14 000. A sample of 1353 subjects was recruited by selecting the second oldest person in each second home within the town. This method obtained a sample with an age distribution mainly within the range 50–65 years. During 1965–66 psychosocial data were recorded from these individuals using a questionnaire and an observation catalogue. Height, weight, and blood pressure were recorded and a note was made as to whether or not the person was a cigarette smoker. Further medical information was recorded during the period 1969–76. Disease occurrence and diagnosis on any death certificates was identified 10 years after the start of the study. A total of 117 males and 87 females developed cancer during the course of the study. In the men this was mainly cancer of the lung, stomach, rectum and prostate gland, whilst in the women it was predominantly the breast, uterus and cervix which were affected. The study was replicated in Heidelberg using a random sample of 1026 subjects.

The results showed a significant relationship between several psychosocial dimensions and the development of cancer. These psychosocial dimensions were:

1. The number of traumatic life events evoking chronic helplessness.
2. Rational and anti-emotional behaviour.
3. A tendency toward self-abnegation for the sake of harmonious social relationships.

4. Lack of hypochondriasis.
5. Absence of psychopathological symptoms such as anxiety.
6. A lack of positive emotional contact.

There was also a significant negative association between the development of cancer and the number of traumatic life events evoking chronic excitement.

The authors of this study concluded that cancer victims appear to strive to fulfil the expectations of those who are significant in their lives. They have a tendency to idealize the person closest to them whilst showing low self esteem and lack of assertiveness themselves. They are well adjusted on the surface, but have a strong need for harmonious relationships. This need is intensified at times of conflict. These individuals have a tendency to deny that they inhibit emotional expression and are socially conformist.

Clearly then, it is important to examine ways in which psychosocial variables could influence the physiological changes which result in cancer. Research in which animals have been used as models supports the view that, in some species of animal at any rate, some types of tumour do respond to events such as handling, type of housing, mildly aversive stimuli, and intermittent rotation (Levine and Cohen, 1959; Ader and Friedman, 1965; Ebbessen and Rask-Nielson, 1967; Riley, 1981).

Cox (1984) has discussed the mechanisms by which psychosocial events could affect cancer development. He has proposed a model in which stress is one of the links between psychosocial events and tumour growth via the immune system.

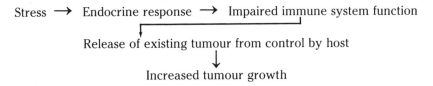

'In order for cancer to develop, essentially two changes must occur. First, normal cells must be transformed to malignant ones, as a result of genetic coding, spontaneous mutation or exposure to a carcinogen. Secondly there must be failure of the host's defences against this cellular proliferation.' (Irwin and Anisman, 1984.)

Fox (1978) also suggests two primary cancer causing mechanisms. The first of these, carcinogenesis, is 'the production of cancer by an agent or mechanism overcoming existing resistance of the body', whilst the second mechanism is 'lowered resistance to cancer which permits a potential carcinogen normally insufficient to produce cancer, to do so'.

Fobair and Cordoba (1982) suggested factors which appear to be involved in the initial transformation of a normal cell into a malignant one. One of these is heredity. Some cancers run in families and virtually all cancers in humans have been shown to occur in both a heritable and in a non-heritable form. Heritable cancers could arise from a genetic change in the cell or they might be present at birth. Some tumours undoubtedly occur as a result of an interaction between genetic and environmental factors. Those tumours which involve a heritable component tend to occur at an earlier age and at multiple sites more frequently than do non-heritable tumours. Ageing, on the other hand, allows the possibility of greater exposure to environmental carcinogens. Hormonal changes and changes in immunological competence also occur with age.

Environmental factors which have been cited as potential carcinogens include viruses, ionizing radiation and chemical substances such as asbestos, and components of cigarette smoke. These carcinogenic substances probably interact with hereditary information in cells.

Irwin and Anisman (1984) were quoted above as arguing that not only must there be an influence which triggers a malignant change but that for that change to become a malignant growth there must also be a failure of the host system which defends against abnormal cell proliferation. In other words an initial malignant change is a necessary but not a sufficient condition for a malignant tumour to grow. The immune system is known to be involved in the destruction of malignant cells and this role will now be discussed.

It is believed that within the immune system it is cytotoxic T-cells, macrophages, antibodies and natural killer (NK) cells which specifically act against malignancy. One model of the mechanism by which malignant cells are destroyed has been suggested by Burnet (1971). In his immune surveillance hypothesis it is suggested that one of the functions of cytotoxic T-cells is to recognize and destroy mutant cells which might potentially develop into tumours. This model has been heavily criticized (Irwin and Anisman, 1984).

A more recent interpretation of the mechanism of the defence against malignancy is a two-phase model of immune surveillance (Herberman and Ortaldo, 1981). Here it is suggested that an initial broad-ranging defence system reacts against foreign cells and substances, controlling them until a more specific immune response is possible. In particular, these workers suggest a role for NK cells and interferon in the specific response. NK cells are a particular kind of the lymphoid cells present in normal individuals. NK cells react against a variety of tumour cells and some normal cells, destroying them. This cytotoxic action is augmented in the presence of interferon.

It is suggested that in stress, psychosocial stimuli affect hormone levels which in turn can depress the immune response and this releases tumour growth from control. Adrenocortical hormones have been shown to reduce both interferon levels and NK cell activity (Rytel and Kilbourne, 1966; Herberman and Holden, 1978). It is also known that macrophages and polymorphonuclear cells are sensitive to changes in glucocorticoid levels. These cells show spontaneous activity against tumour cells.

However the significance of these effects of adrenocortical hormones in life has been challenged, since it appears that pharmacological levels are required to suppress the normal immune system rather than those levels of adrenocorticoids which are within the physiological range. On the other hand no hormone ever exists or produces physiological effects in isolation and other hormones are known to affect the immune system. These are growth hormone, thyroid hormones, testosterone and catecholamines. Secretion levels of all these hormones have been shown to be affected by psychosocial stimuli.

Here we have traced a possible pathway by which stress could influence tumour growth, although there is still no proof that it does do so. In a review of relevant work in this field Cox (1984) argues:

> If it is accepted that the hormonal environment is a determinant of immune system effectiveness then it remains possible that effects of stress on that environment may be of some significance. However, even accepting this, two important questions remain. First, how biologically significant are these immunological effects in animals for cancer production? Second, how far can these effects be generalised to man? These questions remain largely unanswered.

However, Cox (1984) does suggest that stress exerts a very real effect upon the onset of cancer through behaviour such as cigarette smoking and drinking alcohol. These are behaviours which are frequently employed by individuals coping with stress (see Chapter 2). Other behaviour during stress, such as carelessness in handling chemical substances, might also lead to malignant changes. Cox (1984) offers the following model.

Stress $\rightarrow$ Coping behaviour $\rightarrow$ Exposure to carcinogens $\rightarrow$ Cancer

Cox also argues that changes in behaviour and life style which are advocated to prevent cancer are easier to comply with if stress-related problems are dealt with first.

Given such a nebulous chain of events between stress and the development of cancer, health professionals may wonder about the relevance of such a discussion to their work. We believe it is worth knowing, however, that there is a strong possibility that a patient who develops cancer has already undergone recent stress, and that their coping style may be to inhibit emotional reaction on the one hand, and to engage in what we have called palliative coping on the other hand. Such knowledge could be of use in helping the patient to cope with further stressful events.

There are many extremely stressful events associated with cancer and its treatment. These are:

- coming to terms with the diagnosis
- an operation which may involve changes in body image and severe interference with normal function
- radiotherapy treatment
- treatment with cytotoxic drugs (chemotherapy)
- uncertainty associated with the prognosis.

It is these events with which the remainder of this chapter is concerned.

11.2 ATTITUDES TOWARD CANCER: DIAGNOSIS

The importance of attitudes toward and beliefs about cancer within the general (and professional) population cannot be overestimated. They shape people's health behaviour in important ways. For example

1. The individual's willingness to attend screening tests for the detection of cancer.
2. The length of delay in seeking help when an individual believes he/she may have cancer.
3. The psychological impact of being told one has cancer.

The attitudes which people hold toward cancer are overwhelmingly negative (Cox, 1984):

> For most people cancers are among the most feared of diseases: they have been reported as the diseases which are 'most serious' or 'most worrying'. . . Their incidence is generally overestimated and survival rates are markedly underestimated.

Negative attitudes toward cancer are apparent in children as shown by a study reported by Charlton (1981). In a survey of four large secondary schools using questionnaires she obtained 3500 responses from children aged 11–18 years. Nearly half of the respondents (49%) believed that cancers are never curable.

Brooks (1979) argued that the fear component in an individual's attitude toward cancer includes some or all of the following components:

- fear of the medical world in general
- fear of separation from the family including loss of independence, loss of social interaction, death
- fear of the disease including pain, social stigma, deformity/mutilation, disability, helplessness, death

From an examination of studies of public attitudes toward cancer published in the western world, Brooks (1979) concluded that they showed:

- a tendency for respondents to exaggerate the number of deaths caused by cancer
- a tendency to underestimate the number cured of cancer
- a strong tendency to view cancer as the most worrying of all diseases
- a belief that smoking is implicated in lung cancer
- a knowledge of other 'causes' for which some scientific evidence exists
- a knowledge of some bona fide early warning signs of cancer
- a tendency to reject the evidence that early treatment leads to improved prognosis
- a recognition of the non-contagious nature of cancer

One of the problems about holding such attitudes toward cancer is that it could deter people from seeking medical help for cancer. This can lead to delay in going to the doctor if the individual worries that symptoms he or she is experiencing are due to cancer. It could also lead individuals to resist medical screening which might reveal the presence of cancer.

In relation to breast screening, Hobbs (1981) carried out a study to identify women's willingness to undergo mammography for the detection of asymptomatic breast cancer. A sample of women aged 40 or over from a group practice were invited to attend for mammography. The percentage who accepted the invitation decreased with age. For example, in the age group 40–49 years, 71% accepted, whilst only 43% did in the age group 70–79 years. Women could also request mammography and so it was possible to interview a random sample both of this self-referred group and of those who had been invited to attend.

Asked what they would think if a friend told of finding a lump in her breast, responses varied.

In the self referred group:
34% said cancer; 24% said non-malignant.

In the group who accepted the invitation to undergo mammography:
40.7% said cancer; 22% said non-malignant.

Among the group who refused the invitation to undergo mammography:
54% said cancer; 16.7% said non-malignant.

The same respondents were asked 'Do you think cancer can ever be cured?' Results can be seen in Table 11.2.

Table 11.2   Response to the question 'Do you think cancer can ever be cured?'

Responses	Self-referred group	Acceptance of mammography	Rejection of mammography
Usually, sometimes	52%	44.7%	31.3%
If treated early	48%	37.2%	30.7%
Doubtful	0%	5.3%	14.0%
Never	0%	12.7%	24.0%

Hobbs argues that

> there are in the community at one end of a continuum, women who believe in screening and health checks as a general principle and who, in relation to cancer, know that there are possibilities for cure and that early treatment can be beneficial. Such women do not wait to be invited to breast screening. They ask for it. At the other end (of the continuum) are those who avoid or are unenthusiastic about health checks and screening and who, although they may register a health message do not really accept it.

She suggests that between these two extremes are women who are not enthusiastic about screening but who will participate if someone takes the initiative and invites them, if administrative obstacles are reduced or eliminated and if health messages fit their preconceptions.

However, an alternative explanation of the data is that greater fear of cancer is associated with greater reluctance to present for screening. Such fear is also implicated in the case of individuals who delay in seeking professional help when fearing they have cancer.

Delay in seeking professional help in cancer

In the light of a number of studies which have shown that early diagnosis of cancer results in improved prognosis as measured by the five-year survival rate, Brooks (1979) claims that factors implicated in delay in seeking help are of great importance to the prognosis of malignant tumours affecting the treatment which is appropriate:

> The importance of this point about delay, therefore, is not simply the cold language of mortality statistics but its influence on the quality and quantity of living with cancer and quite possibly the quality of death from it.

In a longitudinal study of 22 women with breast cancer reported by Gyllenskold (1982) she discusses the psychology of delay. When a woman becomes aware of the lump in her breast, consciously or unconsciously she links its significance to cancer. Cancer represents such a powerful threat that the connection is dismissed by defence mechanisms to the unconscious. This makes it impossible to act appropriately, and she now links the lump with 'rheumatism', 'it's nothing', 'it will go away', 'it will have gone tomorrow, there are so many irregularities in the breast'. The woman keeps reality at a distance, but bit by bit gathers and uses her inner strength to meet what has happened, restructuring reactions and working through the situation.

Gyllenskold found that there was a statistically significant association between delay and having close relatives who had had cancer, especially breast cancer. There was also a significant association between delay and using defence mechanisms against the cognitive as well as the emotional dimensions of the concept of cancer.

Gyllenskold's (1982) study illustrates the use of mental defence mechanisms as a method of coping with the threat posed by the suspicion of the diagnosis of cancer. It is not an appropriate coping mechanism as she has pointed out. Others faced with the same suspicions cope by seeking medical help as soon as possible. Fortunately in the case of a lump in the breast at any rate, the vast majority turn out to be benign in nature. What about the minority of people whose fears are realized that they do turn out to have cancer? How do they cope at the time of diagnosis?

Coming to terms with the diagnosis

To many, including not insubstantial numbers of doctors, the issue of communicating the diagnosis is a simple one. It is seen in relation to a biological model, within which the doctor carries out tests, makes a diagnosis and then prescribes treatment for combatting the illness and restoring the patient to health. According to such a model the patient's role is to co-operate and to play a relatively passive role (Haan, 1980).

This relatively simple picture is problematic, however. First of all the issue of restoring the patient to health is an uncertain one when the diagnosis is cancer. Secondly, in coming to terms with the diagnosis the patient needs to engage in an active process of coping. This may be suppressed by the relatively passive role expected if the doctor subscribes to the biological model. Thirdly, the meaning the diagnosis has to the patient is a psychosocial factor which may well interact with the biological aspects of the disease affecting its severity and outcome (Engel, 1977). Fourthly, communicating the diagnosis to the patient may be traumatic for the doctor to such an extent that he/she fails to give information at all, or uses such indirect methods to soften the blow that patients fail to understand, although the doctor believes they do (Haan, 1980).

Klein and Lindemann (1961) suggest that for the patient diagnosis can be likened to a psychological crisis, 'a sudden alteration in the field of social forces within which the individual exists, such that the individual's expectations of himself and his relationships with others undergo change'.

This is illustrated by some quotes from the sample of patients with breast cancer interviewed by Gyllenskold about how they felt on being told the diagnosis.

When I was told, it didn't feel as horrible as I thought. . . it felt worse.

It feels as if everything gets blurred. Everything collapses on top of you.

But you can't see that I'm ill. Of course I'm frightened when I look at myself in the mirror and think I'm quite unlike myself. It's probably just an emotional thing. Being terrified of myself.

Haan (1980) argues that doctors communicating the diagnosis are bearers of bad news which causes stress for them. However they are taught in medical school to cope by emotional detachment but this is not necessarily effective as it creates impoverished social understanding. Indeed this emotional detachment was illustrated by Gyllenskold's study, since the doctors gave the diagnosis to the patients in a conference where they were on display and the object of discussion for about twenty doctors and other health professionals. The setting protected the doctor but must have added considerably to the distress felt by the patients. Indeed, one of the patients said,

> First you kind of have to be prepared for having cancer and then you have to listen to what they say and how you're supposed to behave and what you should do. There is so much to keep in your head at once.

Some of the defence mechanisms used by patients to protect against the impact of the diagnosis are illustrated in Gyllenskold's study.

Denial was one of the mechanisms employed but not all denied the disease completely; some employed partial denial whilst others denied in relation to their family for example, but not to medical staff. Depersonalization was used by some and indeed an element of that appears to be present in one of the quotes above. This process is illustrated well in excerpts from what two of the patients said.

> I don't know what I'm trying to say, someone else walking outside me. Because I suddenly realised it was cancer. I thought I was walking beside myself.

> Because I was sort of two people, for a time at the beginning, one who was standing watching myself. But it's come together now.

Both repression and suppression were used, particularly in relation to emotional distress and tears. There was a fear of emotion. 'One would collapse.' Patients also believed that it didn't help to cry. Gyllenskold remarks however that energy locked up in maintaining defences can be released by crying and then used constructively to cope actively and constructively with the disease and treatment.

Patients also isolated and separated their emotions from their conscious intellectual acceptance of the disease. This resulted in patients discussing their disease in an impersonal and calm way.

Displacement also occurred and this is illustrated by a patient who dwelt exhaustively upon a traumatic accident which had taken place years before. She expressed aggression against staff who had looked after her then.

Many patients did consciously associate the diagnosis of cancer with death.

It's obvious that the word cancer is absolutely terrifying, in any case it makes you frightened. You feel. . . like people must have felt in the past when they heard the word plague. That's what it feels like.

Gyllenskold's study clearly reveals that being told the diagnosis does conform to a crisis state, leading to difficulty in defining or formulating reasons for distress and in framing questions to gain the information which is needed for coping.

Rusk (1971) suggested that the application of crisis intervention principles could help. These are:

1. Helping patients to express their feelings about the diagnosis may help them to assess and organize their reactions and feelings.
2. Empathy gives validity to feelings about the diagnosis.
3. Emphasis on the positive aspects of the situation and the patient's own strengths helps the recognition and assessment of coping skills.
4. Helping patients to criticize the counsellor's interpretation contributes to the patient's own appraisal of their condition and supports them as an agent in coping.
5. An attitude of hope and calm confidence taken by the counsellor communicates that others feel the patient's problems are soluble.

Rusk (1971) also stresses the need to avoid making the patient passive. 'Do for others that which they cannot do for themselves and no more.' To do more is to rob them of their sense of self-determination, whilst to do less is to abandon them.

Futterman and Hoffman (1973) believe that counselling at the time of diagnosis should remind patients of the essential and natural commitment to life as well as of the necessity to re-define the meaning of life.

Unfortunately doctors are not trained to communicate the diagnosis in a way which would mobilize coping. Indeed the interaction between doctor and patient at that time has been labelled as one of moral imbalance (Engel, 1977; Haan, 1980) in which the doctor gives all and takes all responsibility. This means he expects to gain gratitude and compliance to redress the balance. Ill patients in crisis are seldom in a position to give much back and indeed compliance may be severely reduced by the patient not taking in any of the instructions he is given, since high anxiety interferes with memory (Ley and Spelman, 1967).

Part of the moral responsibility taken on by doctors is making a decision about whether or not to tell a patient the diagnosis at all, and if he tells, whether or not to communicate the prognosis. One would expect therefore that if this moral responsibility is taken seriously, individual patient characteristics would determine the information given. It also suggests that the information given would better match patients' needs the more the doctor knows about the patient. That this is not the case is suggested by an important observational and interview study carried out by McIntosh (1977) in a cancer ward. Its specific aims were (1) to investigate the ways in which patients conceived of and responded to their illness, and (2) to examine the structure and organization of what was communicated to patients.

In total 80 patients took part in the study; 52 women and 28 men. Interviews with staff were also carried out. At the beginning of the study of each patient, he or she had been diagnosed but had not been told the diagnosis.

McIntosh (1977) found that the doctors believed that the great majority of patients should not be told their diagnosis. This was based on a concern that above all patients should be left some hope, and that they did not want to know the truth and would react badly if they were told it. It was recognized, however, that some patients genuinely did wish to know what was wrong with them. Doctors believed this group should be told provided they could be relied on not to react unfavourably.

The major problem for all concerned was uncertainty. Doctors could not be absolutely certain of the diagnosis and were less certain of the prognosis. They were uncertain about what to tell patients and did not know what patients wished to know or how they would react. In the face of this the doctors adopted a policy of not disclosing the truth unless it was absolutely necessary. What communication was engaged in with patients was routinized so that problems did not appear. Routines were geared to very limited disclosure of information. Only if a patient persistently demanded information or refused treatment was he or she told the truth.

As for the patients, an overwhelming majority either knew or suspected they had cancer on admission to the ward. Few knew their prognosis and so they too were subject to great uncertainty but few sought to find out the truth. McIntosh found that almost 70% of those who suspected malignancy did not want confirmation. Fewer still wished to know their prognosis. They preferred uncertainty, since it gave hope. This group did seek out information however, but information of a kind which would reinforce optimism. Such patients appeared to work at seizing upon cues and then interpreting favourably anything which could sustain hope.

For those patients who did want the truth, the routinization of information made it extremely difficult, since in any case staff assumed that in fact they did not really wish to know. Thus the truth was given in euphemisms and ambiguities.

McIntosh (1977) included a table in his report which summarized patients' wishes for the truth (see Table 11.3).

It would be interesting to find out if few patients wish to know the truth today. However in the light of Gyllenskold's study, crucial aspects of which will be discussed further, it could be that people's desire for the truth varies rapidly with time, since her findings suggest that defence mechanisms such as denial are used in a rapidly fluctuating manner.

It is not at all surprising that individuals find the diagnosis 'cancer' stressful, since research has shown that stress is less well coped with when (Haan, 1980):

- it is not anticipated or it is overanticipated
- the expectation is of something better
- it is a stressor similar to stressors coped with badly in the past
- the stressor is ambiguous
- the individual is already distressed before the onset of the present circumstances
- they are unable to get vital information about the situation
- there is little the individual can do to control or change the stressor
- the stress is prolonged
- the individual has little experience in dealing with stress

Table 11.3   Patients' wishes regarding diagnosis and prognosis in cancer*

Number of patients	Awareness of diagnosis	Wanted to know diagnosis	Wanted to know prognosis
32	suspected	no	no
9	suspected	yes	no
14	knew	–	no
6	suspected	yes	yes
3	knew	–	yes
1	knew	–	–

*Note: 6 patients did not suspect; 3 were misled into believing they did not have cancer; in 6 cases, diagnosis was benign and prognosis was unproblematic. After McIntosh (1977).

11.3 COPING WITH CANCER AND ITS TREATMENT

The experience of having cancer is perhaps best regarded as an ongoing process with several stages each of which pose their own particular problems (Mages and Mendelsohn, 1980).

Uncertainty associated with the prognosis of the disease has already been mentioned but the extent and degree of this uncertainty should be emphasized. It may be many years before the patient can be sure whether or not he or she has been cured. The individual, therefore, must continue to live with uncertainty, fearing each physical upset which could be a symptom of the spread or progression of cancer. Not surprisingly, cancer patients regard the disease as a major discontinuity in their lives and report permanent changes in the way in which they view themselves and their future (Mages and Mendelsohn, 1980).

There are certain times during the process of having cancer when fear and anxiety is greater than at other times. This could be anticipated from a know-ledge of investigations and treatment. However, it has been shown empiri-cally in a retrospective study of patients who had undergone laryngectomy for cancer (Fasting, 1981).

During a home visit with 26 patients and their relatives, an interview was carried out and a questionnaire administered. The data collected allowed the course of the illness to be charted and allowed the researcher to pinpoint the times at which the risk of the development of crisis was greatest. Data were also collected from a prospective study of 22 patients undergoing laryn-gectomy. In the course of the prospective study the researcher acted as a participant observer. Her role in particular was to act as a counsellor for the patient.

Results showed that the 'worst' times (and thus the times of greatest risk of crisis) for the patient were:

1. Immediately before the first consultation with the doctor.
2. Immediately after radiotherapy was completed until patients were told whether or not they were to have an operation.
3. At the time of discharge from hospital which involved confronting the everyday environment which the patient must learn to cope with anew.

There were other findings of interest. One was that patients came into contact with a large number of different professional workers during the course of treatment, each of whom had differing goals for the patient, in spite of the fact that they were all working toward the same end. This increased uncertainty for the patient, since the treatments and care to which he or she was exposed appeared arbitrary. In general, the researcher felt that staff knew too little about the patient's lifestyle to be able to help the patient to cope with problems and changes which had to be faced. The relatives felt left out and poorly prepared physically and psychologically for their role in care.

In this study (Fasting, 1981), most patients knew their diagnosis. The author advocates open communication with cancer patients, but she also points out that unless patients have fully talked out their anxiety, the information given to them is not fully taken in and understood. She argues that the goal of com-munication is not that of telling the patient the diagnosis but rather to give the opportunity of expressing anxiety by getting the patient to talk about his/her cancer.

Health care professionals will understand that the treatment of cancer may involve radiotherapy, operation or chemotherapy. In many cases a combination of two or even all three methods may be used. The order in which treatments are given may also vary. In the case of the laryngectomy patients discussed above, radiotherapy was given prior to operation. To turn now to the patients with breast cancer studied by Gyllenskold, some of these patients had operation alone, some had radiotherapy before operation and the remainder underwent radiotherapy post-operatively.

Coping with radiotherapy

Whilst there is a large literature on the psychosocial aspects of undergoing operation (see Chapter 8), the literature in relation to radiotherapy is sparse. For this reason Gyllenskold's interviews with patients who underwent radiotherapy will be reported fairly extensively here.

Although a part of this study has already been quoted above, the method used has not yet been explained. The study was carried out in Sweden and involved long interviews with each of 21 patients. These interviews were conducted along conversational lines but the researcher had a checklist of topics to be covered in each. Each interview was taped and the tapes were subsequently transcribed and analysed. These conversations occurred at set times in relation to the cancer process, namely: at the time patients were told the diagnosis; 1 week later; 3 weeks after operation; and at 6 months, 1 year, and 2 years after diagnosis. Patients who had radiotherapy were also interviewed at the conclusion of the treatment. Three patients dropped out during the course of the study.

The interviews were analysed within a psychoanalytical framework with a particular focus upon the operation of defence mechanisms. Interestingly, the researcher subjected her own contributions to the conversation to the same type of analysis and this makes the research report a particularly insightful one. It is a study which has particular relevance within the framework of this book, since the analysed conversations make a fascinating record of the use of defence mechanisms in coping with stress.

One of the important findings of the study in respect of the 12 patients who underwent radiotherapy was the need for information about the treatment. Indeed, 2 of the patients had never even heard of anyone who had had radiotherapy.

The information which the patients needed was very basic (see Table 11.4).

In practice, 3 patients did work part-time throughout their course of radiotherapy in spite of discouragement from the doctor. Patients were frightened of the radiotherapy and expressed their fears in the interview both directly and indirectly. For example:

Well you wonder if it is going to damage you or something. (*Direct*)

Table 11.4 Information needed by patients undergoing radiotherapy

1. Whether the treatment would hurt or leave a scar
2. How long each treatment session would be
3. How long a course of treatment is
4. Whether treatment has psychological effects such as depression
5. Whether treatment has physical effects such as sterility
6. Whether the patient is dangerous to others, including her family, during the course of treatment
7. Whether it was possible to bathe or sunbathe during the treatment course
8. Whether it was possible to work during the course of treatment
9. Whether care is transferred to a different doctor during radiotherapy
10. How it will feel during treatment
11. The patient's role during treatment

> She [patient's sister] thought it was dreadful. She was very depressed every time. (*Indirect*)

Perhaps the lack of knowledge noted already was, in part, related to fear, since the defences aroused by fear included a claim of knowing nothing about radiotherapy and a desire to know nothing.

The word 'radiation' was associated with the idea of the spread of effects to the whole body. Whilst patients realized that it was a force which is constructive if controlled, they also realized its potential for destruction. Obviously patients could see the skin changes caused by the radiotherapy and this made them worry about what was happening to deep tissue, the heart, for example. The idea of exposing themselves day after day to a destructive force in order to get well was a worrying one.

Most patients experienced feelings of panic during a session of radiation treatment. This was often during the first session or perhaps on an occasion when the patient's position had been moved so that the apparatus appeared closer than usual. Panic feelings subsided, however.

> It was horrible the first time. I almost panicked, but one had to remember to breathe calmly. . . Well, I think the reason was that it was so big and it hung. . . it was on the ceiling and came so close. . . and then that noise which boomed on but in any case it was just knowing that I had to lie still like that for so many minutes and I was not allowed to move, it's a bit too much of a strain.

One of the problems was being alone whilst receiving the treatment. This aroused feelings of loneliness, fear of helplessness and separation anxiety, even though the patients were supervised by TV. They were frightened of being forgotten or of receiving excessive doses of radiotherapy because of something going wrong. Consequently staff became important, seeming omnipotent, because they could deal constructively with a destructive force. Some patients became particularly attached to an individual member of staff and then became distressed and frightened when that person had a day off.

The therapy itself was physically stressful. Fatigue, skin reactions and sickness occurred. Fatigue in particular could be extreme.

During the conversations about the treatment, Gyllenskold learned how mobile mental defence mechanisms were. They were able to help patients to cope with difficult situations precisely because of their mobility. At the same time patients had a need to express and share difficult experiences with an empathetic individual whilst those same experiences were still fresh.

Defence mechanisms which were used included denial and projection, suppression, reaction formation and incorporation. Gyllenskold interpreted the patients' expressed view that they 'scatter-brained' as indicating the struggle between suppression and conscious realization of feelings and knowledge concerning what they were going through. Reaction formation was illustrated by two patients who claimed that they felt generally more healthy throughout the radiation treatment. Incorporation was concerned with the destructive elements of the treatment. Some patients believed that the radiation lingered in their body, becoming a property of themselves. The patient had become as it were stigmatized with omnipotence and potentially destructive in the way radiation was.

Gyllenskold (1982) believes that it is important to understand and recognize defence mechanisms, since that gives a better chance of being able to identify with the patient and act supportively. Understanding allows the patient the chance to express the thoughts and feelings against which the defence exists. Understanding can be communicated even if the difficulty is not expressed clearly, but only in the form allowed by the defence mechanism. Questions which would be distressing and painful can be avoided by a counsellor who understands.

Gyllenskold (1982) argues that listening to the patient is more important than speaking, since active listening means really sharing experiences, thoughts and feelings.

Interestingly, she believes that there are no rules about what to say or how to behave in conversation with patients. All the therapist can do is to test out whether the patient is able to talk about experiences and whether or not he or she is willing to do so.

This Swedish study suggests that information given before radiotherapy treatment starts could help patients in their coping. Gyllenskold listed information which could be included in a pamphlet to be given to patients. This was:

1. What 'radiotherapy' means.
2. How treatment is organized.

3. The importance of initial skin marking and the maintenance of these marks throughout the treatment.
4. How the patient is summoned for treatment.
5. Possible side effects and how to cope.
6. Possible long-term effects.
7. Instructions the patient should follow during treatment.
8. That the treatment is harmless to others in contact with the patient.

The study allowed comparison between the three groups of patients, namely: those who underwent operation only; those who had radiotherapy first and then operation; those who had the operation before radiotherapy. Patients in each of these groups regarded their own situation favourably compared with those in the other groups. For example, those who underwent radiotherapy first were very frightened of the tumour and wished to get rid of it as quickly as possible. However, they assured themselves that those who were undergoing operation must have a very dangerous tumour which had to be removed rapidly. On the other hand, patients who had operation only felt that the radiotherapy was an additional safety measure and undergoing it meant that the tumour was much worse than their own. Those patients who were operated upon before having radiotherapy felt that if radiotherapy was given first it meant that the tumour was such that it would be inoperable without the radiotherapy.

Undergoing operation for breast cancer

Although psychosocial aspects of surgery have been discussed in Chapter 8, some of the reactions in the special case of surgery for cancer will be included here.

In Gyllenskold's study all the patients who underwent surgery were said to be in the reaction phase of crisis. This phase lasted throughout the active treatment period and for varying periods of time afterwards.

During this reaction phase the women appeared completely absorbed in their concern about cancer. They 'had cancer in the back of their mind' whatever they were doing. Whilst waiting for the operation they worried that the cancer might spread. Patients felt a need to feel that they had taken part in the decision that the breast was to be removed. Indeed, some patients actually believed they had shared in the decision even though the reality was different.

For some of the women the reaction phase was very long drawn out and they suffered deep depression. Even two years after diagnosis some were still only in the transitional phase between reaction and reparation, functioning only with the aid of defence mechanisms and special, even neurotic interpretations of the significance of breast loss.

This study was concerned with breast cancer for which the operative treatment was removal of the breast. The breast has a special significance for women and some of the psychological reactions were concerned with body image changes and grief for the loss of the breast. Some of the women studied suffered phantom breast sensations.

After two years some patients began to question whether they had had cancer at all. Perhaps the loss of the breast had been unnecessary? The researcher interpreted this as meaning that after the initial crisis and thoughts of death the women began to re-evaluate the price they had paid. This questioning of the diagnosis was both a form of denial and displacement of aggression on to the doctor.

Gyllenskold concludes that patients undergoing this experience would benefit from group psychotherapy which included their relatives as well, to work through the emotional stresses. However there is little doubt from the report of the study that the conversations with the researcher were therapeutic for the patients and served as psychotherapy.

McGuire (1975, 1980) in the UK has also studied women undergoing breast surgery for cancer. In one study of 450 women with breast lumps (McGuire, 1975) he found that staff seriously underestimated the patients' distress at the time they saw the surgeon in the clinic. Staff failed to pick up the indirect cues of distress which were present. Women themselves, however, were reluctant to reveal their worries directly, since these might appear silly and overburden busy staff.

Even when patients became in-patients for operation it was still the case that many staff were reluctant to talk with or listen to the women express their feelings. Some patients felt that the possibility of mastectomy was never properly discussed with them and that they were given little or no opportunity to talk the operation over with their husbands.

On recovering from the anaesthetic the first thing they did was to check whether the breast was still there or not. Patients who were not psychologically prepared for mastectomy were extremely shocked and some were bitter and angry. Over a third of the patients were very anxious and depressed but little of this distress was noticed by staff. In another study (McGuire, 1980) focusing on communication between staff and patients, 20 in-patients with breast cancer were visited several times a day by trained observers. It was found that only 5% of communications were concerned with the women's emotional well-being, or psychological reactions to illness and surgery. Few of these communications involved explicit enquiries by nursing staff or disclosure by the patients. Most interactions were focused upon instrumental concerns. McGuire suggested that both patients and staff conspired to pretend that the patients were coping.

McGuire (1980) also followed up cancer patients for sometime after diagnosis. He found that 20–40% of women having mastectomy develop a depressive illness, anxiety neurosis or sexual problems within twelve months of the surgery. Colostomy for anorectal cancer appears equally stressful, since 23% of these patients similarly develop psychiatric problems post-operatively.

The work of both Gyllenskold and McGuire points to the value of psycho-therapy as a method of helping patients to cope with the stress associated both with the knowledge that they have cancer and its treatment. Psycho-therapy is only one of a number of methods available to help people in coping during stress (see Chapter 2).

The **Simonton technique** (1980) incorporates a number of coping strategies.

1. Patients are trained in muscular relaxation and breathing regulation. This is accompanied by mental imagery in which the patient learns to visualize their own white blood cells acting upon the malignancy.
2. Counselling is aimed at encouraging assertiveness, especially in relation to the expression of emotion. It also helps patients with goal setting, guided fantasy and clarification of their underlying beliefs and fears.
3. Education in the benefits of physical exercise.

Use of this technique appears to induce better survival rates in cancer than the baseline statistics suggest.

Grossarth-Maticek *et al.* (1984) have devised a set of methods of helping patients to cope in cancer, based on the findings of their Yugoslavian and Heidelberg studies mentioned earlier in this chapter. This set of methods is called **Creative Novation Therapy (CNT)**.

Creative Novation Therapy was tested in two experimental studies. In the first of these, 175 women with breast cancer and metastases who were to be treated with chemotherapy were invited to undergo psychotherapy at the same time; 17 refused psychotherapy and 56 refused chemotherapy. Matched groups of patients were formed as follows: 25 patients received psychotherapy alone; 25 received chemotherapy alone; 25 underwent both psychotherapy and chemotherapy; 25 had neither treatment.

Three different types of psychotherapy were used; the 50 patients who had psychotherapy being further subdivided for assignment to one of these forms of psychotherapy which were as follows:

1. Behaviour therapy in which desirable behaviour was encouraged and undesirable behaviour discouraged.
2. Depth psychotherapy involving classical psychoanalysis with an emphasis on traumatic incidents in early childhood.
3. Creative Novation Therapy which was designed to enable the patient to express psychological needs which were normally inhibited. They were also helped to engage in more satisfying social interactions. Conflicting needs were analysed and alternative interpretations offered. Alternative behaviour was suggested. Relaxation and suggestion were used to

emphasize alternative interpretations. The patient was encouraged to work on concrete behaviour changes at home.

Of the 50 patients undergoing psychotherapy, 24 had CNT, 12 depth psychology and 14 behaviour therapy. Half of these patients in each case also received chemotherapy whilst the remainder had psychotherapy alone. Effectiveness of therapy was evaluated by using the mean survival time of patients.

Results were as follows: The mean survival time of all 100 patients was 15.7 months. Those who received neither chemotherapy nor psychotherapy survived a mean of 11.25 months. The patients who received chemotherapy alone had a mean survival time of 14.08 months. With psychotherapy alone patients survived a mean 14.92 months. Chemotherapy and psychotherapy together were associated with a mean survival time of 22.4 months. This suggested a synergistic relationship between chemotherapy and psychotherapy, each enhancing the value of the other.

A comparison of the three methods of psychotherapy showed that CNT was associated with the longest average survival time of 25.54 months. The survival time mean was 15.29 months for those who had received behaviour therapy and 12.82 months among the group receiving depth psychology. The researchers believed that the depth psychology may have given the patients insight into their psychological problems without helping to resolve them.

General analysis of the effects of psychotherapy showed that it increased the drive to live, self-esteem and anxiety. There was a decrease in blocking of emotional expression. Interestingly, psychotherapy was also associated with a less negative response to the side effects of chemotherapy and an increase in the lymphocyte count.

Overall, the study could be interpreted as suggesting that psychotherapy in general, and CNT in particular, might have a valuable effect upon the prognosis in breast cancer.

A second study was carried out by Grossarth-Maticek et al. (1984) to evaluate the effects of CNT. This involved 98 patients with regional lymphatic metastases who were undergoing radiotherapy. Two groups were formed from matched pairs of patients. One group acted as control, and the other group received psychotherapy of twenty hours duration in addition to the radiotherapy. The psychotherapy group was further subdivided: 13 patients (Group 1) were given CNT by its originator; 13 patients (Group 2) were also given CNT but by a therapist who had had 100 hours training in the technique; 13 patients (Group 3) received conventional psychotherapy by a therapist who had had 8 hours' training in CNT; 10 patients (Group 4) received depth psychotherapy or behaviour therapy from a therapist who knew nothing about CNT.

Results (Table 11.5) suggested that CNT had had a positive effect upon the

Table 11.5 Evaluation of the effects of Creative Novation Therapy

Group	Patient numbers	Mean survival	Mean difference*
1	Therapy $n = 13$ Control $n = 13$	55.15 months 45.77 months	+ 9.39 months
2	Therapy $n = 13$ Control $n = 13$	52.08 months 45.31 months	+ 6.77 months
3	Therapy $n = 13$ Control $n = 13$	48.85 months 44.00 months	+ 4.84 months
4	Therapy $n = 10$ Control $n = 10$	30.80 months 45.00 months	− 14.20 months

*Therapy survival time minus control survival time. After Grossarth-Maticek et al. (1984).

survival time of patients with advanced cancer. It appeared that survival was improved further still if the therapist was experienced in CNT.

Changes in patients which were associated with an improved prognosis were an improvement in social interactions, an increased will to live and an increase in emotional expression.

On extremely detailed analysis of data collected during the course of the study the authors suggested that the positive effects of CNT seemed to be due to psychosocial changes which occurred before treatment had started. They speculated that the possibility of therapy gives patients new hope, replacing hopelessness and depression. Using that explanation, however, makes it difficult to understand the results for the patients in Group 4, unless it is that therapists who have been trained in Creative Novation Therapy have much greater credibility than the therapist working with Group 4 who had not undergone such training.

Systematic desensitization

A study in which systematic desensitization was used to help patients to cope with chemotherapy treatment in cancer was reported by Morrow and Morrell (1982). Specifically this study was concerned with helping patients to cope with anticipatory nausea and vomiting. This symptom seems to occur in 25% of patients undergoing chemotherapy treatment and is resistant to anti-emetic drugs.

For this study, 500 patients having chemotherapy for cancer were screened for anticipatory nausea and vomiting: 120 had suffered this prior to previous treatment and from these, 60 were chosen to take part in the study. There was no difference in the characteristics of those who took part in the study compared with the 60 who did not. The 60 patients remaining in the study were assigned into three groups of 20 patients. One group underwent systematic desensitization; one group had counselling; and the third group had no psychological treatment at all.

Between the fourth and fifth chemotherapy treatments patients in the systematic desensitization group were exposed to two 1-hour sessions of psychological treatment. This involved learning a progressive relaxation technique, following which they constructed a hierarchy of situations in which they suffered progressively worse anticipatory nausea and vomiting. In deep relaxation they were asked to imagine each of the scenes in the hierarchy for 20 seconds. Provided they remained relaxed imagining a particular scene twice they then proceeded to the next scene in the hierarchy. Each patient was treated individually.

The counselling group of patients also underwent therapy between the fourth and fifth chemotherapy treatments. They were given individual therapy by the same experimenter as the desensitization group but the therapy in this case was Rogerian counselling.

Effectiveness of the treatment was measured by subjective reports of anticipatory nausea and vomiting submitted by the patients. In addition, State-Trait Anxiety and Health Locus of Control inventories were completed by patients in all groups. Patients in the two treatment groups also rated the credibility of the investigator and their expectation of results.

In practice, results were significantly in favour of the systematic desensitization procedure over counselling and the omission of psychological treatment. Fewer patients in the group receiving systematic desensitization suffered anticipatory nausea compared with the counselling group ($p < 0.05$) and the no-treatment group ($p < 0.01$). Similar results occurred in relation to anticipatory vomiting. Furthermore the effect was sustained for two chemotherapy treatments subsequent to the intervention.

In spite of the lack of change on the Health Locus of Control measure the researchers speculated that treatment may have had its effects through giving the patient a feeling of control over a symptom in relation to which they experienced helplessness.

The study does show the usefulness of a behavioural technique in helping patients to cope with a physical problem in relation to cancer treatment.

Although only a few different types of psychological methods have been discussed here, there is sufficient evidence to encourage workers to try a variety of different psychological measures in helping cancer patients with their coping.

11.4 SOCIAL ASPECTS

Social comparison processes in coping with cancer

Much of the work on the psycho-social aspects of cancer has thrown up the problem of the uncertainty associated with prognosis and the patients' consequent need for therapeutic communication and information. What happens, however, if patients fail to obtain the psychological support they need from professionals? Obviously patients do not exist in isolation and they will turn to non-professionals. In particular, fellow patients may well be seen as an important source of potential help in such circumstances. A study which was concerned with the extent to which fellow patients were perceived as sources of support was carried out in seven out-patient departments in the Netherlands (Molleman *et al.*, 1986). The researchers based their work upon social comparison theories propounded by Festinger (1954) and Gruder (1977) that social comparison stems from a need to reduce uncertainty.

During the course of this study 565 patients over the age of 16 years and with diagnosed cancer were approached in out-patients; 506 of these were given a questionnaire and asked to complete it anonymously at home. The questionnaire was concerned with: uncertainty and the need for information; accessibility or otherwise of information from expert professionals; preferred sources of information; the need for social comparison; preferred comparison persons; and the affective consequences of interaction with fellow patients. A modified version of the State-Trait Anxiety Scale was included in the questionnaire.

In practice, 418 completed questionnaires were returned from 257 male patients and 181 females. The average age of respondents was 53.7 years with a range of 21–78 years.

Results showed that patients clearly preferred to obtain information about aspects of the illness and treatment from professionals compared with non-experts. However, if the experts appeared inaccessible, then patients expressed a need for social comparison with fellow patients. Surprisingly, there was no relationship between uncertainty and the need for social comparison but fellow patients were seen as more informative as uncertainty became greater. Not all fellow patients were seen as equally informative. The more similar the fellow patient was to the respondent, the more he or she was seen as informative. A fellow patient who was perceived as being much worse off than the respondent was considered the least informative. There was also a marked preference for interaction with fellow patients who were considered similar to the patient or only very slightly better off. As anxiety in relation to the situation was greater so was the expressed need for social comparison up to a moderate level of anxiety. Above that level the expressed need for social comparison diminished.

The researchers concluded that social comparison processes do play a role in helping patients to cope with uncertainty and anxiety. This not only has theoretical implications but also has important practical ones, since patients are likely to rely more on information from fellow patients or other non-expert sources if information from professionals is not readily available. Health care staff need to be aware of this. However, even if patients do feel that their informational needs have been met by professionals, fellow patients may still play an important role in helping the patient to evaluate his/her own emotional responses.

Cancer patients and their coping on return to work

So far this chapter has focused upon the stress suffered by the cancer patient in relation to the diagnosis, prognosis and treatment of the disease. However, there is another important source of stress, and that is the reactions of other people within the social world of the sufferer from cancer. For many people, contact with someone known to have cancer may evoke fear and negative attitudes. This kind of reaction will have a great impact on the cancer sufferer who encounters it, and it can occur on the individual's return to work. The problems which cancer sufferers face at work has been studied by Feldman (1984).

In three studies he showed that adverse reactions to cancer were not unusual within the workplace. Patients who fared best were those who avoided playing the sick role, and without denying the diagnosis or treatment presented themselves as 'well and able'. Interestingly some hospitals refused access to the researcher for study, since they argued that work had nothing to do with cancer.

A total of 344 patients were involved in the three studies and a 20% sample of employers was also interviewed. Interviews with patients took place 18–30 months after diagnosis in two studies and 2–5 years after diagnosis in the third study which was concerned with young people aged 13–23 years at diagnosis.

The main initial concerns of the patients in relation to work were worry about money, their physical ability to hold down the job and workplace friendships. Men worried about how they would fill their time if they could not work and women were concerned about being bored and missing the social life and fulfilment associated with work.

Some respondents did not see work as problematic since they regarded their illness as a purely private concern. A few used their diagnosis to justify not working.

Many respondents had no expectation that their return to work would pose difficulties and, indeed, this frequently proved to be the case. At the time of the study 90% of the white collar respondents and 83% per cent of the blue collar respondents were working. The remainder for the most part were trying to find work.

Almost 66% of respondents reported positive experiences at work, having been helped in their adjustment by workmates or employers. Nonetheless 50% of the white collar workers, 80% of the blue collar workers and 50% of the young group had experienced problems at work. The source of stress varied with the site of cancer and the age of the individual. In particular those over the age of 45 years reported problems, as did those with cancer of the rectum or colon. Undoubtedly some problems were a consequence of the respondents' own attitudes.

However, negative attitudes within the workplace did lead to dismissal, transfers, or being placed on less popular shifts or locations. Some patients were demoted or failed to get salary increases. There was a problem in some cases that their group health or life insurance was terminated. Excessive solicitude from fellow workers also posed a difficulty in some cases.

Those of the sample who experienced problems in getting a new job or in the case of the younger people a first job, sometimes attributed this to prejudice. It was frequently, however, because the company doctor noted that the applicant had not been symptom-free for five years.

Methods of coping

Apart from instrumental reasons for returning to work, most patients wished to do so as an outward sign of their wellness and their ability to control their own lives. Many respondents wished to work to 'prove' themselves and to channel their emotional distress into productive directions. They compensated for their illness by intense efforts to improve quality and productivity and in avoiding absence. Indeed some had exceeded their physical limits.

Those who suffered hostility at work made the best of it if they failed to succeed in finding a new job. Many of this group had recurring depression. Self pity and denial were used by some as coping methods. Feldman argues that depression deserves special attention since it appears to be a stressor, a response to stress and a coping device.

In general the respondents' ability to cope with work was associated with intellectual endowment, personality, characteristic ways of handling stress before the illness, strength of motivation and family, formal and informal social support.

Clearly to have cancer stretches an individual's coping resources to the limit and the demands made do not cease when treatment finishes. Uncertainty continues, and the attitudes of others may be problematic. 'Cancer almost inevitably produces enduring personal change, which, to be fully understood, should be viewed in the context of the individual's life stage and previous history' (Mages and Mendelsohn, 1980).

11.5 SUMMARY

Cancer is an important topic for a book on stress since the word itself is associated with negative attitudes and emotions even for those who do not suffer from the disease. Nonetheless it is a widespread condition in Britain, and is the second most frequent cause of death in the developed world. To consider cancer as a single entity, however, is inaccurate, as it is really a group of rather different diseases varying in degree of malignancy, site and tissue of origin.

The possibility that stress is implicated in the causation of cancer has been discussed, together with a critique of study methods used to establish such a link. A possible mechanism was traced by which psycho-social factors could adversely affect the physiology of the body allowing malignancy to develop.

The remainder of the chapter has been concerned with psycho-social problems arising from the disease itself. Negative attitudes toward cancer mentioned above may affect early diagnosis both through the individual's reluctance to undergo screening and through delay in attending for medical opinion when there is suspicion that symptoms might be due to cancer.

Being told that one has cancer appears a major stressor not only for the victim but also for the doctor who is responsible for telling the patient. Medical staff may protect themselves from open communication not only about the diagnosis but also the prognosis which is associated with a great deal of uncertainty. Lack of open communication may suit the expressed wishes of some patients who suspect they have cancer, but probably severely hinders the development of coping strategies in many. However, being told one has cancer has been likened to a major psychological crisis.

The treatments available for cancer, namely radiotherapy, surgical excision and chemotherapy, are also extremely stressful. There is evidence that the hospital medical and nursing staff may block patients from expressing their feelings during treatment. However, counselling and psychotherapy appear helpful, and there is evidence that a wide range of mental defence mechanisms are used frequently and flexibly by patients in coping. Nonetheless psychiatric disorder has been reported in about 25% of sufferers from cancer at some sites, some one to two years after diagnosis.

Other methods of helping patients to cope include the Simonton technique and Creative Novation Therapy. These both include a range of methods of psychological help, for example, imagery, relaxation, assertion training, help in expressing emotions and help in changing interaction patterns. A study of systematic desensitization showed that this, too, may have a role, particularly in symptom control. Social comparison with other patients may also be used by patients as a method of coping.

Finally a study of the difficulties faced by patients on return to work and their coping strategies suggests that the 'cancer process' is a long and arduous one.

REFERENCES

Ader, R. and Friedman, S. R. (1965) Differential early experience and susceptibilities to transplanted tumours in the rat. *J. Comp. Physiol. Psych.*, **59**, 361–4.

Brooks, A. (1979) Public and professional attitudes to cancer. *Proc. Nursing Mirror Intern. Cancer Nursing Conference 1978*, pp. 151–6.

Burnet, F. M. (1971) Immunological surveillance in neoplasia. *Transplant Rev.*, **7**, 3–25.

Caplan, G. and Grunebaum, J. (1967) Perspectives on primary prevention. *Archives of General Psychiatry*, **17**, 331–46.

Charlton, A. (1981) She'll die, won't she, Miss? – teaching children about cancer, in *Cancer Nursing Update* (ed. R. Tiffany), Baillière Tindall, London, pp. 51–3.

Cox, T. (1984) Stress: a psychophysiological approach to cancer, in *Psychosocial Stress and Cancer* (ed. C. C. Cooper), J. Wiley, Chichester, pp. 149–69.

Cox, T. and Mackay, C. (1982) Psychosocial factors and psychophysiological mechanisms in the aetiology and development of cancers. *Soc. Sci. Med.*, **16**, 381–96.

Crisp, A. H. (1970) Some psychosomatic aspects of neoplasia, *Br. J. Med.*, **45**, 313–31.

Donaldson, R. J. and Donaldson, L. J. (1983) *Essential Community Medicine*. MTP, Lancaster.

Ebbessen, P. and Rask-Nielsen, R. (1967) Influence of sex-segregated groupings and of innoculation with subcellular leukemic material on development of non-leukemic lesions in DBA/2 BALB/C and CBA mice *J. Natl. Cancer Inst.*, **39**, 917–32.

Engel, G. L. (1977) The need for a new medical model: a challenge for biomedicine. *Science*, **196**, 129–36.

Fasting, U. (1981) 'Communication problems in the nursing care of patients before and after laryngectomy', in *Cancer Nursing Update* (ed. R. Tiffany), Baillière Tindall, London, pp. 94–100.

Feigenberg, L. (1970) Erfarenheter som psykiater vid en tumörklinik. *Läkartidningen*, **67**, 5641–9.

Feldman, F. L. (1984) 'Wellness and work', in *Psychosocial Stress and Cancer* (ed. C. L. Cooper), J. Wiley, Chichester, pp. 173–200.

Festinger, L. A. C. (1954) A theory of social comparison processes. *Human Relations*, **7**, 117–40.

Fobair, P. and Cordoba, C. S. (1982) Scope and magnitude of the cancer problem in psychosocial research, in *Psychosocial Aspects of Cancer* (eds J. Cohen, J. W. Cullen and L. R. Martin), Raven Press, New York, N.Y.

Fox, P. Y. (1978) Premorbid psychological factors as related to cancer incidence. *J. Behav. Med.*, **1**, 45–133.

Futterman, E. H. and Hoffman, I. (1973) 'Crisis and adaptation in the families
of fatally ill children', in *The Child in His Family: The Impact of Disease and
Death* (eds E. J. Anthony and C. Koupernik), J. Wiley, New York, N.Y.

Grossarth-Maticek, R., Schmidt, P., Vetter, H. and Arndt, S. (1984) Psychotherapy research in oncology, in *Health Care and Human Behaviour* (eds
A. Steptoe and M. Mathews), Academic Press, London, pp. 325–41.

Gruder, C. O. (1977) Choice of comparison persons in evaluating oneself. (eds
J.M.F. and R. Miller) cited in Molleman, E. Pruyn J. and Van Knettenber, A.
(1986) Social comparison process amongst cancer patients in *Bri. J. Soc.
Psych.*, **25**(1), 1–13.

Gyllenskold, K. (1982) *Breast Cancer: The psychological effects of the Disease
and its Treatment*, translated by Patricia Crampton, Tavistock Publications, London.

Haan, N. G. (1980) Psychosocial meanings of unfavourable medical forecasts,
in *Health Psychology – A Handbook* (eds G. C. Stone, F. Cohen, N. E. Adler
et al.) Jossey-Bass, San Francisco, CA, pp. 113–40.

Herberman, R. and Holden, H. (1978) Natural cell-mediated immunity.
Advances in Cancer Research, **27**, 305–77.

Herberman, R. and Ortaldo, H. T. (1981) Natural killer cells: their role in
defenses against disease. *Science*, **214**, 24–30.

Herzlich, C. (1973) *Health and Illness: A Social-Psychological Analysis*, Academic Press, New York.

Hobbs, P. (1981) Acceptors and rejectors of breast screening, in *Cancer Nursing Update* (ed. R. Tiffany), Baillière Tindall, London, pp. 53–6.

Irwin, J. and Anisman, H. (1984) Stress and Pathology: immunological and
central nervous system interactions, in *Psychosocial Stress and Cancer* (ed.
C. L. Cooper), J. Wiley, Chichester, pp. 93–147.

Klein, D. C. and Lindemann, E. (1961) Preventive interaction in individual and
family crisis situations, in *Prevention of Mental Disorders in Children* (ed. G.
Caplan), Basic Books, New York, N.Y.

Lee, P. R. and Franks, P. E. (1980) Health and disease in the community, in
Primary Care (ed. J. Fry), Heinemann, London.

Levine, G. and Cohen, C. (1959) Differential survival to leukaemia as a function of infantile stimulation in DBA/2 mice. *Proc. Soc. Experimental and
Biological Medicine*, **104**, 180–3.

Ley, P. and Spelman, M. S. (1967) *Communicating with the Patient*, Staples
Press, St Albans.

Mages, N. L. and Mendelsohn, G. A. (1980) Effects of cancer on patients' lives:
a personological approach, in *Health Psychology* (eds G. C. Stone, F.
Cohen, N. E. Adler *et al.*), Jossey-Bass, San Francisco, CA, pp. 255–84.

McGuire, P. (1975) The psychological and social consequences of breast cancer. *Nursing Mirror* (April 3), 54–7.

McGuire, P. (1980) A conspiracy of pretence. *Nursing Mirror* (January 10), 17–19.

McIntosh, J. (1977) *Communication and Awareness in a Cancer Ward*, Croom Helm, London.

Molleman, E., Pruyn, J. and van Knippenbor, A. (1986) Social comparison processes among cancer patients. *Brit. J. Soc. Psych.*, **25**, 1–13.

Morrow, G. R. and Morrell, B. S. (1982) Behavioural treatment for the anticipatory nausea and vomiting induced by cancer chemotherapy. *New England J. Medicine*, **307**(24), 1476–80.

Riley, V. (1981) Psychoneuroendocrine influences on immunocompetence and neoplasia. *Science*, **212**, 1100–9.

Rosch, P. J. (1984) Stress and cancer, in *Psychosocial Stress and Cancer* (ed. C. L. Cooper), John Wiley, Chichester, pp. 3–19.

Rusk, T. N. (1971) Opportunity and technique in crisis psychiatry, *Comprehensive Psychiatry*, **12**, 249–63.

Rytel, M. W. and Kilbourne, E. F. (1966) The influence of cortisone on experimental viral infection. *J. Exp. Medicine*, **123**, 767–75.

Senescu, R. A. (1963) The development of emotional complications in the patient with cancer. *J. Chronic Diseases*, **16**, 813–32.

Senescu, R. A. (1966) The problem of establishing communication with the seriously ill patient. *Annals of the New York Academy of Science*, **125**, 696–702.

Simonton, O. C., (1980) Psychological intervention in the treatment of cancer. *Psychosomatics*, **21**, 226–33.

Simonton, O. C., Matthews-Simonton, S. and Sparks, T. F. (1980) Psychological intervention in the treatment of cancer. *Psychosomatics*, **21**, 226–33.

Temoshok, L. and Heller, B. W. (1984) On comparing apples, oranges and fruit salad: a methodological overview of medical outcome studies in psychosocial oncology, in *Psychosocial Stress and Cancer* (ed. C. L. Cooper), J. Wiley, Chichester, pp. 231–60.

Wellisch, D. K. (1981) Intervention with the cancer patient, in *Medical Psychology: Contributions to Behavioural Medicine* (ed. C. K. Prokop and L. A. Bradley), Academic Press, New York, pp. 224–39.

CHAPTER TWELVE

Change in body image: dying, bereavement

In the final chapter of this section we have chosen to discuss what might seem at first to be widely disparate concepts; namely, change in body image, dying and bereavement. However they are all examples of significant loss, and the process of adaptation through which the individual comes to terms with the loss is similar in each case. Indeed the adaptation process has already been touched on in previous chapters, particularly in the chapter on cancer, since both a change in body image and fear of dying assume great importance in cancer.

Loss is a basic concept which underlies all change throughout an individual's life. Change may well mean that gains are made, but alongside the gains there are always losses, even though the loss may be of something we wish to get rid of. Bower (1980) believes that loss is an inevitable part of life and that each maturational development involves loss. For example, becoming an adult also involves leaving behind the role of 'child'. However not all writers define loss quite as broadly as that. Roberts (1986) for example defines loss as 'any change in the individual's situation that decreases the probability of achieving implicit or explicit goals'. She also argues that loss is the deprivation of an object, person, possession or ideal that was considered valuable and in which there was an investment of self. According to Roberts (1986) loss may be actual, potential or symbolic. Bower argues that the way in which a person responds to loss is determined by their previous experience with loss or death. Each loss not only reflects back on previous loss but also carries a threat of further loss in the near or distant future (Bower, 1980).

Personal loss is defined as the permanent loss of a significant person which requires adaptation. The term 'significant person' implies a relationship with or attachment to that person. Such personal loss attacks the roots of an individual's security and may pose a threat to survival. It may bring about a sense of abandonment and extreme loneliness. Personal loss can come about through the death of a significant person, divorce, abortion, stillbirth, estrangement, and in the case of a child, by being sent to boarding school or hospital.

Loss of self image (Bower 1977a, b) is also of great significance, since it means that an important part of the individual is lost, namely the mental image of their total personality. Such loss might involve abstractions such as ideas of one's attractiveness, lovableness, or worth. Social constructs such as loss of social role, independence and control also contribute to negative changes in self image.

The effect of loss is to evoke a process of grief or mourning, but grief is discussed later in relation to bereavement.

12.1 BODY IMAGE

Self image incorporates the body image, and the latter is extremely important in relation to health and ill health. The body image is probably subject to change, albeit only temporarily, every time an individual becomes a patient. Change in body image, especially if significant in degree, will affect the patient and the way he/she copes with the condition even though the changes may remain at an unconscious level as far as the patient is concerned and be completely unrecognized by health professionals.

The concept of body image can be traced to Head (1920) who described it as 'a unity in the sensory cortex developed from past and current body sensations'. From this somewhat mechanistic definition by a neurologist, the concept has developed in richness and meaning. Schilder (1935) defined it as 'a tridimensional image involving interpersonal, environmental and temporal factors'. He described body image as developing from the beginning of self-awareness through input from all sensory modalities, but in particular visual, tactile, proprioceptive and kinaesthetic sensations. He argued that these experiences of our own body combine with our observations of others and our perceptions of the reactions by other people to ourselves.

Shontz (1974) elaborated the functions of the body image. According to him it acts as a sensory register, selecting, recording, integrating and storing data from sense organs. Thus it is an essential component of perception, learning and memory, acting both to promote action and to set the limits on action. Body image is a source of motivational drives and a stimulus both to oneself and others. Whilst body image is an intensely private concept, at the same time it may also be used as an expressive instrument.

Norris (1970) defined body image as

the constantly changing total of conscious and unconscious information, feelings and perceptions about one's body in space as different and apart from all others. It is a social creation, developed through the reflected perceptions about the surfaces of one's body and responses to the sensations originating from the inner regions of the body as the individual copes with a kaleidoscopic variety of living activities. The body image is basic to identity and has been referred to as the somatic ego.

Norris argues that the body image acts as a frame of reference which influences the way in which the individual perceives self as well as influencing one's ability to carry out actions and perform skills. Ultimately, she says, body image is an intrapersonal organization of the individual's feelings and attitudes toward his or her own body. However, much of this process is subconscious and no one can describe their own total body image.

Norris lists the following aspects of body image as an operational definition of the concept. However, she warns that this is an oversimplified definition of a complex phenomenon.

1. It is a social creation.
   (a) Normality is judged by appearance, ways of gesturing or posturing and other ways of using the body that are prescribed by society.
   (b) Painful sanctions are imposed for deviations from normality, either behavioural or structural.
   (c) Approval and acceptance are given for normal appearance and proper behaviour.
   (d) Body image emerges out of an almost infinite variety and number of approvals and sanctions and an individual's response to them. Experience is integrated into the personality in terms of the satisfaction or dissatisfaction that the individual has had with it.
   (e) Body development continually enlarges the individual's world, his mastery of it, his interaction with it and his ability to respond to the wide variety of experience it offers.
   (f) This integration, which is highly unconscious, is constantly evolving and can be identified in the person's values, attitudes and feelings about himself.
2. There is a very close interdependence between body image and personality, ego, self image and identity.
3. Body image is an important determinant of behaviour.
4. The impact of any experience on the human being is determined by the interplay of its meaning in reality; the amount of conscious fantasies and feelings about it and unconsciously motivated fantasies and feelings.

Esberger (1978) claims that there are four characteristics of body image:

1. It is the totality of perceptions regarding one's own body and its performance.
2. It serves a definite function for each individual, influencing most aspects of daily living. Elements of the body image can be identified as values, attitudes and feelings.
3. Body image is dynamic, constantly changing.
4. It includes elements both of reality and of the ideal identity. Thus each

individual has a mental image of their own appearance which may or may not be consistent with actual body structure. For example, as ageing occurs, the individual's body image may resemble their younger self rather more than the actual self. In general a person's body as perceived and evaluated by themself plays an important role in the maintenance of a sense of self-esteem and security.

Bower (1977a) identified three levels of body experience:

1. The innermost somatic experience which forms the core body image. Neurological, metabolic, endocrine and hormonal elements contribute to this.
2. Behavioural body experience, contributing to which are motor actions, perceptual, cognitive and personality factors.
3. Topological body experiences which emanate from the surface boundary of the body and include direct sensory experiences of the world in terms of pain, pressure, sound and temperature, as well as the reflections of the reactions of other people toward the individual's appearance.

Developmental aspects of body image

O'Brien (1980) considered that the body image continues to develop throughout the life span.

As a baby the individual does not at first perceive himself as separate from the rest of the world responding to inner and outer experiences at the same sensory level (O'Brien, 1980). Through learning and maturation the infant moves to the behavioural level of bodily experience. Exploration of space, his own body, and solid objects in the environment provide the kinaesthetic and tactile sensations which contribute to the neural model of the body image. By responding to stimuli and exploration the child begins to differentiate self from non-self. Experiences begin to relate one to another within developing sensori motor schemata (Piaget, 1954). Alongside these experiences the development of mastery of his own body occurs (Norris, 1970). As the individual grows, motor development allows more wide ranging exploration of a changing environment, but this consolidates the experience of his own body as a constancy. Although a constant this latter experience is far from static. It is continuously differentiated, re-integrated and modified.

As age progresses, social experience increases and the topological body image develops (Bower, 1977a). It is through social interaction that the individual learns those aspects of cultural norms and values related to concepts of the body. The norms and values of the culture are initially transmitted to the child by a parent (or parent substitutes). It is this which determines whether the individual regards his body as good, bad, clean, or dirty etc., and indeed his attitude toward particular bodily functions (Pettit, 1980).

Adolescent experiences contribute significantly to the individual's ideal body image and the extent to which his actual body image conforms with this. Conflict may arise if the discrepancy is too great. The value placed by society and the individual on being 'handsome', 'beautiful', 'athletic', 'feminine', 'slim', and so on may ultimately determine the degree of conflict aroused by trauma or illness affecting the body image (Kolb, 1959).

However, the mature individual is one who has integrated and worked through the three levels of bodily experience successfully. Such an individual learns to accept his or her body without undue distress in respect to appearance, function, or control (Norris, 1970). For the mature person the body image moves to the background and development in relation to self-actualization predominates.

Nonetheless the body image is dynamic, and constantly integrates and reintegrates changes in structure and experience throughout life. Changes such as puberty, pregnancy, childbirth and the menopause are major, whilst others are much less significant. McDaniel (1976) argued that any change in stimulation from within the body must be evaluated and if significant it is incorporated into the body image and modifies it. Corbeil (1971), however, argued that body image change is related not so much to actual bodily change but more to perceived bodily change. Age, speed of the change and its visibility all play a part in the individual's perception of bodily change (Bower, 1977a). Bower argues that a change in body image will be perceived differently at different stages within the lifespan.

Body image changes associated with illness or injury

Illness or injury usually involves a change in body structure and/or function which may be temporary or permanent. Roberts (1986) argues that this forces the individual into a body image change. Frequently more than one bodily change takes place at the same time, such as a change in appearance, a change in functional ability, a change in control over one's actions. New sensations may occur of a type never before experienced (Norris, 1970). An example of this is the phantom limb sensations which frequently follow limb amputation.

Emotions which are experienced as a result of a change in the body image include anxiety and depression, shame, hopelessness and fear (Norris, 1970; Stone, 1976; Henke, 1979; Roberts, 1986). Since the body image is so basic to our identity any change in it is a threat. However, the subjective and objective meaning of a particular change to the individual concerned may increase the level of threat experienced. For example, aphasia may well have a different meaning for a teacher or politician than for a manual labourer. Hysterectomy might pose a greater threat to a childless woman anxious for a family than to one who has already completed her family. Loss of hair may be an enormous threat to a model.

Temporary threats to the body image associated with illness or injury have rarely been studied, but invasive procedures such as an enema, vaginal examination, catheterization or tracheal section certainly create temporary changes of the body image. Indeed such change could well be of a more permanent nature, since the part of the body affected and represented in the body image may assume an importance never before perceived.

Several authors have attempted to describe and/or classify conditions in which a permanent change in body image occurs.

Shontz (1974) classified changes of body image as follows:

1. From brain damage.
2. From damage to other parts of the nervous system, especially if posture and movement are affected.
3. From dismemberment.
4. Associated with toxic or metabolic disturbance.
5. In conditions in which there is great psychological impact from the body changes, e.g. in obesity, arthritis.
6. When there is faulty personality development as in neurosis/psychosis.

Bower (1977b) suggests a different classification, using a developmental framework.

1. The innermost bodily experience is affected. Examples are diabetes mellitus, change in acid–base balance, hormonal imbalance, changes of body chemistry due to drugs. Bower argues that since this category of body image change is poorly understood the changes can be very frightening.
2. The behavioural level of body image is affected. Examples here are multiple sclerosis, mental illness and cerebral palsy.
3. The topological level of body image is affected. Here the way in which the individual experiences the world outside himself is affected. Examples include blindness, deafness.

It is worth noting that many of the most obvious conditions which affect body image involve more than one of Bower's levels. An example is limb amputation in which innermost bodily experience may be affected. Behaviour and topological body image certainly will.

Norris (1970) gives the following classification of body image changes.

1. Loss of a part of the body.
2. Surgical procedures in which relationship between parts of the body is disturbed, e.g. colostomy, ileostomy, gastrostomy, intestinal resection.
3. A loss of internal body parts. Examples are gastrectomy, hysterectomy, lung lobectomy, cholecystomy.

4. Changes due to pathophysiology. This includes such conditions as obesity, emaciation, acromegaly, hirsutism in women, Addison's disease, dermatitis.
5. Loss of function as in paraplegia, for example.
6. Problems associated with body parts which are symbolically important. Examples are myocardial infarction, asthma.

However, it could be argued that each of these classificatory schemes is unsatisfactory. Part of the reason for this has already been mentioned, and that is that any one illness or injury will involve many different levels of body image. In any case it is probably more helpful in relation to the care of patients to identify the body image change in relation to the particular patient concerned.

Adaptation to altered body image

The circumstances in which a change in body image occurs vary considerably and the time which an individual has to prepare for the change also varies, depending upon whether the change results from a long drawn-out illness, a planned operation or sudden trauma.

For a patient who is to undergo surgery which will result in altered body image, adaptation begins pre-operatively (Norris, 1970). Family support is important in this adaptation and three types of family reaction have been described (Dyk and Sutherland, 1956). The first of these is positive, and the family give the patient every support and encouragement, hiding their own anxieties. A second type of family response is less helpful. Here the family members feel threatened and in turn become threatening toward the patient, attempting to force him or her into having immediate surgery, warning of dire consequences as a result of any delay. The third type of family response is also unhelpful. Here the family members become frightened and withdrawn, leaving the patient to cope (psychologically) alone.

Pre-operatively, the patient needs to engage in preparatory coping and adaptation. A normal preoperative response is that of concern and anxiety. Norris (1970) argues that absence of anxiety, joking about the surgery or treating it matter-of-factly are potential signs of maladaptation. It may be that the patient is repressing extreme anxiety which will overwhelm the defence mechanism post-operatively, manifesting itself as panic.

Not all changes of body image of course are a result of planned surgery, but may occur in injury, illness, or sudden catastrophes such as myocardial infarction, or stroke. Here the patient has no opportunity for appraisal and preparatory coping. Under such circumstances not only may the body image change be sudden but it may also be extensive. This is highly threatening to the individual who may respond with denial. Such denial may be manifest as physical symptoms of a psychosomatic type. Anger and guilt may be experienced. Any loss of control consequent upon physical changes may be accompanied by shame.

Adaptation begins when the individual begins to acknowledge the change by asking to see the part of the body concerned. He or she may not ask, but may peep at the site for increasing periods of time. Testing the staff and/or relatives may occur. The individual may ask if they have seen the site, or wish to do so, whilst watching their reactions very closely for signs of revulsion. The person's own reactions may fluctuate between fascination with the site and revulsion. Not all body changes affecting the body image are visible of course. Positive coping is signalled by a willingness to discuss feelings about the change and to begin looking to the future.

Adaptation to body image has also been described as a process with several phases (Roberts, 1986). These phases are: Impact, Retreat, Acknowledgement, Reconstruction.

Impact

This occurs at the time of the initial physical change. It is manifest by numbness and dissociation from what has occurred. Despair, depression and extreme passivity may occur. Frustration and feelings of forced dependency and immobility may add to the depression experienced.

Retreat

This is a period during which the individual begins to handle the impact of the physical change psychologically. Denial may occur. Threat is felt and the individual may be very tense and anxious. Grief and mourning occur and the future may be perceived as very much worse than the reality.

Acknowledgement

During this phase, the individual begins to go over the events which led up to the change. This may be a mental activity or it may be discussed overtly with staff or relatives. In an attempt to make sense of what has happened the patient may try to identify cause and effect relationships between the body image change and the events immediately preceding it. Self esteem may be very low during this time. The patient has a need to communicate his or her uncertainty about the future.

Reconstruction

During this phase the patient begins to come to terms with the altered body image and to the reality of life in the future. Full re-integration within the family is important.

Nursing role

During the impact phase, especially when body image change has been sudden, it is important for staff to assess the patient's perception of what has happened. There may well be a need to define for the patient what has happened, where he is, and the location and extent of any body damage. Respect for the patient as an individual requires that he or she is allowed time and privacy to mourn and grieve. As the patient begins to adapt, it is helpful to examine openly his or her coping strengths and assets. If the physical change is an obvious one, he or she should be encouraged to look and examine, slowly and in privacy. Later, the patient can be encouraged to interact with others who have the same problem. Staff should be open to cues which reveal that the patient wishes to discuss his/her feelings and be prepared to listen. Relatives need support so that they can respond positively to the patient. The individual's self-esteem should be boosted by praising any progress made and stressing the individual's strengths. Realistic encouragement is needed throughout.

Staff also need to be alert to the possibility of non-adaptation and lack of progress. In this case professional psychotherapy may be needed.

Stigma

Body image change has been discussed above as an example of loss. However, body image change may be associated with stigma, in which case the individual has additional psychological and social factors to contend with. Goffman (1963) has discussed stigma. He states that stigma occurs when the reality of an individual's appearance and social identity is negatively different from what is expected. If the stigma is obvious to others during interaction then the individual is said to be discredited. If it is not obvious then the person is said to be discreditable, i.e. they are potentially discredited should the stigma become known.

A stigmatized individual poses a challenge to the majority of the population's concept of normality. The reaction to this challenge according to Goffman is to assume that the discredited person is less than human. This reduces the threat inherent in a challenge to the concept of normality which has been developed within a particular culture and society. In turn, the new 'less than human' stigmatized individual may become labelled by words with negative connotations such as cripple, amputee, etc. 'Normals' go on to attribute a wide range of imperfections on the basis of the original imperfection. Stereotyping occurs.

Once the body image has adapted to change, a stigmatized person will feel 'normal' to him/herself and thus expect to be treated normally. At the same time he or she will recognize the difference and fear the reactions of others. Even kindly people may patronize the discredited, addressing them without a proper introduction, asking impertinent and personal questions, treating adults as if they were children or dogs. Examples are: adults in wheelchairs being patted on the head; the disabled being talked over as if they were dumb or mentally handicapped. Indeed a British radio programme for and about the disabled draws attention to this phenomenon by its title *Does He Take Sugar?*

Goffman has identified two groups of people who are of positive significance to the discredited. These are the 'own' and the 'wise'. The own are those who are stigmatized in the same way as the individual. An example would be someone who also has a facial scar. The wise are normals who have become knowledgeable and understanding about the condition. These may include those who are part of the same primary family or social group as the stigmatized person. Blackwell (1970) calls these the intimate wise. Doctors, nurses and social workers who are professionally knowledgeable have been called the professional wise by Blackwell (1970).

Social interaction between the stigmatized person and normals creates tension for the discredited person and indeed for the discreditable person. The stigmatized individual copes by attempting to control information about the stigma, choosing carefully those to whom he or she will disclose information. Examples of stigmatizing conditions are:

- Spinal cord injury leading to paraplegia or quadriplegia
- Stroke
- Amputation
- Mastectomy
- Laryngectomy
- Burns
- Skin disease, e.g. eczema, dermatitis
- Stomata

The implication of stigma is that for some groups of patients adaptation to change in body image does not end their problems. Stigma makes every subsequent social exchange with strangers a potent stressor which has to be managed.

12.2 THE THREAT OF IMPENDING DEATH

To most of us the time and place of our death is unknown and quite unpredictable. The knowledge that one will die within weeks or months and that one can to a large extent determine where that death will take place is considered extremely stressful in our society. This is perhaps paradoxical since being able to control and predict events normally reduces the stress inherent in many life events, a view which can also be taken about death (see Nabokov, 1963).

However, what has perhaps been insufficiently explored in the stress literature is the importance of the concept of hope. Roberts (1986) argues that hope
is a basic need of all individuals and that without hope neither a patient nor
the family will be able to cope with a current illness. A similar finding can be
inferred from the research of people with cancer (see Chapter 11; MacIntosh,
1977).

Thus whilst control and predictability reduces stress for most events, there
is implicit evidence that in the case of the most feared events, not knowing
and so being able to maintain an element of hope is the preferred option.
Amongst examples of such highly feared events are the diagnosis of cancer
and being given only a short time to live. However, when such events are
accepted as inevitable then predictability and control reduce their inherently
stressful nature.

It is the management of the conflict between maintaining a vestige of hope
and accepting the reality of highly feared events which is the task of coping
for the patient who is dying. Kubler-Ross (1969) argues that the patient with a
fatal condition needs hope and that telling the person his prognosis should be
done in such a way that hope can be maintained.

Many doctors believe they should not tell a patient about their impending
death since that abolishes hope. Kubler-Ross (1969) discussed the issue of
whether or not to tell a patient he or she has a fatal condition. She argued that
the question is not whether to tell but how to tell. In practice, she has found
that in the case of doctors who claim that patients do not wish to know it is the
doctor's attitude toward death which is a problem, rather than the patient
truly not wishing to know. This is because there is plenty of evidence that
patients come to know they are dying by picking up cues from those around
them, and so if they are not openly told, they exist in a state of suspicion
awareness (Glaser and Strauss, 1965). Closed awareness is particularly stressful for all concerned.

In discussing the issue of telling or not telling the patient he or she has a fatal
illness, Glaser and Strauss (1965) have classified what they term awareness
contexts.

Closed awareness

This is where the patient fails to recognize that he or she is dying, even
though the staff know and usually the relatives know as well. Here, the
staff and relatives see their task as preventing the patient from becoming
suspicious.

Suspicion awareness

This is where the patient suspects that he/she is dying but does not know this
for sure. Staff and relatives know the true situation but the doctor does not

wish the patient to know. The situation becomes one of a verbal fencing match in which the patient attempts to trap staff into revealing the truth and the staff try to prevent the truth from slipping out. Here the greatest problem is posed for the most junior staff who frequently spend the most time with the patient, are the least sophisticated in coping and who are seen by the patient as the most likely to be trapped into telling the truth.

Mutual pretence

This is the situation in which the patient knows he is dying but has not been told this openly. Staff and relatives know, but all behave implicitly as if the patient does not know he is dying and is going to live. All parties are pretending.

Open awareness

This occurs when staff, relatives and patient all know the patient is dying and the knowledge is open. Discussion about the impending death can take place and the patient can obtain the support he or she needs.

Kubler-Ross (1969) carried out a now classical study of the psychological process undergone when patients know that they are dying. She advises that patients should not be given a time limit to indicate how long they have to live. She takes this view because leaving the question open gives hope and in any case no one can predict the time of death accurately. Kubler-Ross (1969) also argues that when talking to a patient about death the most important thing is to convey empathy and to share the information in a simple way, in privacy and with an assurance that everything possible will be done for the patient.

From her study of dying patients, Kubler-Ross (1969) has described the process of coping with the knowledge of one's own impending death. She has described this as a series of consecutive stages. These should not be taken too literally, however. Not everyone displays each stage and the order may not be as described by Kubler-Ross. Other evidence (Parkes, 1975; Gyllenskold, 1982) also suggests that people's emotions and psychological defence mechanisms during acute stress are labile and can change very rapidly and within short time spans.

The initial reaction on being given the news is described by Kubler-Ross as one of shock and denial. A temporary state of shock and numbness is not characteristic in every case but most people appear to deny the fatal nature of their condition for a time which can be brief or much longer. Kubler-Ross suggests that denial gives the individual time to come to terms with the situation and to develop other coping strategies.

Anger is said to occur as the second stage; what Kubler-Ross describes as

'Why me?' This is a particularly difficult stage for those who are caring for the patient, since anger and resentment may frequently be displaced on to the healthy people around: doctors, nurses and relatives. There is envy and rage and frequently whatever others do is wrong. If the patient is left alone this is a sign that others do not care, but if they are with the patient the patient is annoyed because he or she cannot be left alone. It is particularly important for professional staff to understand this anger reaction so that they can not only continue to support the patient but also can give help and advice to the relatives. Helping the patient to gain as much control as possible over his or her life may contribute enormously to the quality of the remaining time. It will prevent the patient from feeling that he or she is finished.

The third stage is described as one of bargaining. This means that the individual feels that if only he or she promises something in the way of a particular form of behaviour, more time will be granted before death occurs. Such bargaining may be private or more public in conversation with the chaplain, relatives etc.

Depression is another stage which has been described. Kubler-Ross considers that an element within the depression is reactive as a response to actual losses already suffered by the patient. These losses are a consequence of illness and possible hospitalization and include the loss of job, role, and separation from family and friends. Part of the loss suffered is associated with lowered self-esteem. Some of these losses can be compensated for to some extent by encouraging contact with family and friends, boosting the patient's self-esteem and giving him or her as much control as possible. However, Kubler-Ross also suggested that some of the depression is preparatory grief for the loss to come. The individual can be helped with grief by silent empathy, sitting and holding the patient's hand and giving the patient a chance to talk about feelings, past achievements and memories.

Acceptance is a stage that all dying patients would reach if given enough time. It is therefore a goal toward which they can be helped, but some patients will need a great deal of time spent with them before they can come to acceptance.

Older patients after a long and fulfilling life may feel completed and that they have found meaning and contentment in their own life. There is a sense of achievement when they look back over their past life. Such people may come to acceptance with little or no help.

Hope is part of acceptance. Kubler-Ross found that hope equates to a feeling that suffering has some meaning and that it will pay off eventually if it can be endured a little longer. It is a sense of mission in life. On the other hand it may be a form of temporary denial.

Ideally a patient works through the stage of acceptance, a sense that their life has been worthwhile and that the tasks of life are completed. Emotionally there is calm and a certain degree of disengagement from the concerns and worries of day-to-day living. However, a feeling of being able to control as much as the patient wishes to control should be maintained to the end.

Kubler-Ross (1969) describes the patient at this stage as feeling physically tired and weak and requiring to sleep for increasing periods of time. It is during this period that the relatives and friends may need the most help and support since the patient may well wish to be physically alone in addition to the emotional and cognitive disengagement. A request by the patient for short visits from few people at a time may hurt and upset those close to the patient and they need to have explained to them the process through which the patient is progressing – non-verbal communication through touch; quietly sitting by the patient's side may be what he or she most needs.

The Hospice Movement pioneered in this country by Saunders (1980) provides an environment in which the dying patient is given physical, psychological and spiritual care, leading to the stage of acceptance and a peaceful death. Relatives are supported and in particular the patient is kept pain-free.

12.3 BEREAVEMENT

Grief is a process which occurs as a response to all significant loss but our concern so far in this chapter has been with the loss which is associated with severe health problems. When health problems result in loss the response seen is partially the response to loss but it is frequently confounded by being also a response to illness, disability or trauma.

Grief in a severe but relatively unconfounded form can be seen in bereavement suffered by the survivor of a very close relationship. Parkes (1975) studied grief during bereavement and his reason for doing so was partly because the grief process is so obvious following the death of a loved one. Society expects grief from a new widow or widower. Indeed many societies institutionalize grief at such a time. The causal relationship between the death and the grief of the survivor is very easy to identify.

Bereavement is a severe stressor and interestingly Parkes (1975) characterized grief as like a physical injury or blow followed by gradual healing. Like physical injury grief may occasionally be so severe that it is associated with the death of the bereaved individual. A further stressor during the grief process can delay recovery. On the other hand, Parkes argues that for those who come through it successfully, the experience of grief can be an agent of maturity and strength.

The pain of grief is an integral part of life, as fundamental as the joy of love. Indeed the two are related. Earlier we defined loss as being related to attachment and this implies the close link between attachment and grief.

A fundamental point made by Parkes (1975) is that grief is a process and not a state, and so it can be expressed in different ways at different points in the process. The misconception that it is a state can lead to confusion and arid argument as to the characteristics of that state (e.g. is grief characterized by anxiety or depression? As a process both occur).

Parkes (1975) also pointed out that the loss experienced on the death of a spouse is by no means a single loss. The various roles which any individual performs may mean that for the survivor of a suddenly severed relationship many secondary losses occur in addition to the primary loss. A great change in role must be mastered by the surviving partner. For example the loss of a husband may also mean the loss of a sexual partner, companion, helper with the children, provider of money, fellow music-lover etc.

Stigma may add to the problem faced by the recently bereaved widow or widower. This is because the newly bereaved individual challenges society's concept of normality. Not only society in general but the immediate social circle has become used to the 'couple' being the normal state. Where such stigma occurs it is likely to fall more severely upon a widow than a widower. The ultimate example comes from societies where new widows are expected to commit ritual suicide.

Death in bereavement

Bereavement has already been likened to a physical injury and attention drawn to the fact that grief may be so severe that death ensues. There is evidence to support this from an increase in mortality during the first year of bereavement, particularly amongst widowers. Young et al. (1963) found an increase of almost 40% in the death rate of newly bereaved males aged 50 years or more compared with non-bereaved males of the same age. The most common cause of death following bereavement is coronary heart disease.

Death from coronary heart disease during grief is an extreme reaction but other physical illnesses are also more common during the first year of bereavement. Examples are cancer, ulcerative colitis, asthma, headache, digestive upset and rheumatism. The work of Holmes and Rahe (1967) confirms the link between life events and ill health. Bereavement is a prime example of a major life event, scoring a large number of life change units on their scale.

The grief process in bereavement (Parkes, 1975)

Parkes' work was based upon a study of 22 widows under the age of 65 years over a period of rather more than a year, who exhibited what appeared to be a normal grief reaction (the London Study). He interviewed the widows toward the end of the first month of bereavement and then at 3 months, 6 months, 9 months and 13 months. He also studied a group of psychiatric patients whose psychiatric condition was attributable to bereavement. These were said to display 'atypical grief'.

Parkes uses a model of the grieving process in which he describes a number of phases. It is important to recognize that these are not consecutive phases through which the mourner passes but that the individual can vary rapidly between these phases.

The first phase described by Parkes is alarm.

1. Alarm

This is a sign of extreme stress according to Parkes (1975). 'In the London Study it was clear that for most of the widows the world had become a threatening and potentially dangerous place' (Parkes, 1975). During the first month the widows reported that they felt very restless. There were signs of high arousal (severe enough on occasions to approach panic) and increased muscle tone. The women lost their appetite and this was accompanied by weight loss. They had difficulty in sleeping at night. Digestive disturbance was accompanied by dryness of the mouth and a sense of fullness in the epigastrium. Often heartburn occurred. There were also palpitations, headache and muscular aches and pains.

2. Searching

Parkes (1975) identified the most characteristic feature of grief as the occurrence of acute and episodic pangs and a 'pang' he defined as an incidence of severe anxiety and psychological pain during which the loss is very strongly felt and the sufferer sobs or cries. These episodes began within a few hours or days of bereavement, reaching a peak of severity in 5–14 days. They occur during the same time as the alarm phase described above. The bereaved individual may exhibit a characteristic expression on the face in which there is raising of the inner aspect of the eyebrows, wrinkling of the forehead and base of the nose with depression of the angles of the mouth.

Searching for the lost person is a cognitive aspect of grief. The bereaved individual mistakes passing strangers for the lost one. One of the widows in Parkes' (1975) study said 'I can't help looking for him everywhere. I walk around searching for him'.

The griever holds a particularly clear perception of the deceased and memories preoccupy the mind. Parts of the environment associated with the deceased assume special significance.

Lindemann (1944) drew attention to the behaviour of individuals during the searching associated with grief.

> The activity throughout the day of the severely bereaved person shows remarkable changes. There is no retardation of action and speech; quite

to the contrary, there is a rush of speech, especially when talking about the deceased. There is restlessness, inability to sit still, moving about in an aimless fashion, continually searching for something to do. There is, however, at the same time, a painful lack of capacity to initiate and maintain normal patterns of activity.

3. Mitigation

The commonest way of mitigating the pain of grief seems to be the maintenance of a feeling that the deceased is nearby and this is comforting. Rees (1970) in a sample of 227 widows and 66 widowers found that 39% had a sense of the presence of the deceased and 14% experienced hallucinations and illusions of the deceased's presence. This group experienced greater loneliness than the rest but felt helped by the nearness of the deceased and they suffered less sleep disturbance than the remainder of the sample.

Bereavement dreams occurred amongst the widows. In these the deceased was alive but the dreamers retained an awareness of the death in a concealed or non-concealed form.

During mitigation, ways of coping with grief are developed. These enable the pain to be avoided. One of the most frequent of these is not to believe in the loss. Many widows in Parkes' study felt they were waiting for their husbands to come back after a temporary absence. One said, 'It's like a dream. I feel I'm going to wake up and it'll be all right. He'll be back again'.

Some avoid thoughts of the loss by filling their lives with activities. They put away photographs and personal effects but avoid sorting out clothing of the deceased. Selective forgetting occurred but the clarity of the remembered image of the loved one persisted. Many widows tended to stay at home, not going out in case they met people who were sympathetic and would cause control to break down. At home they only wished to admit people with whom they felt secure.

Parkes (1975) described two opposing tendencies which occurred in oscillation. One of these was characterized by inhibition, repression, avoidance and holding back disturbing ideas. The other tendency was facilitative and comprised reality testing in which perception of the deceased's image and thinking disturbing thoughts occurred.

This can be seen as the operation of defence mechanisms, allowing coming to terms with the problem gradually and in a relatively safe way. The individual gains control over how quickly they are going to come to terms with loss.

Bereavement involves major changes in identity (Parkes, 1975) and the individual buys time against complete realization by the use of defence mechanisms. Provided the balance of facilitation and inhibition is right, inappropriate behaviour diminishes and ceases and new behaviour is developed.

Reminiscences of the time leading up to the bereavement occurs and there is a need to 'get it right', to make sense of what has happened, to classify it and to make it fit the individual's expectations of the world.

This is a process which occurs retrospective to the death but which is similar to the worry work described pre-operatively by Janis (see p. 190). Freud called this **grief work** and suggested that energy is used in order to let go of each memory connected with the deceased.

Parkes (1975) suggested that bereavement is so overwhelming an event that the normal pre-event appraisal fails to occur even if the death is expected, and so appraisal takes place after the death.

Grief work includes:

1. Preoccupation with thoughts of the lost person. This is associated with the urge to search.
2. Painful repetitious recollections of the loss which must occur if the loss is to become fully accepted as irrevocable.
3. An attempt to make sense of the loss by getting it to fit into one's assumptive world (one's basic ideological model of the world). This may mean a change in the assumptive world to accommodate the realization of the loss.

As time passes the intensity of pining is mitigated and recollection is experienced as bitter-sweet nostalgia.

Anger and guilt

Among Parkes' London widows exhibiting normal grief there was the experience of feelings of anger intense enough to be reported at interview. These were experienced as episodes of anger in between which repressive withdrawal was associated with apathy. This latter depressed mood became more dominant as time passed.

Episodes of anger were associated with restlessness and tension but the impulse to action was rigidly controlled, often resulting in a fine tremor or a stammer. Widows said 'I feel in a turmoil inside', 'Stupid little things upset me'. Relatives trying to induce the widow to stop grieving might have the anger directed at them. Sometimes the death became personalized as something done to the griever. The bereaved might seek someone to blame for the death; this could be the deceased, or turn to self blame. The anger could also be displaced and expressed in relation to trivial matters. Amongst Parkes' sample of widows it was the most socially isolated who experienced the most anger. They also felt guilty about their anger. Self-reproach means an examination of their own behaviour to identify the cause of the death.

Guilt and self-reproach were experienced to a much greater extent by those who needed psychiatric help after bereavement than by those who went through bereavement 'normally'.

One aspect of bereavement is giving up the old identity and taking on a new role. The characteristic emotion associated with this is depression, according to Parkes (1975). Depression is not a clean-cut phase, but it occurs again and again.

It takes time for the individual to realize and to accept the change consequent upon major loss. A widow in Parkes' study said,

> I think I'm beginning to wake up now. . . I'm starting to live instead of just existing. It's the first time I've had a positive thought. I feel I ought to plan to do something. I feel as if I was recovering from a major illness. . . you suddenly wake up. I felt I was hollow inside as if my heart had been torn out and left a ragged hole.

During the first year of bereavement time 'gets out of joint' and the year may be looked upon as a limbo of meaningless activity.

Atypical grief

Parkes' description of atypical grief was derived from his study of bereaved individuals who broke down and were referred for psychiatric help. He studied a group of 35 individuals; of these, 26 were depressed, 4 had become alcoholics, 5 developed hypochondriacal symptoms and 4 developed phobias.

They all suffered more or less the same grief process as the normal group and only guilt and self-reproach were more marked. However in the atypical group grief was prolonged and the reaction to bereavement was delayed considerably.

All the patients seen had at some time developed depression and in some grief was so intense that any distinction between delayed grief and chronic grief was lost. Hypochondriacal symptoms often resembled the symptoms suffered by the deceased during their fatal illness. Two features which were exhibited by all in this group were intense separation anxiety and strong but only partially successful attempts to avoid grief.

Parkes (1975) identified a large number of determinants of the outcome of bereavement and he classified these determinants as antecedent, concurrent or subsequent.

Antecedent determinants

- Childhood experiences (especially the loss of a significant person)
- Later experiences (especially the loss of a significant person)
- Previous mental illness (especially depressive illness)

- Life crises prior to bereavement
- The relationship with deceased in terms of kinship, strength of attachment, security of attachment, degree of reliance, and the intensity of ambivalent emotions (love/hate)
- The mode of the death in terms of timeliness, previous warning, ability to prepare for bereavement, need to hide feelings from the dying individual

Concurrent determinants

- Sex
- Age
- Personality in terms particularly of grief proneness and inhibition of feelings
- Socio-economic status
- Nationality
- Religion
- Cultural and familial factors influencing the expression of grief.

Subsequent determinants

- Social support or isolation
- Secondary stresses
- Emergent life opportunities, i.e. options which are available

Parkes (1975) discussed the possibility of anticipatory grief occurring in the bereaved individual in circumstances where the death could be predicted and there was time to come to terms with it. He argues that if both the dying individual and the close relative can share their grief they often both reach a state of contented calm which persists to the end. The surviving spouse is then likely to look back upon this period of time with satisfaction rather than distress.

Parkes described three patterns in the expression of grief as a result of his study.

The first pattern is one in which there is severe disturbance within the first week of death which persists throughout the first and second month but has become much reduced by the third month.

A second pattern comprises moderate emotion in the first week followed by severe grief in week two but this is rapidly over and in general this pattern is associated with a comparatively fast recovery.

In the third pattern, the immediate response in week one is to experience no emotion. By the fourth week there is moderate disturbance but in the third month there is disturbance which is more severe than in either of the other patterns at this time. Improvement follows but there is greater disturbance in this group at the time of the first anniversary of the death.

Amongst widows showing the third pattern of grief there was a higher incidence of physical symptoms in the first month. The group had an average age nine years younger than the groups showing other grief patterns. Their husbands had died suddenly and unexpectedly.

Helping the bereaved

Parkes (1975) discussed the ways in which newly bereaved individuals could be helped. He argued that initially the grieving individual who is in a state of numbness needs help with the simplest decision. Relatives and friends can help by looking after the new widow or widower, and take over or help with the administrative tasks associated with the death, such as the registration of death, funeral arrangements and the notification of other friends and relatives. Over-protection or possessiveness should be avoided however. Help with such decisions gives the bereaved person time to take in what has happened and to organize ideas.

Rituals attending the death may help and the funeral brings family and friends together so that they can plan to support the bereaved widow or widower.

The peak of grief may occur in the second week of bereavement and it is helpful if time is available to allow full and free grief to occur. What is most valuable at this point is a close friend or relative who can quietly get on with the day-to-day business making few demands upon the bereaved person. Understanding may be needed since anger may be directed at the helper. If the griever can be allowed to express their feelings at this time, it is beneficial to them, but time is needed since grief work cannot be hurried. It is reassuring to the widow or widower if those around also show their grief and sadness. The sense of isolation is reduced.

Conventional but sincere expressions of sympathy help, but pity should be avoided. Visits of sympathy express the worth of the deceased to those around. Great comfort can be derived from quiet communication of affectionate understanding.

Worden (1983) has discussed the professional counsellor's role in helping the bereaved individual. He uses the concept of tasks of mourning to elaborate the process following loss from the death of a loved one. He reserves the term grief to signify the subjective experience of the bereaved individual.

Four tasks make up the tasks of mourning. These are:

1. Accepting the reality of the loss.
2. Experiencing the pain of grief.
3. To adjust to an environment in which the deceased is missing.

4. To withdraw emotional energy and to re-invest it in another relationship.

   Mourning is finished when these tasks are completed, but this is a very long-term process. For Worden (1983) a benchmark of recovery is when the bereaved person is able to think of the deceased without pain, although sadness probably always persists.

   Worden (1983) has catalogued the manifestations of normal grief reported by Parkes (1972) but using a different classification from that of Parkes (1975), as follows:

A. Feelings

These include:

- sadness
- guilt and self-reproach
- loneliness
- helplessness
- yearning
- relief and numbness
- anger
- anxiety
- fatigue
- shock
- emancipation

B. Physical sensations

These are:

- hollowness in the stomach
- tightness in the throat
- a sense of depersonalization
- weakness in muscles
- dry mouth
- tightness in the chest
- over-sensitivity to noise
- breathlessness
- lack of energy

C. Cognitions

- disbelief
- preoccupation
- hallucinations.
- confusion
- a sense of the presence of the deceased

D. Behaviour

- sleep disturbance
- absent-minded behaviour
- dreams of the deceased
- searching and calling out
- appetite disturbances
- social withdrawal
- avoiding reminders of the deceased

- restless overactivity
- visiting places or carrying objects which remind the survivor of the deceased
- sighing
- crying
- treasuring objects belonging to the deceased

Worden (1983) uses the tasks of mourning as a basis for the goals of grief counselling, which are:

1. To increase the reality of the loss.
2. To help the bereaved to deal with both expressed and latent emotion.
3. To help the bereaved to overcome impediments to readjustment after loss.
4. To help the bereaved to make a healthy emotional withdrawal from the deceased and to feel comfortable reinvesting emotion in another relationship.

Principles of counselling are related firmly to these goals.

First, Worden argues, the survivor should be helped to talk about the loss. This can be encouraged by asking questions about the circumstances surrounding the death and the funeral.

Secondly the identification and expression of feelings can be helped by asking what they miss about the deceased and what they do not miss. This helps to elicit felt anger, but balance between positive and negative feelings should be maintained and the individual should be left with positive feelings.

Guilt feelings will yield to reality testing.

Sadness can be helped by encouraging crying. In anxiety and helplessness the individual can be helped to identify their preferred coping strategies and strengths and to plan coping strategies for the future. It may help if the individual can be helped to talk out their own death fears.

The third principle is to help the bereaved individual to begin the task of living without the deceased. Problem-solving techniques are useful to help decision making. The widow or widower should be prevented from making major life-changing decisions too soon, however.

The fourth principle again should not be followed too soon, but it involves encouraging new relationships.

Overall, time is needed to allow grieving and this may have to be explained to friends and relatives of the bereaved. Rather critical times in grieving are at around three months after the death since family support tends to be withdrawn at about that time. The first anniversary of the death is also a difficult time and so is holiday time. The client should be encouraged to anticipate the problems at these times and to plan ahead.

Further principles of counselling are:

- to interpret the normal experiences of grief by explaining their normality

- to examine mental defence mechanisms and coping styles and to suggest other ways of coping if the clients' preferred styles are ineffective.

12.4 SUMMARY

In this chapter the main issue has been the effect of significant loss upon the individual and the ways in which the individual copes with such loss. Whilst all change involves loss (Bower, 1980) significant loss is associated with an investment of self within the object which is lost.

One such significant loss is associated with changes in body image, since along with such change goes a loss of the previous body image. In turn the body image is a crucial aspect of self. Body image change is of particular concern to health professionals. We have discussed the concept of body image and its development, as well as the circumstances in which a change in body image occurs.

Frequently the changed body image may bring stigma with it. Stigma adds considerably to the stress experienced by the individual. The concept of stigma was discussed briefly.

Another significant loss is one's own death. Kubler-Ross's (1969) classical work on the coping mechanisms employed by the individual who knows of their own impending death was also referred to.

The impact of body image change and impending death is confounded by other problems faced by the individual. These may be physical problems associated with illness or trauma, or psychological and social problems.

Thus the major discussion of coping with significant loss in this chapter concerned the newly bereaved individual who has suffered the death of a loved one, i.e. one with whom there was a relationship of attachment.

Parkes (1975) carried out a major study of bereavement and his work has formed the basis of the last part of this chapter. Bereavement is a major life event as defined by Holmes and Rahe (1967). The chapter ends with a brief account of grief counselling following bereavement.

REFERENCES

Blackwell, B. (1970) Stigma, in *Behavioral Concepts and Nursing Intervention* (ed. Carolyn E. Carlson), Lippincott, Philadelphia, PA, pp. 317–29.
Bower, F. L. (1977a) *Normal Development of Body Image*, J. Wiley, London.
Bower, F. L. (1977b) *Distortions of Body Image in Illness and Disability*, J. Wiley, London.
Bower, F. L. (1980) *Nursing and the Concept of Loss*, J. Wiley, London.

Corbeil, M. (1971) Nursing process for a patient with a body image disturbance. *Nursing Clinics of North America*, **6**(1), 156–7.

Dyk, R. B. and Sutherland, A. M. (1956) Adaptation of the spouse and other family members to the colostomy patient. *Cancer*, **9**, 123.

Esberger, K. (1978) Body image, *J. Geront. Nursing*, **4**(4), 35–8.

Glaser, B. G. and Strauss, A. L. (1965) *Awareness of Dying*, Aldine, Chicago, IL.

Goffman, E. (1963) *Stigma: the Management of a Spoiled Identity*, Pelican, London.

Gyllenskold, K. (1982) *Breast Cancer: The Psychological Effects of the Disease and its Treatment*, translated by Patricia Crampton, Tavistock Publications, London.

Head, H. (1920) *Studies in Neurology*, Vol. 2, Oxford University Press, London.

Henker, F. D. (1979) Body image conflict following trauma and surgery, *Psychosomatics*. **20**(12), 812–20.

Holmes, T. H. and Rahe, R. H. (1967) The social readjustment rating scale. *J. Psychosom. Res.*, **11**, 213–18.

Kolb, L. (1959) Disturbances of the body image, in *American Handbook of Psychiatry*, vol. 1 (ed. Silvane Arieta), Basic Books, New York, N.Y., pp. 750–68.

Kubler-Ross, E. (1969) *On Death and Dying*, Macmillan, New York, N.Y.

Lindemann, E. (1944) Symptomatology and management of acute grief. *Amer. J. Psychiatry*, **101**, 144–8.

McDaniel, J. W. (1976) *Physical Disability and Human Behaviour* (2nd edn), Pergamon Press, Oxford.

McIntosh, J. (1977) *Communication and Awareness in a Cancer Ward*, Croom Helm, London.

Nabokov, V. (1963) *Invitation to a Beheading*, Penguin Books, Harmondsworth.

Norris, C. M. (1970) The professional nurse and body image, in *Behavioral Concepts and Nursing Intervention* (ed. Carolyn E. Carlson), Lippincott, Philadelphia, PA, pp. 39–65.

O'Brien, J. (1980) Mirror, mirror, why me?, *Nursing Mirror* (April 24th), **150**, 36–7.

Parkes, C. M. (1972) Bereavement: *Studies of Grief in Adult Life*. International Universities Press, N.Y.

Parkes, C. M. (1975) *Bereavement: Study of Grief in Adult Life*, Penguin, Middlesex.

Pettit, E. (1980) Body image. *Nursing*, **16**, 690–92.

Piaget, J. (1954) *The Construction of Reality in the Child*, Basic Books, New York, N.Y.

Rees, W. D. (1970) The Hallucinatory and Paranormal Reactions of Bereavement, MD Thesis (cited by Parkes, 1975).

Roberts, S. L. (1986) *Behavioural Concepts and the Critically Ill Patient* (2nd edn), Appleton-Century-Crofts, Norwalk, CT.

Saunders, C. (1980) St Christophers Hospice, in *Death: Current Perspectives*, 2nd edn, (ed. E. S. Schneidman), Mayfield, Paulo Alto, CA.

Schilder, P. (1935) The image and appearance of the human body, in *Psychological Monograph*, London, George Routledge & Sons. Reprinted 1950 by International Universities Press, New York, N.Y.

Shontz, F. C. (1974) Body image and its disorders. *International Journal of Psychiatry in Medicine*, **5**, 461–72.

Stone, S. K. (1976) Emotional reactions to alterations in body image. *Journal of Practical Nursing*, **26**, 24–6.

Worden, J. W. (1983) *Grief Counselling and Grief Therapy*, Tavistock Publications, London.

Young, M., Benjamin, B. and Wallis, C. (1963) Mortality of widowers. *Lancet* **ii**, 456.

PART FOUR

CONCLUSIONS

CHAPTER THIRTEEN

Stress and coping:
A summary

It might be helpful to the reader if this chapter takes the form of a discussion between the two authors.

MC Now that we have finished reviewing the literature relating to stress and coping, you looking at that which applies to nurses, and I at that relating to patients, I think it might be useful to re-assess the cognitive–phenomenological–transactional (CPT) model, don't you? To what extent do you go along with it, and how do you rate it now?

RB Well, for the studies that I've reviewed and certainly for the studies that you've reviewed, the CPT as we've called it has been a useful model because it's given us a very rich range of possible explanations; where some of the models of the past have really been quite limited in terms of the understandings they provide. Firstly then, it's a very rich model for providing explanations and it opens up other areas that we hadn't thought of before.

MC Yes, that's right. I agree with you that the CPT model is very rich and I think that it's very good for interpreting events that have happened, so to speak. On the other hand, one of the things that worries me a little about the model is that in some respects it's not that scientific. What I mean is, it seems to be able to explain virtually everything in retrospect but it doesn't help in making predictions which are very precise.

RB No, that is one of its clear limitations; that it is not so good as a predictive model, but that is a limitation that many other models have as well. In choosing a model as a framework for reviewing these studies we examined many others and they all have this problem. Basically the question is really whether in spite of all the work carried out on stress and coping we know enough yet to refine prediction. However, it is true to say that we probably do need a reformulation of the concepts of stress and coping. Can I just say one other thing? The CPT model clearly has got an advantage in that it can be used with the single case study and it has a tremendous amount to offer nursing.

MC Yes, I agree wholeheartedly with your last point, because when we're talking about nursing and particularly when we're talking about patients, we're not really wanting prediction to any precise degree. It seems to me that what we want is the ability to help and to understand people. In this respect I personally believe that the whole stress and coping framework is particularly useful in bringing us to a better understanding of people so that we can help them. That, I think, is what we wanted to show in this book. Now, in terms of your literature review, was there anything that came out of it that you were surprised about, or any highlights that you want to mention?

RB There were a couple of highlights. One would be this. As you said, the CPT model is very useful for individuals but something it doesn't take account of sufficiently is the culture or the social construction of the reality of nursing. We need to keep that in mind because when that's operational then a number of common factors are bound to affect nurses. The CPT model (or others for that matter) doesn't do much to help us to appreciate that. What it does do is to help us to make sense of the interpretations and reactions of individuals. Another point really, is something you've mentioned, and that is the place of defence mechanisms. There seems to have been a trivialization of them going on but they need to have their place. I don't know what you feel about that.

MC Well certainly one of the startling things that has been drawn to my attention a good deal more than when I started reviewing the literature is the extent to which people who are physically ill do use defence mechanisms and that they seem to be positively helpful. A lot of the literature within general psychology and psychiatry seems to give defence mechanisms a very negative connotation, whilst the medical psychology literature shows them in a positive light. The other thing is that when you read Freud you develop a concept of defence mechanisms as being very stable and lasting, perhaps for years and years, but in much of the literature I've looked at, there is evidence that defence mechanisms may be used in a very mobile and labile way. A person can be using defence one minute and accepting reality the next. This came out particularly in that study of breast cancer patients by Gyllenskold. I think if nurses can realize that, it may be very useful for understanding and caring for patients. Perhaps the defence mechanism the patient is using right now will shift and the patient will come to a different understanding very quickly indeed.

RB I know that Lazarus has come very squarely now to paying much more attention to defence mechanisms and the role they play in helping people rather than preventing them from dealing with problems. You can really see this, though as a break with the Freudian view. What you are really saying is that defence mechanisms are useful up to a point and have some purpose for the person dealing with their own problems.

MC Yes, that's right. I think we did bring this out briefly in the beginning part of the book on theory. Defence gives the person time and that is obviously very important.

RB Yes. Can I just make a plea about the importance of mentioning this in any reformulation of stress and coping? Going through the literature I found a number of themes beginning to come out, like the role of control and its relationship to the human organism. There seems to be a dynamic relationship between defence, equilibrium and control and the role of significant events. In fact, one thing which does come from the literature is the importance of events which are significant to the individual. What are the characteristics of these? That's something we might want to develop further. Maybe we can draw up some pointers for future research. All this is pointing to a review or reconsideration of theory.

MC So we are really thinking that we have come round to an idea that we need to develop the conceptual framework further from the one we had when we started.

RB Yes, I think that would be very useful.

MC Certainly, this is a very important area for nursing. You know, earlier, we talked about the use of the CPT model in helping to understand people but the other aspect we must bear in mind is that, I think, it actually helps one to self knowledge as well. I hope it brings one to a better level of coping. Certainly it is my wish that nurses reading our book could begin to apply the concepts to themselves as well as their patients and find it a positive help in their own coping. If it has done that it will at least have made some small contribution to nursing.

Stress and coping –
a proposed synthesis
the concept of an individual
psychological constellation
of beliefs

One important aspect of human functioning which we believe has been neglected somewhat in the stress and coping literature is the psychological background which the individual brings to a new situation and against which demands and coping take place. To reinforce the view of human functioning as proactive not merely reactive we consider that demands and coping are a particular category or type of transaction with the environment. The environment can be defined as the physical, psychological and social external and internal bodily states which contribute to our total experience and within which we behave and act.

In emphasizing the psychological background which is brought by the individual to a transaction we wish to promote the viewpoint that from birth the human being is engaging in much activity in relation to the environment. It is from these transactions within the individual's personal history that the individual's psychological background is derived. (This is entirely compatible with Piaget's work (1954); Flavell (1963).) Whilst the infant's activities result in the collection of information about the environment, what is crucial is the use to which this information is put. It is used in the creation of individual knowledge of the environment. However this creation of knowledge is a more active process than the mere collection of information. Human beings impose structure and meaning upon the environment which thus becomes an individual construction, which is used in turn to formulate expectations and beliefs about the future. Much of the structure and meaning imposed upon the environment derives from the individual's language and culture.

It is important to recognize that in the crucial early years of life our environment is interpreted to us through our family or other caregivers who transmit a highly specific culture at the same time. A similar situation pertains in later life when subgroups such as school, university, or school of nursing interpret and transmit the subcultural values to us.

Thus we come to incorporate in our individual construction of the environment beliefs in such concepts as simple cause–effect relationships; concepts of fairness; rewards for good behaviour and punishment for bad behaviour. We come to look for cause and effect relationships amongst random events. We develop expectations about the pattern of our future life and formulate life goals which we pursue. We could be said to be in a state of dynamic synthesis or in Allport's terms (1955) to be engaged in a process of 'becoming'.

We wish to label this process as the 'individual's psychological constellation of beliefs', which we define as the individual dynamic synthesis of beliefs, values, world view, expectations about the future and life goals.

It is against this individual psychological constellation of beliefs that we wish to consider stress and coping. A point which should be made clear is that experiences of stress and coping come to be incorporated within the individual's psychological constellation of beliefs which in turn is brought to new demands and coping. Thus the individual psychological constellation of beliefs is far from being static but is dynamic, continually being revised, differentiated and developed. We will return to this concept later but first we wish to reconsider stress and coping.

SIGNIFICANCE THEORY

One of the things which has been emphasized throughout this book is that an event affects someone only if it has significance and meaning for them. Therefore significance is a prime concept and we wish to explore what we will call **significance theory**. We also wish to call a sequence of related events occurring in the present a scenario, so that the present comprises a multitude of scenarios ranging from those which are similar to one another to those which are unique. It is in this wide range of different scenarios that the appraisal of demands, stress, coping and outcomes take place. This is entirely consistent with the CPT model which we have supported throughout the book. All the studies we have discussed reveal how appraisal plays a central role in stress and coping.

What we wish to do now is to establish the basic precepts underlying significance theory. These are:

A. Degree of control
B. Degree of change
C. Present scenario

This can be presented diagrammatically (Fig. A1), together with the

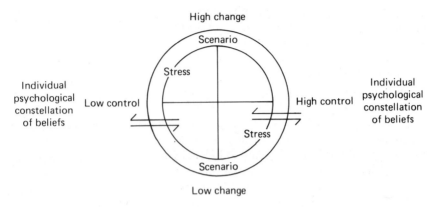

Figure A.1 The basic precepts of significance theory.

relationship to the individual psychological constellation of beliefs mentioned above.

A scenario in which there is high control and low change is likely to be stressful unless change can be induced. Similarly a scenario in which there is high change and low control is highly likely to be stressful. The arrows identify the dynamic relationship between the scenario and the individual psychological constellation of beliefs in that the latter is brought to the scenario and affects both appraisal and coping. In turn demand and coping experience is incorporated into the individual psychological constellation of beliefs (IPCB).

Precepts of significance theory

A. Degree of control

The degree of control can vary from being very low to being very high. The particular degree of control in any scenario arises from one or some combination of the following:

1. Personal coping competence
2. Collective coping through social, psychological, physical support
3. Organizational systems for coping (policies and practice) ·

The organizational system can reinforce the individual's coping or make it more difficult. Included within the organizational policy will be a value system and legal and statutory constraints. These latter may reduce the range of coping available to an individual. On the other hand they may prescribe coping which, if the scenario is amenable to the prescribed coping, will enhance control.

B. Degree of change

The degree of change should not be seen in isolation but in its dynamic relationship within the background environment. For example, a nurse who is working in an accident and emergency department will relate the degree of change occurring in a current scenario (e.g. dealing with a major accident) to the amount of change which occurs within the 'normal' scenarios for that accident and emergency department.

C. Present scenario

The degree of control and change takes place within the present scenario. A scenario is an interrelated set of significant circumstances occurring in the present and lasting for a finite period of time.

For example, a patient admitted for surgery encounters a series of scenarios, each of which is relevant to his/her well-being. Coping takes place in relation to these scenarios. In each the degree of change and the degree of control achieved may vary. It is through coping, achievement of control, and optimum levels of stress that health outcomes are experienced.

Significance and synthesis

The central assumption in our theoretical proposal is the significance of events to those experiencing them. It is the significance of each transaction within any scenario which forms the keystone of stress and coping. Degree of control and degree of change should be seen in relationship to the significance attributed to each scenario. Therefore although in any scenario the objective conditions of change and control may be present, the mechanism which initiates the experience of stress and coping is *significance*.

An example can show what we mean. James, a 47-year-old businessman was admitted to a coronary care unit. Objectively he no longer had control over his business. However, this particular scenario was no longer of significance to James; it caused him no stress. The significant scenario was his health and physical well-being.

Maintenance of harmonious synthesis

This could be said to be the purpose of individual functioning. Harmonious synthesis is an important concept, since it implies change rather than the absence of change. We wish to emphasize the point that stress and coping function to allow change within the individual who uses this change to elaborate the IPCB referred to above, into more complex forms of expression. However such synthesis should be harmonious. This means that the change arising from the stress and coping function should be compatible with the IPCB and should not be such that it disrupts the IPCB.

Disruption of individual psychological constellation of beliefs

One of the circumstances which we have yet to account for is the devastating effect of some health problems which completely disrupt the individual's psychological continuity.

We talked of control within a scenario above, but what happens if the scenario is of enormous significance and it is completely incompatible with the IPCB brought to the scenario. We should bear in mind that the IPCB summarises all that the individual has experienced so far and expects to experience in the future. Scenarios which may bring about such disruption include natural disasters (e.g. landslides, earthquakes, eruption of volcanoes), having a well-known and loved 'significant other' act in a way which is opposite from all one knows about them, the death of a loved one, developing cancer, facing one's own impending death at an unexpectedly young age, sudden paralysis, loss of a part of the body. These are events which cause a major discontinuity in the individual's existence and a devastating loss of control. All the IPCB is lost. The individual's task becomes a complete building up of a new IPCB from scratch.

It is in such circumstances we would argue that defence mechanisms are particularly useful, since they give the individual the comfort of the old IPCB and thus control whilst allowing time for the building of a new IPCB.

REFERENCES

Allport, G. W. (1955) *'Becoming'. Basic Considerations for a Psychology of Personality*, Yale University Press, New Haven.

Flavell, J. H. (1963) *The Developmental Psychology of Jean Piaget*, D. Van Nostrand, Princeton, New Jersey.

Piaget, J. (1954) *The Construction of Reality in the Child*, Basic Books, New York.

INDEX